WORKBOOK TO ACCOMPANY DELMAR'S
COMPREHENSIVE MEDICAL ASSISTING

Administrative and Clinical Competencies

Fourth Edition

Gerry A. Brasin, AS, CMA (AAMA), CPC
Corporate Education Coordinator
Premier Education Group
Springfield, MA

Barbara M. Dahl, CMA (AAMA), CPC
Program Director
Whatcom Community College
Bellingham, WA

Comprehensive Examination by:
Tricia Berry, MATL, OTR/L
Assistant Dean of Clinical Placement
School of Health Sciences
Kaplan University
Johnston, IA

DELMAR
CENGAGE Learning

Australia • Brazil • Japan • Mexico • Singapore • Spain • United Kingdom • United States

DELMAR
CENGAGE Learning

**Workbook to Accompany Delmar's
Comprehensive Medical Assisting:
Administrative and Clinical Competencies,
Fourth Edition**
**Gerry A. Brasin, Barbara M. Dahl, and
Tricia Berry**

Vice President, Career and Professional Editorial:
Dave Garza

Director of Learning Solutions: Matthew Kane

Senior Acquisitions Editor: Rhonda Dearborn

Managing Editor: Marah Bellegarde

Senior Product Manager: Sarah Prime

Editorial Assistant: Chiara Astriab

Vice President, Career and Professional Marketing:
Jennifer McAvey

Executive Marketing Manager:
Wendy E. Mapstone

Senior Marketing Manager: Nancy Bradshaw

Marketing Coordinator: Erica Ropitzky

Production Director: Carolyn Miller

Senior Content Project Manager: Stacey Lamodi

Senior Art Director: Jack Pendleton

Production Technology Analyst: Tom Stover

Library of Congress Control Number: 2008930399

ISBN-13: 978-1-4354-1915-5

ISBN-10: 1-4354-1915-4

Delmar
5 Maxwell Drive
Clifton Park, NY 12065-2919
USA

Cengage Learning is a leading provider of customized learning solutions with office locations around the globe, including Singapore, the United Kingdom, Australia, Mexico, Brazil and Japan. Locate your local office at:
international.cengage.com/region

Cengage Learning products are represented in Canada by Nelson Education, Ltd.

To learn more about Delmar, visit **www.cengage.com/delmar**
Purchase any of our products at your local college store or at our preferred online store **www.ichapters.com**

For your lifelong learning solutions, visit **delmar.cengage.com**
Visit our corporate website at **www.cengage.com**

Notice to the Reader

Printed in the United States of America
3 4 5 6 7 12 11 10

CONTENTS

This workbook is part of a dynamic learning system that will help reinforce the essential competencies you need to enter the field of medical assisting and become a successful, multiskilled medical assistant. It has been completely revised to challenge you to apply the chapter knowledge from *Delmar's Comprehensive Medical Assisting: Administrative and Clinical Competencies*, Fourth Edition, to develop basic competencies, use critical thinking skills, and integrate your knowledge effectively.

WORKBOOK ORGANIZATION

The Chapter Assignment Sheets are divided into the following sections: Chapter Pre-Test, Vocabulary Builder, Learning Review, Certification Review, Learning Application, Chapter Post-Test, and Self-Assessment. The content of the workbook has been designed to give you a creative and interpretive forum to apply the knowledge you have learned, not simply to repeat information to answer questions. Realistic simulations appear throughout the workbook that reference the characters in the textbook. This gives the material a real-world feel that comes as close as possible to your future experiences in an ambulatory setting. Clinical principles, such as infection control or communication and patient education, are repeatedly reinforced through simulation exercises that require the ability to use your knowledge effectively and readily.

COMPETENCY ASSESSMENT CHECKLISTS

Competency Assessment Checklists are designed to set criteria or standards that should be observed while a specific procedure is being performed. The procedural steps are listed in the textbook, and the Competency Assessment Checklist scoring reflects the major milestones, or outcomes, of following the specific procedural steps. As you perform each procedure, the evaluation section of this checklist can be used to judge your performance. The instructor will use this checklist to evaluate your competency in performing this skill. Your instructor may combine some Competencies and adjust others to suit individual program schedules. These checklists are provided for guidance.

A master Competency Assessment Tracking Sheet is also provided for you prior to this section of the workbook to use as an overview of all competency assessment checklists. This tracking sheet can serve as a table of contents for all checklists, as well as a guide to easily view your performance on the assessment checklists.

The format of the Competency Assessment Checklists is designed to provide specific conditions, standards, milestone steps, and evaluation and documentation sections for essential skills necessary for an entry-level medical assistant. Forms are provided on the Student Online Companion for use with the competency assessment checklists as you complete the procedures in your textbook. To access the Student Online Companion, use the instructions on the tear-out Access Card in your book to create your account and log in.

COMPREHENSIVE EXAMINATION

Feel certain that each procedure and concept you master is an important step toward preparing your skills and knowledge for the workplace. A final comprehensive examination is presented at the conclusion of the workbook, covering all the essential topic areas that medical assisting graduates must master. This examination has 200 questions and provides excellent practice for national certification examinations.

v

FINAL THOUGHTS

The textbook, software CDs, workbook, and online companion have all been coordinated to meet the core objectives. Review the performance objectives at the beginning of each chapter in the textbook before you begin to study; they are a road map that will take you to your goals.

Remember that you are the learner, so you can take credit for your success. The instructor is an important guide on this journey, and the text, workbook, student software CD, and practicums are tools, but whether or not you use the tools wisely is ultimately up to you.

Evaluate yourself and your study habits. Take positive steps toward improving yourself, and avoid habits that could limit your success. Do family responsibilities and social opportunities interfere with your study? If so, sit down with your family and plan a schedule for study that they will support and to which you will adhere. Find a special place to study that is free from distraction.

Because regulations vary from state to state regarding which procedures can be performed by a medical assistant, it will be important to check specific regulations in your state. A medical assistant should never perform any procedure without being aware of legal responsibilities, correct procedure, and proper authorization.

As you pursue a wonderful career in medical assisting, make the most of your education and training.

Chapter Assignment Sheets

CHAPTER **1**

The Medical Assisting Profession

CHAPTER PRE-TEST

Perform this test without looking at your book. If an answer is "false," rewrite the sentence to make it true.

1. Circle all that apply: Are medical assistants licensed, registered, or certified?

2. True or False? Anyone can take the AAMA medical assisting examination without going through a special program.

   _____

   _____

3. True or False? Medical assistants are allowed to work only in the clinical area of the office.

   _____

   _____

4. True or False? Medical assistants can become office managers.

   _____

   _____

5. Circle all that apply: Medical assistants work as administrative medical assistants in such positions as medical bookkeepers, medical insurance coders and billers, transcriptionists, office managers, and as clinical medical assistants in such positions as laboratory assistants, surgical assistants, phlebotomists, electrocardiography technicians, patient educators.

6. True or False? Choosing to attend an accredited medical assisting program is not as important as getting trained as quickly as possible so you can find employment.

   _____

   _____

7. True or False? Medical assistants do not have to be credentialed to work in their profession.

   _____

   _____

VOCABULARY BUILDER

Misspelled Words

Find the words below that are misspelled; underline them, and then correctly spell them in the space provided.

acredits	complience	integrate
ambulatory care setting	credential	licensure
associate's	disposition	liscensed
attributes	empathy	litigous
certify	facilitates	practicums
competancy	improvising	versatile

_____   _____   _____

_____   _____

Fill in the Blanks

From the vocabulary list below, select the term that best fits in the blank in each sentence. (Hint: not all terms will be used.)

accreditation	CMAS	practicum
ambulatory care facilities	competency	RMA
CCMA	compliance	scope of practice
certification examination	credential	versatile
certify	diploma	
CMA (AAMA)	litigious	

1. The medical assistant is a _____ health care professional.

2. The medical assistant performs many clinical and administrative duties in providers' offices and _____ _____.

3. In today's _____ society, health care consumers are demanding educated, skilled health care professionals.

4. The AAMA and AMT provide national _____ examinations which certify the skills of medical assistants at entry level.

5. Medical assisting programs undergo _____ processes that prove they are covering the appropriate curriculum and are properly serving the education/learning needs of their students.

6. When you graduate from your medical assisting program, you will be given a _____ (sometimes called a certificate), which proves that you have taken all the courses necessary to graduate from the program.

7. Upon successfully passing the AAMA's certification examination, you will be credentialed as a _____.

8. The American Medical Technologists offers examinations to become an _____ and/or _____.

9. The National Healthcareer Association offers an examination to become a _____.

Word Search

Find the words in the grid below. They may go in any direction.

```
B L E C O M E C E R T I F I E D Z B E C G O
M I P I H S N R E T X E E I N L I C E N S E
V T O L V E D Q Y C N E T E P M O C I C O S
N I T C I N I U E E L E A R N I N T G S Z I
B G C L E E T N Z M Z W Q M Z K T K H C P V
M I D H J R C L T R P Y V M T E K D L O R O
N O L T X X T N G E R A F Q S A R M R P O R
O U D V N K L I A G G A T E B R M D N E F P
I S W Z G N C L F I C R R H J R E O Q O E M
T P J R W M F X J I L A A G Y L R D L F S I
A R J K A M K B L P C P X T A F W D D P S L
T R L Y X R J I I Y P A M I E B P I E R I N
I D B R R X T H R R M Z T O K R T S T A O D
D T J V R A S O A Y T N P I C Q M P A C N Y
E R T Q T N T C K P E W N C O C C O V T A V
R F K E R A T T P D Z K P R W N Z S I I L Y
C Z W E L I R V E F N D G F K L M I T C I F
C Y T U C M W R X K Q P N A D N Z T L E S N
A N B U L T C T N H L K N R M R T I U D M V
I M M T T R W R N D H K V M R R Z O C J M R
A M B Y H A T T R I B U T E V Y D N Z Q K Z
G D E X T E R I T Y Y R A T E I R P O R P K
```

Accreditation	Cultivate	License
Ambulatory care setting	Dexterity	Litigious
Attribute	Diploma	Practicum
Certification	Disposition	Professionalism
Certified	Empathy	Proprietary
CMA (AAMA)	Facilitate	RMA
Competency	Improvise	Scope of practice
Compliance	Integrate	
Credentialed	Internship	

LEARNING REVIEW

True or False

Mark a true statement with a T *and a false statement with an* F. *If an answer is "false," rewrite the sentence to make it true.*

____ 1. Medical assistants are licensed by each state.

_____

_____

——— 2. All medical assisting programs are accredited by either CAAHEP or ABHES.

_____

_____

——— 3. Anyone can call himself or herself a medical assistant, but professional medical assistants have graduated from an accredited program and obtained a credential to prove their competency.

_____

_____

——— 4. If you graduate from a medical assisting program and get a diploma or certificate, then you are automatically credentialed.

_____

_____

——— 5. Medical assistants continue their education by attending seminars, workshops, and professional meetings.

_____

_____

——— 6. Individuals with RMAs and CMA (AAMA)s are required to obtain continuing education units (CEUs) to recertify.

_____

_____

——— 7. Medical assistants must be either CMA (AAMA)s or RMAs to join the AAMA or the AMT.

_____

_____

——— 8. The AAMA "owns" the CMA (AAMA) credential, and individuals may not call themselves CMA (AAMA)s unless they have passed the national AAMA certification examination.

_____

_____

——— 9. Possessing empathy is not considered important in the health care profession.

_____

_____

——— 10. It is extremely important that medical assistants demonstrate a positive attitude toward the patient.

_____

_____

——— 11. Emotionalism can sometimes cloud the medical assistant's judgment.

_____

_____

_____ 12. When dealing with a patient, in certain circumstances it is acceptable for the medical assistant to demonstrate an unpleasant disposition.

_____

_____

_____ 13. Certification is mandatory for medical assistants to become employed.

_____

_____

_____ 14. The CMA (AAMA) exam is a computer-based examination offered on a continuous basis throughout the year.

_____

_____

_____ 15. Two agencies that accredit medical assisting programs are ABHES and CAAHEP.

_____

_____

_____ 16. Becoming certified or registered depends solely on the accrediting body of the institution where the student is enrolled in the program.

_____

_____

_____ 17. All CMA (AAMA)s who are currently employed must have current status as CMA (AAMA)s to use the credential.

_____

_____

_____ 18. The AAMA does not encourage continuing education for medical assistants.

_____

_____

_____ 19. The NHA offers several allied health certifications, including CCMA, CMT, and MLA.

_____

_____

_____ 20. The federal government and most states require a medical assistant to be registered or certified to practice the profession.

_____

_____

_____ 21. Neither the CMA (AAMA) or the RMA is higher than the other.

_____

_____

_____ 22. Another profession the AMT certifies is that of certified medical administrative specialist.

_____

_____

Matching

A medical assisting curriculum should provide a variety of clinical, administrative, and general skills courses. Write a C next to each clinical course, an A next to each administrative course, and a G next to each general course.

_____   1. Medical Records

_____   2. Medical Law and Ethics

_____   3. Urine and Blood Testing in the Laboratory

_____   4. Insurance, Billing, and Coding

_____   5. Pharmacology

_____   6. Medical Terminology

_____   7. Word Processing

_____   8. Anatomy and Physiology

_____   9. Appointments and Scheduling

_____   10. Electronic Medical Records

_____   11. Patient Education

_____   12. Infection Control

_____   13. Temperature, Pulse, Respirations, and Blood Pressure

_____   14. Drawing Blood Samples

Web Search

Search the Web and find the site for both the AAMA, the AMT, and the NHA. List the Web site, address, and phone number for each.

American Association of Medical Assistants

_____

_____

American Medical Technologists

_____

_____

National Healthcareer Association

_____

_____

The Nines

The following word bank consists of the nine attributes of a medical assistant. Choose the word that best describes the listed attribute and fill in the blank.

Ability to communicate   Desire to learn   Flexibility

Attitude   Empathy   Initiative

Dependability   Ethical behavior   Professional appearance

_____ 1. Considering the patient's welfare and being kind

_____ 2. Helping your patients feel more at ease by portraying a warm and friendly disposition and possessing a sense of humor

_____ 3. Being punctual; limiting absences from work

_____ 4. Being willing and able to work independently, being observant of work to be done, and taking the action to complete the tasks

_____ 5. Being adaptable and developing alternative action plans

_____ 6. Acquiring information and updating knowledge and skills

_____ 7. Having an appearance that reflects good health habits

Write a sentence for each attribute describing how each contributes to better patient care and the development of good relationships with both coworkers and employers.

1. Ability to communicate

_____

_____

2. Empathy

_____

_____

3. Flexibility

_____

_____

4. Dependability

_____

_____

5. Attitude

_____

_____

6. Desire to learn

_____

_____

7. Ethical behavior

_____

_____

8. Initiative

_____

_____

9. Physical attributes

_____

_____

Short Answer

1. Name four reasons why the medical assisting profession has grown to require more formal, skilled education and credentialing for medical assistants.

_____

_____

_____

_____

_____

2. The U.S. Department of Labor, Bureau of Statistics, lists medical assisting as the fastest-growing allied health profession. Name eight settings where medical assistants are usually employed.

_____

_____

_____

3. What is the purpose of the CARE bill?

_____

_____

_____

4. State the significance of being credentialed.

_____

_____

_____

_____

5. State the benefits of graduating from a program accredited by either CAAHEP or ABHES.

_____

_____

_____

6. Define the profession of medical assisting.

   _____

   _____

   _____

7. List at least four benefits of the practicum experience.

   _____

   _____

   _____

   _____

   _____

8. What are some of the benefits that medical offices receive as a result of being a practicum site?

   _____

   _____

   _____

   _____

9. Define the acronym CAAHEP and state its purpose.

   _____

   _____

   _____

   _____

10. Membership in the AAMA is at three levels. Name them.

    _____

    _____

11. List at least six components that constitute the professional appearance of a health care provider.

    _____

    _____

    _____

    _____

12. List the three terms used to define the transition period between the classroom and actual employment.

    _____

    _____

13. Circle all that apply. The Occupational Analysis for the CMA (AAMA) and the AMT's Medical Assisting Task List are lists of competencies compiled by practicing medical assistants. These competencies can be used by medical assisting program directors to develop curricula that ensure:

   a. certification

   b. employment preparedness

   c. continuing education

   d. high-quality medical assisting education

CERTIFICATION REVIEW

These questions are designed to mimic the certification examination. Select the best response.

1. Medical assistants may take the AAMA examination to obtain which credential?

   a. CMAS

   b. RMA

   c. CMA (AAMA)

   d. CPC

   e. AMT

2. Select the following statement(s) that best describes the professional medical assistant.

   a. Has good written and oral communication skills

   b. Looks and acts professional at all times

   c. Is aware of the scope of practice and stays within the legal boundaries

   d. Assists the provider in all areas of the ambulatory care setting

   e. All of the above

3. Good medical assistants portray their professional attitude by:

   a. discussing their personal lives at work because it is therapeutic for them

   b. talking with their coworkers to help them with their problems

   c. reminding their providers that they work only 7.5 hours per day

   d. helping patients in a friendly and empathetic manner

   e. doing a basic workload

4. To become involved with their professional organization, medical assistants could:

   a. attend local chapter or state meetings

   b. attend a national conference or state convention

   c. join their national organization

   d. offer to serve on a local, state, or national committee

   e. do all of the above

5. A system of values that each individual has that determines perceptions of right and wrong is called:

   a. laws

   b. ethics

   c. attributes

   d. attitudes

6. Stepping into a patient's place, discovering what the patient is experiencing, then recognizing and identifying with those feelings is:

   a. sympathy

   b. association

   c. flexibility

   d. empathy

7. Which of the following contribute to a professional appearance?

   a. Good nutrition and exercise

   b. Healthy looking skin, teeth, and nails

   c. Daily showering and use of deoderant

   d. All of these answers

8. Courses in a professional medical assisting program include a complement of general knowledge classes such as anatomy and physiology and:

   a. assisting with minor surgery

   b. CPR

   c. medical terminology

   d. computer applications

9. The type of regulation for health care providers that is legislated by each state and is mandatory in order to practice is:

   a. licensure

   b. registration

   c. certification

   d. a and c

LEARNING APPLICATION

CASE STUDY 1

During your course of studies to become a medical assistant, you have an opportunity to volunteer to help out at a multiprovider urgent care center downtown in a large city to gain some firsthand experience in a professional setting.

CASE STUDY REVIEW QUESTIONS

1. Would this opportunity be interesting to you? Would you want to volunteer in this professional setting?

   _____

   _____

   _____

   _____

2. Even though you are a volunteer, why is it important to look and behave like a professional?

   _____

   _____

   _____

   _____

   _____

   _____

   _____

   _____

CASE STUDY 2

Michelle Lucas is preparing for her practicum. Michelle is an excellent student, detail oriented, responsible, and professional in her dress and attitude. Michelle is eager to experience her practicum with a large general practice or clinic with open hours built into the schedule for emergency patients, such as Inner City Health Care. Michelle is intrigued by the idea of working with a group of providers and a diverse patient population where she can really work on improving her screening skills. Michelle, however, is shy and quiet; she has difficulty meeting new people and relies on a core group of friends.

CASE STUDY REVIEW QUESTIONS

1. Is Michelle really suited to practicum at Inner City Health Care? What are the potential advantages or disadvantages of this practicum placement?

_____

_____

_____

_____

_____

_____

_____

2. What would be some ways in which Michelle could overcome the difficulty she experiences when meeting new people?

_____

_____

3. Being able to work with diverse populations is just a small part of being a health care professional. What suggestions would you offer Michelle in reaching her goal of professional growth?

_____

_____

4. Consider your own short- and long-range goals. How important is it to challenge yourself, personally and professionally, with experiences that contribute to your growth and knowledge? How can you use your practicum placement to work toward fulfilling your goals?

_____

_____

CHAPTER POST-TEST

Perform this test without looking at your book. If an answer is "false," rewrite the sentence to make it true.

1. True or False? Medical assistants may be either licensed, registered, or certified.

   _____

   _____

2. True or False? The AAMA medical assisting certification examination is available to anyone, even people who have not been formally trained.

   _____

   _____

3. True or False? Medical assistants work in only the administrative part of the office.

   _____

   _____

4. True or False? The position of office manager is a career option for a medical assistant.

   _____

   _____

5. Circle all that apply: Medical assistants work as administrative medical assistants in such positions as medical bookkeepers, medical insurance coders and billers, transcriptionists, office managers, and as clinical medical assistants in such positions as laboratory assistants, surgical assistants, phlebotomists, electrocardiography technicians, patient educators.

6. True or False? Getting trained as quickly as possible is more important than attending an accredited medical assisting program.

   _____

   _____

7. True or False? Medical assistants may work in their profession even without being credentialed.

   _____

   _____

SELF-ASSESSMENT

1. As you begin your education as a medical assistant, you may not be sure whether you want to work in the administrative and clerical area or in the clinical and laboratory areas. What are some ways for you to explore the various options?

   _____

   _____

   _____

2. For each of the attributes listed in your textbook to describe a professional, identify individuals from your family, circle of friends, work, or community who possess one or more of those traits. Explain why you chose them.

_____

_____

_____

3. Imagine your first day in your practicum. What will you wear? How will you prepare the night before? How will you look? Would you change your hairstyle? Makeup? Jewelry?

_____

_____

_____

_____

_____

_____

C H A P T E R **2**

Health Care Settings and the Health Care Team

CHAPTER PRE-TEST

Perform this test without looking at your book. If an answer is "false," rewrite the sentence to make it true.

1. True or False? Providers who work in sole proprietorships work alone and employ no other providers.

   _____

   _____

2. True or False? When two or more providers join under legal agreement, a partnership is formed.

   _____

   _____

3. True or False? Urgent care centers are like emergency rooms and do not offer routine care services.

   _____

   _____

4. True or False? Medical assistants do not generally work in urgent care centers.

   _____

   _____

5. True or False? An HMO is one example of a managed care operation that hosts a network of providers within a defined geographic area.

   _____

   _____

6. True or False? Providers are licensed to practice nationally so they can move freely from state to state.

   _____

   _____

7. True or False? Doctors of chiropractic medicine work only on the musculoskeletal system.

_____

_____

8. True or False? Acupuncturists treat pain in a variety of disorders in the gastrointestinal, urogenital, gyneco-logic, circulatory, respiratory, neuromusculoskeletal, and many other systems.

_____

_____

VOCABULARY BUILDER

Misspelled Words

Find the words below that are misspelled; circle them and correctly spell them in the spaces provided. Then insert the correct vocabulary terms from the list that best fit the descriptions below.

accupuncture	homeopathy	prefered provider organization (PPO)
ambulatory care settings	independent provider association (IPA)	screening
concerge	intagrative medicine	urgant care
frindge benefits	managed care options	
health maintainance organizations (HMOs)		

_____   _____   _____

_____   _____   _____

_____

1. _____ Organizations designed to provide a full range of health care services under one roof or, more recently, through a network of participating providers within a defined geographic area

2. _____ Advantages added to the terms of employment, such as health insurance and vacation time

3. _____ An independent organization of providers, whose members agree to treat patients for an agreed-upon fee

4. _____ Treatment using highly diluted doses of certain substances derived from plants, animals, or minerals that are manufactured by pharmaceutical companies under strict guidelines

5. _____ Medical setting that provides services on an outpatient basis

6. _____ A form of oriental medicine where sterile fine needles are inserted in specified sites of the body

7. _____ Organizations in which providers network to offer discounts to employers and other purchasers of health care

8. _____ Alternative forms of health care increasingly perceived as complements to traditional health care

9. _____ A for-profit center that provides services for primary care, routine illnesses, and injury, as well as minor surgery

10. _____ Another avenue of health care that provides exclusive services for fees ranging from $2,000 to $6,000.

11. _____ Assessment of patient needs to determine the priority of medical action

12. _____ A standard of patient care that seeks to provide quality care while containing costs

LEARNING REVIEW

Short Answer

1. How has managed care changed medical settings as the health care profession works to offer high-quality, cost-effective care to patients? What is the medical assistant's role in contributing to the efforts of the health care team in an era of managed care?

   _____

   _____

   _____

   _____

   _____

   _____

   _____

2. Since medical assistants are often patients' first contact with the facility and the provider, what attributes must medical assistants possess?

   _____

   _____

   _____

3. Name six administrative duties of the medical assistant as a member of the health care team.

   _____

   _____

   _____

4. Name five clinical duties of the medical assistant as a member of the health care team.

   _____

   _____

   _____

   _____

5. In the medical field, the abbreviation Dr. is used, and the title of doctor is addressed to the person qualified by education, training, and licensure to practice medicine. List the medical degree associated with each of the following credentials, and define each specialty.

M.D. _____

_____

D.P.M. _____

D.C. _____

_____

N.D. _____

_____

D.O. _____

_____

O.D. _____

_____

D.D.S. _____

6. Using a medical dictionary or encyclopedia to help you, define the following eight medical and surgical specialists. Refer to your textbook for a complete listing of medical and surgical specialties.

Radiologist _____

_____

Obstetrician/gynecologist _____

_____

Ophthalmologist _____

Pediatrician _____

_____

Allergist and Immunologist _____

_____

Dermatologist _____

Cardiologist _____

7. Medical assistants are only one of many allied health and other health care professionals who form the health care team. Although medical assistants may not work directly with each professional, they are likely to come into contact with many of them through telephone, written, or electronic communication. List six of those types of professionals.

_____

_____

_____

_____

_____

8. In an effort to receive alternative therapies, many health care providers and patients are pursuing integrative medicine as a complement to traditional health care. Name eight alternative forms of health care that may be currently perceived to supplement traditional health care.

_____

_____

_____

9. List at least five services that a so-called boutique or concierge medical practice offers.

_____

_____

_____

_____

10. What is the role of the physician assistant? How does a physician assistant relate to a medical assistant?

_____

_____

_____

_____

_____

11. What are the licensure requirements for a physician assistant?

_____

_____

_____

_____

_____

Medical Settings Activity

For each of the three forms of medical practice management, list appropriate medical settings. Describe the patient's experience with care under each form of medical practice management. Note how patient experiences may differ and why this is possible.

1. Sole Proprietorships

   Medical settings: _____

   Patient experience: _____

   _____

   _____

2. Partnerships

   Medical settings: _____

   Patient experience: _____

   _____

   _____

   _____

3. Corporations

   Medical settings: _____

   Patient experience: _____

   _____

   _____

CERTIFICATION REVIEW

These questions are designed to mimic the certification examination. Select the best response.

1. The form of medical practice management that states that personal property cannot be attached in litigation is a:

   a. partnership

   b. sole proprietorship

   c. corporation

   d. group practice

2. The minimum amount of time it takes to become an M.D. without specialization is:

   a. 6 years

   b. 8 years

   c. 12 years

   d. 4 years

3. In the ambulatory care setting, the medical assistant may prefer what tasks?

   a. Educating patients

   b. Administration such as coding and billing

   c. Performing various laboratory tests

   d. All of the above

4. The American Society of Clinical Pathology is the professional organization that oversees credentialing and education in what allied health area?

   a. Nurses

   b. Medical laboratory

   c. Registered dietician

   d. Physical therapy

5. The specialty that is based on the belief that the cause of disease is violation of nature's laws is called:

   a. chiropractic

   b. osteopathy

   c. podiatry

   d. naturopathy

6. A branch of the healing arts that gives special attention to the physiologic and biochemical aspects of the body's structure, including manipulation of the spine, is:

   a. acupuncture

   b. chiropractic

   c. massage

   d. oriental medicine

7. HMOs are organizations designed to:

   a. provide a full range of health care service under one roof

   b. employ providers who network to offer discounts to employers and other purchasers of health care

   c. include environments such as a medical office and a primary care center

   d. serve as an emergency room

8. In order to practice medicine, a physician must:

   a. go to college

   b. pay a fee

   c. take online courses

   d. obtain a license to practice from a state or jurisdiction of the United States

9. Another name of the organization where providers network to offer discounts to employees and other purchasers of health insurance is:

   a. IPA

   b. HMO

   c. PPO

   d. group practice

10. Another term for assessing the patient's needs is:

   a. screening

   b. prescribing

   c. taking vital signs

   d. monitoring

LEARNING APPLICATION

CASE STUDY 1

Abigail Johnson is an older woman in her 70s with mature-onset diabetes. She is having trouble managing her diet; she lives alone but craves social contact and seems to enjoy her visits to the family provider's office. She has an appointment today for dietary counseling.

CASE STUDY REVIEW QUESTIONS

1. How can Mrs. Johnson be encouraged to consider herself part of the health care team?

   _____
   _____
   _____

2. What is the role of the medical assistant?

   _____
   _____
   _____

CASE STUDY 2

Herb Fowler is an African American man in his early 50s. Herb is a heavy smoker, is significantly overweight, and has a chronic cough. He believes the cough is caused by bronchitis and stubbornly insists on being prescribed antibiotics. Today, Herb is at the medical office for a preventive medicine appointment.

CASE STUDY REVIEW QUESTIONS

1. How can Mr. Fowler be encouraged to consider himself part of the health care team?

   _____
   _____
   _____

2. What is the role of the medical assistant?

   _____
   _____

CASE STUDY 3

Juanita Hansen is a single mother in her mid-20s with one son, Henry. Juanita arrives at the urgent care clinic for the fourth time in a month. Henry has fallen down the stairs twice, suffered a burn on the hand, and is now refusing to eat. There are bruises on various parts of Henry's body, as well.

CASE STUDY REVIEW QUESTIONS

1. How can the mother be encouraged to consider herself part of the health care team?

   _____

   _____

2. What is the role of the medical assistant?

   _____

   _____

   _____

CASE STUDY 4

Lenore McDonell is a disabled woman in her early 30s who lives independently with the aid of a motorized wheelchair. Lenore functions well in her home environment but has grown fearful of venturing out, even to the provider's office for her routine follow-up examinations. She has canceled three appointments in a row. Today she is in for her yearly physical.

CASE STUDY REVIEW QUESTIONS

1. How can Mrs. McDonell be encouraged to consider herself part of the health care team?

   _____

   _____

   _____

2. What is the role of the medical assistant?

   _____

   _____

   _____

CHAPTER POST-TEST

Perform this test without looking at your book. If an answer is "false," rewrite the sentence to make it true.

1. True or False? Sole proprietors work alone and do not employ other providers.

   _____

   _____

2. True or False? Partnerships are made up of two or more providers who share the total business operation of the practice.

   _____

   _____

3. True or False? Urgent care centers are for emergencies only.

   _____

   _____

4. True or False? Urgent care centers require skills that medical assistants do not generally have.

   _____

   _____

5. True or False? A form of managed care is the HMO, whose providers form a network within a geographic area.

   _____

   _____

6. True or False? Providers are licensed to practice state by state.

   _____

   _____

7. True or False? Chiropractors work on only musculoskeletal conditions.

   _____

   _____

8. True or False? Acupuncture can be helpful when dealing with pain and a variety of disorders in the gastrointestinal, urogenital, gynecologic, circulatory, respiratory, neuromusculoskeletal, and many other systems.

   _____

   _____

SELF-ASSESSMENT

As you were deciding to become a medical assistant, what other career were you considering? List the three reasons you were considering that other career, and then list three reasons you chose medical assisting instead. Keep in mind not just the time, money, and education involved, but also the profession itself, the day-to-day duties, the type of work, the people involved, and so forth. Think about the similarities between the careers. Are there more similarities than differences? Are you going to be using some of the same skills? Is there a way these different careers will come together at any point in the future?

_____

_____

_____

_____

_____

CHAPTER **3**

History of Medicine

CHAPTER PRE-TEST

Perform this test without looking at your book. If an answer is "false," rewrite the sentence to make it true.

1. True or False? The practice of medicine began when we started keeping medical records.

_____

_____

2. True or False? Plants used to be the basis of all medications but are not anymore.

_____

_____

3. True or False? Cultural differences do not and should not influence the way we treat our patients.

_____

_____

4. True or False? Magic was practiced because it was considered an essential ingredient in chasing evil spirits away.

_____

_____

5. True or False? Ancient Eastern treatments included curing the spirit and nourishing the body.

_____

_____

6. True or False? Acupuncture uses the placement of needles in thousands of points on the body.

_____

_____

7. True or False? Women were not accepted as medical doctors in Western culture until the 1800s.

_____

_____

8. True or False? The "father of preventive medicine" was Louis Pasteur.

_____

_____

9. True or False? Edward Jenner developed the smallpox vaccine in the late 1700s.

_____

_____

10. True or False? The Oath of Hippocrates mentions mischief, sexual misconduct, and slaves.

_____

_____

VOCABULARY BUILDER

Misspelled Words

Find the words below that are misspelled; circle them, and correctly spell them in the spaces provided. Then insert the correct vocabulary terms from the list that best fit the descriptions below.

acepsis	malaria	septacemia
acupuncture	opiods	typhis
alopathic	pharmacopoies	yellow fever
bubonic plague	pluralistic	

_____   _____   _____

_____   _____   _____

1. In our _____ society, we rely on several philosophies of medicine that serve an individual's needs by respecting ethnic, cultural, and religious traditions while providing the best standard of care to patients and their families.

2. The piercing of the skin by long needles into any of 365 points along 12 meridians that traverse the body and transmit an active life force called qi is the practice of _____, an ancient Chinese technique thought by many today to be effective in the treatment of chronic pain.

3. That bacteria can enter the bloodstream to cause infection, _____, was observed in the nineteenth century by Hungarian physician and obstetrician Ignaz Philipp Semmelweiss.

4. Since the twentieth century, the discovery of antibiotics, the development of vaccines, and the institution of proper health and sanitation measures have largely contributed to the containment of many infectious diseases, including _____, _____, and _____.

5. _____ physicians treat illness and disease with medical and surgical interventions intended to alleviate the condition or effect a cure.

6. A _____ is a book that describes drugs and their preparation and details plant, animal, and mineral substances as essential ingredients in effecting cures.

7. In the nineteenth century, _____, the process of sterilizing surgical environments to discourage the growth of bacteria, and anesthesia, the process of alleviating pain during surgery, revolutionized surgical practices throughout the world.

LEARNING REVIEW

Short Answer

1. Religion, magic, and science all play a vital part in the history of medicine. Describe each.

   Religion _____

   _____

   Magic _____

   _____

   Science _____

   _____

   _____

2. Name the five methods of treatment important to the practice of medicine according to ancient Chinese tradition. How are these methods relevant for allopathic physicians today?

   _____

   _____

   _____

   _____

   _____

   _____

   _____

   _____

   _____

3. Individual cultures and people throughout history have conferred different, and often changing, status upon women in medicine. For each of the five cultures below, describe the status of women in medicine.

   (1) Primitive societies:

   _____

   _____

   _____

   (2) Chinese:

   _____

   _____

   (3) Muslim:

   _____

   _____

   (4) Italian:

   _____

   _____

(5) American:

_____

_____

4. Trace the progression of medical education by listing the important advances, discoveries, or medical philosophies for each period or century listed. What do you expect for the twenty-first century?

(1) Prehistoric times:

_____

_____

_____

(2) Ancient times:

_____

_____

_____

_____

_____

(3) Seventh century:

_____

_____

_____

_____

(4) Ninth century:

_____

_____

_____

(5) Renaissance:

_____

_____

_____

_____

(6) Nineteenth century:

_____

_____

_____

_____

(7) Twentieth century:

_____

_____

_____

_____

_____

_____

(8) Twenty-first century:

_____

_____

5. Attitudes toward illness have changed throughout the history of medicine and also often differ among cultures. For each situation listed, give both historical and current attitudes toward the sick person. Discuss how attitudes toward illness may, or may not, have changed through history.

(1) Elderly and infirm people are encouraged to end their own lives or are outcast from society.

_____

_____

_____

_____

(2) Individuals with a frightening illness, for which there is no cure, are shunned or quarantined.

_____

_____

_____

_____

(3) Sickness is seen as a moral or spiritual failing of an individual.

_____

_____

_____

_____

(4) Survivors of illness are viewed as heroic individuals.

_____

_____

_____

_____

(5) People with disabilities are valued as individuals and receive care that allows them to function in mainstream society.

_____

_____

_____

_____

6. Name 15 infectious or epidemic diseases that have been controlled in the twentieth century through medical advances and discoveries such as antibiotics, vaccines, asepsis, and insulin.

_____

_____

_____

7. The Hippocratic Oath, which originated in ancient Greece, embodies within it many ethical standards of treatment and care that providers espouse to this day. In contemporary layperson's language, name the five basic standards contained in the oath.

_____

_____

_____

_____

_____

8. Fill in the blanks below with the three epidemics discussed in the chapter, along with descriptions of each and treatment options.

Epidemic   **Description, Causes, Treatment**

_____   _____

                            _____

                            _____

                            _____

_____   _____

                            _____

                            _____

                            _____

_____   _____

                            _____

                            _____

                            _____

Matching I

For each of the following, write an R *if the statement describes a belief in religion, an* M *if the statement describes a belief in magic, or an* S *if the statement describes a belief in science.*

_____ 1. A recent research study involved two groups of patients with AIDS: One group received daily prayers from an anonymous prayer group hundreds of miles away, and the other received no prayers. The group receiving the prayers responded better to treatment.

_____ 2. Trephination was used by prehistoric cultures to release evil spirits responsible for illness.

_____ 3. Chinese acupuncture techniques are used to control pain or treat drug dependency.

_____ 4. Botanicals are effective in treating certain conditions. The Chinese pharmacopoeia is rich in the use of herbs.

_____ 5. Some Native Americans believe that someone recovering from a serious illness might hold extraordinary powers.

_____ 6. Some practitioners throughout history have held to the belief that healing involves not just medical treatment, but attention to the purity of the patient's soul and to the faith of the individual as well.

Matching II

Match the individuals listed below with each of their contributions to the history of medicine.

_____ 1. Andreas Vesalius   A. Developed a vaccine for poliomyelitis

_____ 2. Sir Alexander Fleming   B. "Father of medicine"

_____ 3. W. T. G. Morton   C. Developed smallpox vaccine

_____ 4. Moses   D. Discovered penicillin

_____ 5. Edward Jenner   E. "Father of bacteriology"

_____ 6. Clara Barton   F. Advocate of health rules in Hebrew religion

_____ 7. Louis Pasteur   G. Invented the stethoscope

_____ 8. Elizabeth Blackwell   H. First female physician in the United States

_____ 9. Hippocrates   I. Rendered accurate anatomical drawings of body systems

_____ 10. René Laënnec   J. Wrote first anatomical studies

_____ 11. Robert Koch   K. Laid the groundwork for asepsis

_____ 12. Florence Nightingale   L. Started the American Red Cross

_____ 13. Anton van Leeuwenhoek   M. Founder of modern nursing

_____ 14. Wilhelm von Roentgen   N. Introduced ether as an anesthetic

_____ 15. John Hunter   O. Discovered lens magnification

_____ 16. Elizabeth G. Anderson   P. Discovered X-rays

_____ 17. Leonardo da Vinci   Q. Founder of scientific surgery

_____ 18. Joseph Lister   R. Developed culture-plate method

_____ 19. Jonas Salk   S. Discovered insulin

_____ 20. Frederick G. Banting   T. First female physician

CERTIFICATION REVIEW

These questions are designed to mimic the certification examination. Select the best response.

1. Who of the following was not a scientist who contributed to the study of bacteriology?

    a. Louis Pasteur

    b. Robert Koch

    c. Joseph Lister

    d. John Hunter

2. The first female physician in the United States was:

    a. Clara Barton

    b. Elizabeth Blackwell

    c. Florence Nightingale

    d. Joan of Arc

3. The Oath of Hippocrates:

    a. establishes guidelines for all health care providers

    b. establishes guidelines for the practice of medicine

    c. is a well-known document about the ethics of ancient medicine

    d. was the first scientific journal of significance

4. The ancient culture that believed that illness was a punishment by the gods for violations of moral codes was the:

    a. Chinese

    b. Egyptian

    c. Mesopotamian

    d. Indian

5. Ancient healing priests performed many functions that involved the welfare of the entire community or village and were referred to as:

    a. shamans

    b. chi

    c. lipuria

    d. polypenia

6. Medical education in established universities began in what century?

    a. Second

    b. Fifteenth

    c. Eighteenth

    d. Ninth

7. What country today quarantines everyone who tests positive for HIV, even if they show no signs of the disease?

   a. Africa

   b. Cuba

   c. Korea

   d. Canada

8. In 1922, insulin was established as a treatment for diabetes by:

   a. Lister

   b. Pasteur

   c. Salk and Sabin

   d. Banting and Best

LEARNING APPLICATION

 CASE STUDY

When 52-year-old Margaret Thomas, Martin Gordon's younger sister, begins to experience mild hand tremors and balance problems, Martin suggests that Margaret go see Dr. Winston Lewis. Dr. Lewis is Martin's primary care provider, who had provided treatment for Martin's prostate cancer. Feeling more comfortable with a female physician, Margaret chooses to make an appointment with Dr. Lewis's associate in the group practice, Dr. Elizabeth King. On the day of the examination, she brings her 25-year-old daughter with her to the clinic.

After taking a detailed patient history and undertaking a thorough physical examination of Margaret, Dr. King makes note of signs and symptoms, including a resting tremor, shuffling gait, muscle rigidity, and difficulty in swallowing and speaking. Margaret also complains of a "hot feeling" and odd, uncharacteristic moments of defective judgment when "she just can't keep things straight." Dr. King suspects Parkinson's disease and tells Margaret and her daughter that she would like to refer Margaret to a neurologist for more specific examination and medical tests. Dr. King explains that there are effective drug therapies for controlling the disease, although it has no known cure, and that the neurologist will outline Margaret's treatment options if a diagnosis of Parkinson's is made. Margaret seems to be shaken but takes Dr. King's words in stride.

Dr. King leaves Margaret and her daughter in the examination room with Audrey Jones, CMA (AAMA), who has assisted Dr. King throughout the examination and asks Audrey to be sure to give Margaret the referral to the neurologist. Margaret's daughter asks Audrey if Parkinson's is the disease that has shown promise in fetal tissue research and if her mother might be a candidate. Before Audrey can answer, Margaret becomes visibly distressed. "We're a good Catholic family, I could never consider that. Me—a grandmother." Looking to Audrey, she adds, "Please tell me I won't be involved with such a thing."

continues

CASE STUDY REVIEW QUESTIONS

1. What part does the role of women in medicine and in society play in this situation?

   _____

   _____

   _____

   _____

   _____

   _____

   _____

   _____

   _____

2. How should Audrey, the medical assistant, reply to Margaret and her daughter? What course of action, if any, should she take?

   _____

   _____

   _____

   _____

   _____

3. How do religious beliefs make an impact on the attitude toward illness held by the patient? How might these beliefs affect a treatment plan?

   _____

   _____

   _____

   _____

   _____

4. Discuss the issues that arise when a potential medical breakthrough involves controversial or radical ideas that challenge long-held cultural viewpoints and beliefs.

   _____

   _____

   _____

   _____

   _____

   _____

   _____

CHAPTER POST-TEST

Perform this test without looking at your book. If an answer is "false," rewrite the sentence to make it true.

1. True or False? The practice of medicine began long before we started keeping medical records.

_____

_____

2. True or False? Plants remain the basis of many medications.

_____

_____

3. True or False? Cultural differences do and should influence the way we treat our patients.

_____

_____

4. True or False? Magic has never played a role in medicine.

_____

_____

5. True or False? Ancient Eastern treatments did not include working with the human spirit.

_____

_____

6. True or False? Acupuncture uses the placement of needles in 365 points on the body.

_____

_____

7. True or False? Women were accepted as medical doctors in Chinese culture long before Western cultures.

_____

_____

8. True or False? The "father of preventive medicine" was Joseph Lister.

_____

_____

9. True or False? Edward Jenner developed the smallpox vaccine in the late 1800s.

_____

_____

SELF-ASSESSMENT

1. Make a list of the various ethnic, religious, and cultural groups you and your family members participate in or are descended from.

_____

_____

_____

_____

2. Interview family members to determine how their ethnic, religious, or cultural beliefs make an impact on the kind of medical care and treatment they expect to receive and how attitudes may have changed or evolved from generation to generation. Write a brief summary of your family's beliefs.

_____

_____

_____

_____

3. Write down any folk or home remedies used by your parents or grandparents that may or may not still be used by your family today. Why might these remedies have been more widely relied on by previous generations? Is there a scientific basis for each remedy?

_____

_____

_____

_____

4. An experimental treatment may be the only alternative available for your patient. How would this particular situation affect you, the medical assistant, if it is against your cultural or religious beliefs?

_____

_____

_____

_____

C H A P T E R **4**

Therapeutic Communication Skills

CHAPTER PRE-TEST

Perform this test without looking at your book. If an answer is "false," rewrite the sentence to make it true.

1. True or False? Gestures and expressions have nothing to do with what a person is thinking or feeling.

_____

_____

2. True or False? You can make sick patients "feel better" just by the way you communicate with them.

_____

_____

3. True or False? Everyone enjoys a hug.

_____

_____

4. True or False? Patients should not be encouraged to verbalize their feelings and concerns.

_____

_____

5. True or False? Therapeutic communication can take place without considering the cultural and religious background of the patient.

_____

_____

6. True or False? Personal space is the distance at which we feel comfortable with others while communicating.

_____

_____

7. True or False? It is not necessary to accept the uniqueness in each person.

_____

_____

8. True or False? It is important for the patient to know that the provider will take the time to listen, answer any questions, and talk with the patient openly.

_____

_____

VOCABULARY BUILDER

Misspelled Words

Find the words below that are misspelled; circle them, and correctly spell them in the spaces provided. Then, insert the correct vocabulary terms from the list that best fits the descriptions below.

active listening	defense mechanisms	perseption
biases	denial	prejidices
body language	encode	rationalization
closed questions	hierarcky of needs	regression
cluster	indirect statements	repression
compinsation	interview technikes	roadblocks
congruancy	kinesics	therapuetic communication
cultural brokering	masking	time focus
decode	open-ended questions	

_____   _____   _____

_____   _____

_____   _____

_____   1. Allows patients to feel comfortable, even when receiving difficult or unpleasant information, achieved through use of specific and well-defined professional communication skills

_____   2. The person seems to experience temporary amnesia; forgetting or wiping things out of the conscious memory

_____   3. Knowing how to encourage the best communication between the health care provider and the patient

_____   4. Human needs grouped into five levels, each level being satisfied first before moving on to the next

_____   5. Types of questions that require only a yes or no answer

_____   6. Verbal or nonverbal messages that prevent patients from expressing themselves

_____   7. The study of nonverbal communication, which includes unconscious body movements, gestures, and facial expressions

_____ 8. Statements that turn a question into a topic of interest that allows the patient to speak without feeling directly questioned

_____ 9. Being aware of what the patient is not saying or the ability to pick up on hints by the patient's body language regarding the real message

_____ 10. Personal preferences slanting toward a particular belief

_____ 11. An opinion or judgment that is formed before all the facts are known

_____ 12. Nonverbal communication that conveys expression or feelings

_____ 13. Types of questions that require more than a yes or no answer, the patient being required to verbalize more information

_____ 14. An attempt to conceal or repress one's true feelings or real message

_____ 15. Nonverbal messages grouped together to form a statement or conclusion

_____ 16. When a person's nonverbal message agrees with that person's verbal message

_____ 17. Interpreting the meaning of the message to understand it

_____ 18. Creation of a carefully crafted message by a sender to match the receiver's ability to receive and interpret it properly

_____ 19. Conscious awareness of one's own feelings and the feelings of others

_____ 20. Substituting a strength for a weakness

_____ 21. The mind's way of making unacceptable behavior or events acceptable by devising a rational reason for it

_____ 22. Refusal to accept painful information that is apparent to others

_____ 23. Attempt to withdraw from an unpleasant circumstance by retreating to a more secure state of life

_____ 24. Act of bridging, linking, or mediating between groups or persons through the process of reducing conflict or producing change

_____ 25. Statements eliciting a response from the patient without the patient's feeling questioned

_____ 26. Unconscious behavior used to protect the ego from guilt, anxiety, or loss of esteem

Crossword Puzzle

Across

9. Gestures and expressions together with body poses (two words)
11. Moving back to a former stage to escape conflict
12. This "cycle" involves sending and receiving messages, verbal and nonverbal (two words)
13. The art of really hearing another person's message and sometimes verifying with that person what you are hearing
14. The study of body movements
15. Questions that can be answered with a simple yes or no response

Down

1. Opinions or judgments formed before all the facts are known
2. Giving the speaker information about what you are hearing
3. The act of justification, usually illogically, that people use to keep from facing the truth
4. The rejection of or refusal to acknowledge information
5. The position of the body and parts of the body
6. Behavior that protects people from feelings of guilt, anxiety, and shame
7. A slant toward a particular belief
8. Sometimes referred to as temporary amnesia

LEARNING REVIEW

Short Answer

1. List the three listening goals of the health care professional.

_____

_____

_____

2. The four modes of communication most pertinent in our everyday exchange are:

_____

_____

3. Circle the five correct responses. The five Cs of communication are:

clear   coherent   concise

constant   complete   curious

credible   courteous   comment

curt   cooperative   cohesive

4. Understanding Maslow's hierarchy will help medical assistants assess patients' needs and facilitate therapeutic communication. For each level, list a minimum of three needs that meet it.

_____

_____

_____

_____

5. Identify eight significant roadblocks to communication.

_____

_____

_____

6. In order for any type of communication to take place, the patient must trust the health care provider. List the necessary steps in building the patient's trust.

_____

_____

_____

_____

_____

7. How does therapeutic communication differ from normal communication?

_____

_____

8. List and explain the four basic elements included in the communication cycle.

_____

_____

_____

_____

_____

_____

9. Edith Leonard arrives at the clinic for a routine six-month follow-up examination. At her last visit, she had been referred to an ophthalmologist for removal of a cataract in her right eye. Compose (1) a closed question, (2) an open-ended question, and (3) an indirect statement regarding Ms. Leonard's condition.

Closed question:

_____

_____

Open-ended question:

_____

_____

Indirect statement:

_____

_____

10. Time focus relates to whether the patient's attitude toward life is future, present, or past. Fill in the blanks below by explaining what each of these categories mean and list cultures or religions that are oriented to each.

Time focus	Meaning	Cultural or religious groups
Future time focus	_____	_____
	_____	_____
	_____	_____
	_____	_____
Present time focus	_____	_____
	_____	_____
	_____	_____
	_____	_____
Past time focus	_____	_____
	_____	_____
	_____	_____

Matching I

Identify each of the following as high-context communication (H) or low-context communication (L).

_____   1. African-American, Western culture

_____   2. Relies on highly detailed language to communicate ideas

_____   3. Asian culture

_____   4. Native American

_____   5. Relies on relevant phraseology to communicate ideas

_____   6. Caucasian, Western culture

_____   7. Hispanic and Latino cultures

_____   8. Islam

_____   9. Relies on body language to communicate ideas

Matching II

Biases and prejudices common in today's society have the potential to create hostility. Match each difficult situation below to the corresponding bias or prejudice that motivates it. Put a letter in the space provided.

A. A preference for Western-style medicine

B. The tendency to choose female rather than male providers

C. Prejudice related to a person's sexual preference

D. Discrimination based on race or religion

E. Hostile attitudes toward persons with a value system opposite to your own

F. A belief that persons who cannot afford health care should receive less care than those who can pay for full services

_____ 1. Mr. Gordon refuses to accept a referral to an acupuncturist to help alleviate the chronic pain of advancing prostate cancer.

_____ 2. Medical assistant Bruce Goldman mistakenly assumes that patient Bill Schwartz has AIDS when he arrives at the clinic with a gentleman friend, seeking attention for a recurring black mole on his calf.

_____ 3. Rhoda and Lee Au fear they will not receive adequate medical care because they use Chinese as their first language and speak only broken English.

_____ 4. Corey Boyer resists his gym teacher's efforts to get him to the clinic to check out a recurring rash on his arm because his family has no health insurance.

_____ 5. Mary O'Keefe is relieved to find that the practice's OB/GYN is a female physician, Dr. Elizabeth King.

_____ 6. Edith Leonard, a widow in her 70s, counsels medical assistant Liz Corbin that she should settle down and get married instead of pursuing a dream to attend medical school and become a pediatrician.

CERTIFICATION REVIEW

These questions are designed to mimic the certification examination. Select the best response.

1. Which of the following is not part of communication?

    a. Speech

    b. Facial expression

    c. Gestures

    d. Attitude

    e. Body positioning

2. Which is the most basic need in Maslow's hierarchy?

    a. Food

    b. Safety

    c. Status and self-esteem

    d. Need for knowledge

    e. Self-actualization

3. Your patient refuses to accept a diagnosis, claiming the doctor "must be mistaken." Assuming the doctor is correct, which self-defense mechanism is the patient using?

   a. Repression

   b. Denial

   c. Projection

   d. Compensation

   e. Rationalization

4. Congruency in communication can be described as when:

   a. the verbal message matches the body language

   b. the verbal message does not match the gestures

   c. the verbal message can be interpreted in two or more different ways

   d. two different messages are interpreted as the same

5. The conscious awareness of one's own feelings and the feelings of others is:

   a. congruency

   b. perception

   c. bias

   d. masking

6. The founder of humanistic psychology is:

   a. Jacobi

   b. Freud

   c. Erikson

   d. Maslow

7. The grouping of nonverbal messages into statements or conclusions is known as:

   a. assimilating

   b. feedback

   c. clustering

   d. introjection

8. The goal of therapeutic communication at the point of care is:

   a. to collect a blood specimen

   b. to determine the reason for the visit

   c. to explain the treatment plan for the patient

   d. all of the above

LEARNING APPLICATION

CASE STUDY

Wayne Elder arrives at the clinic for an examination to check on a recurrent ear infection that has been treated with antibiotics. Wayne, who is slightly retarded and lives in a group home, is still reporting dizziness and pain in his right ear. He has come to the clinic by himself, taking a bus from his job as a part-time dishwasher. Wayne's boss asked him to return to the clinic because Wayne could not concentrate at work.

Wanda Slawson, who is the medical assistant at the clinic, discovers from Wayne that he has not been taking his medication properly; he stopped taking his pills once his ear began to feel better. She must politely ask Wayne to repeat himself several times before she can clearly understand his slurred speech, and she has difficulty holding his attention or maintaining eye contact.

Wanda conveys Wayne's situation to Dr. Ray Reynolds, who examines Wayne and gives him a new prescription for antibiotics, gently explaining the need to finish the entire prescription to get well. After Dr. Reynolds leaves the examination room, however, it is clear to Wanda that Wayne is still confused about why he must take the medication even after he begins to feel better. Wanda carefully explains to Wayne that the infection will continue to heal even though he no longer feels sick. To be sure he understands, Wanda asks Wayne to repeat to her what he must do and why; she then asks Dr. Reynolds to step in briefly to remind Wayne once more to complete the prescription.

CASE STUDY REVIEW QUESTIONS

1. How does the unequal relationship that exists between patients and health care professionals have an impact on the therapeutic communication between provider, medical assistant, and patient?

_____

_____

_____

_____

_____

_____

2. How must medical assistant Wanda Slawson tailor her verbal and nonverbal messages to meet the abilities of her receivers: the provider and the patient?

_____

_____

_____

_____

_____

_____

continues

3. How does Wanda use active listening? Which interview techniques are the most effective in facilitating therapeutic communication? Does nonverbal communication play a role?

_____

_____

_____

_____

_____

_____

_____

_____

4. Using Maslow's hierarchy of needs, discuss how the health care team meets Wayne's special needs resulting from his disability.

_____

_____

_____

_____

_____

_____

_____

_____

5. Do you think the medical assistant acted appropriately? What else could she have done? What should she not do in this situation?

_____

_____

_____

_____

_____

Role-Play Exercises

Active listening is an important element of therapeutic communication. To practice active listening skills, role-play as a patient and a medical assistant. Have the "patient" say each of the phrases below. The "medical assistant" should then rephrase each of the messages listed for verification from the sender and also include a therapeutic response. When you are finished role-playing, write what you have said in response to each statement below.

1. "I don't know what to do. My father takes so many pills he can't remember which is the right one, so he ends up refusing to take any of them."

_____

_____

_____

_____

_____

2. "I can't give you my insurance card because I lost it and I can't remember the name of the company, either. You've always taken care of this before."

_____

_____

_____

3. "I can't help being worried. The doctor just suggested a referral for treatment at that hospital where somebody had their wrong foot operated on. What do you think?"

_____

_____

_____

_____

4. "I feel dizzy just thinking about having my blood taken. Do you really need to do it?"

_____

_____

_____

CHAPTER POST-TEST

Perform this test without looking at your book. If an answer is "false," rewrite the sentence to make it true.

1. True or False? Gestures and expressions can always tell you what a person is thinking or feeling.

_____

_____

2. True or False? You can make a sick patient "feel worse" just by the way you communicate with her.

_____

_____

3. True or False? Hugs are universally acceptable as a means of communicating.

_____

_____

4. True or False? Patients should not be allowed to say how they feel or what they are concerned about.

_____

_____

5. True or False? In therapeutic communication, it is not necessary to take into consideration the cultural and religious background of the patient.

_____

_____

6. True or False? The distance at which we feel comfortable while communicating with others is called personal space.

_____

_____

7. True or False? The health care provider should not accept the uniqueness of the patient.

_____

_____

8. True or False? Patients must realize that providers are taking the time to listen to them, answer any of their questions, and speak with them openly.

_____

_____

SELF-ASSESSMENT

Think about your own facial expressions and body language. Are you always portraying the message you want to send? List two situations in which you have been misinterpreted through your nonverbal communication, or situations in which you have misinterpreted someone else's message. Then think of what would have been a verbal message to help make the situation more accurate. That is, explain what you could have said to the person to determine if he or she was really hearing the message you meant to send.

_____

_____

_____

_____

_____

_____

CHAPTER **5**

Coping Skills for the Medical Assistant

CHAPTER PRE-TEST

Perform this test without looking at your book. If an answer is "false," rewrite the sentence to make it true.

1. True or False? Stress is always something bad.

_____

_____

2. True or False? Stress is something we cannot prevent.

_____

_____

3. True or False? If you have a lot of responsibility in your job, you cannot avoid burnout.

_____

_____

4. True or False? Setting goals helps relieve stress.

_____

_____

5. True or False? Goal-oriented employees are more effective than those with no goals or future objectives.

_____

_____

6. True or False? Revitalization outside the workplace is not necessary when preventing burnout.

_____

_____

7. True or False? Worry causes stress but does nothing to resolve the problem that is causing the worry.

_____

_____

VOCABULARY BUILDER

Misspelled Words

Find the words below that are misspelled; circle them, and correctly spell them in the spaces provided. Then insert the vocabulary terms from the list next to their definitions below.

burnout   long-range goal   short-range goal
goal   outer-directed people   stress
inter-directed peepel   self-actualzation   stressers

_____   _____   _____

_____   1. Achievements that may take several years to accomplish

_____   2. Fatigue and exhaustion which results from stress and frustration

_____   3. The body's response to change, which may be manifested in a variety of
                          ways, such as increased blood pressure, heart rate, or headache

_____   4. People who decide what to do based on events, environmental factors, or
                          other people

_____   5. Demands to change that cause stress

_____   6. People who decide for themselves what they want to do

_____   7. Achievement toward which effort has been directed

_____   8. Interim goal that helps to achieve a larger goal over a longer period of time

_____   9. Developing your full potential and experiencing fulfillment

Word Search

Find the words in the grid below. They may go in any direction.

```
T  A  K  E  C  A  R  E  O  F  Y  O  U  R  N  S  E  L  E  F
S  R  O  S  S  E  R  T  S  X  K  L  E  G  O  J  D  M  L  Y
L  L  J  C  K  L  K  K  C  Y  F  L  G  M  I  E  X  R  P  T
T  R  T  F  O  L  F  J  R  G  O  P  W  J  T  X  D  R  O  B
K  H  T  P  H  P  S  G  M  R  T  X  E  Z  A  H  R  S  E  H
L  W  G  R  R  T  I  X  X  Y  N  M  J  M  T  A  F  H  P  H
T  T  F  I  R  I  F  N  T  R  I  G  L  J  P  U  H  O  D  S
H  G  C  E  L  C  O  U  G  T  F  M  L  T  A  S  L  R  E  L
R  R  S  I  R  F  O  R  G  S  F  F  Z  X  D  T  B  T  T  A
M  S  R  R  L  N  R  N  I  R  K  J  K  D  A  I  M  R  C  O
N  C  B  M  R  F  I  O  U  T  L  I  Q  R  T  O  K  A  E  G
N  G  T  U  X  G  N  S  T  Q  I  X  L  L  Y  N  P  N  R  E
Y  Q  B  V  A  C  T  O  R  H  R  Z  H  L  K  Q  Z  G  I  G
T  W  J  N  D  R  Z  C  C  P  G  L  I  Z  S  M  Z  E  D  N
C  R  A  J  A  H  F  F  Z  E  R  I  Z  N  T  H  K  G  R  A
W  M  T  T  J  G  D  V  T  V  L  Q  F  T  G  B  Y  O  E  R
H  Y  I  C  O  N  T  R  O  L  T  O  T  H  N  M  R  A  N  G
Z  O  R  R  S  L  A  O  G  Q  N  T  R  C  M  P  T  L  N  N
N  Z  R  T  J  Z  K  H  N  L  C  V  K  Y  N  M  V  S  I  O
O  U  T  E  R  D  I  R  E  C  T  E  D  P  E  O  P  L  E  L
```

adaptation	frustration	prioritizing
burnout	goals	role
control	inner-directed people	role conflict
coping skills	long-range goals	short-range goals
exhaustion	managing time	stress
fight or flight	outer-directed people	stressors

LEARNING REVIEW

Short Answer

1. Han Selye's general adaptation syndrome (GAS) theory proposes that adaptation to stress occurs in four stages. Identify each stage in the order in which it is manifested and describe the physiologic changes that occur during each stage.

_____

_____

_____

_____

_____

_____

_____

_____

_____

2. Identify six changes in your approach to your work environment and lifestyle that will help you to avoid burnout.

_____

_____

_____

_____

_____

_____

3. List and define the five considerations important in determining a goal.

_____

_____

_____

_____

_____

4. Stressors are divided into three categories. List and describe them.

_____

_____

_____

_____

_____

Matching

Burnout is stress-related energy depletion that takes place in the working world. Burnout occurs gradually over a period of continued stress. Place a P *next to those items that promote burnout and an* R *next to those that reduce the risk for burnout.*

____ 1. Keep work separate from your home life.

____ 2. Have regular physical examinations.

____ 3. Work harder than anyone else in the office.

____ 4. Feel a greater need than others to do a job well for its own sake.

____ 5. Prioritize tasks and perform the most difficult ones first.

____ 6. Prefer to tackle projects yourself rather than consult a supervisor.

____ 7. Never stop until you achieve your goals, regardless of the personal cost to yourself or loved ones.

____ 8. Postpone vacation time.

____ 9. Give up unrealistic goals and expectations.

____ 10. Maintain a positive self-image and your self-esteem.

____ 11. Develop interests outside your profession.

____ 12. Procrastinate.

____ 13. Wear loose-fitting, comfortable clothes and shoes.

____ 14. Stretch or change positions. Walk around and deliver charts or laboratory specimens.

____ 15. Know your limits and be aware of your body's needs.

Labeling

Hans Selye's General Adaptation Syndrome (GAS) theory proposes that four stages are involved in adapting to stress. Identify the four stages on the figure, and then explain each stage in the space below.

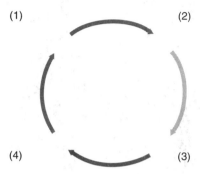

1. _____

_____

2. _____

_____

3. _____

_____

4. _____

_____

CERTIFICATION REVIEW

These questions are designed to mimic the certification examination. Select the best response.

1. The body's response to mental or physical change is called:

   a. stress

   b. adaptation

   c. denial

   d. burnout

2. Which of the following is not part of Hans Selye's general adaptation syndrome?

   a. Exhaustion

   b. Alarm

   c. Fear

   d. Fight or flight

   e. Return to normal

3. The four parts of the process leading to burnout are the honeymoon stage, the reality stage, the dissatisfaction stage, and the:

   a. sad stage

   b. angry stage

   c. retaliation stage

   d. giving up stage

4. In order for the body to survive, the sympathetic nervous system prepares the body for:

   a. fight or flight

   b. sleep

   c. developing a good appetite

   d. exercises

5. Time segments for short-range goals may be:

   a. monthly

   b. quarterly

   c. yearly

   d. all of the above

6. The result of long duration stress could be:

   a. making quick judgments

   b. job related

   c. immune system disorders

   d. an adrenaline rush

7. Stressors can be divided into which category(ies)?

   a. Frustration

   b. Conflicts

   c. Pressure

   d. All of the above

8. Needlessly worrying is an example of which type of stress?

   a. Short-term stress

   b. Episodic stress

   c. Long-term stress

   d. Intermediate stress

9. A common cause of stress in an organization would be:

   a. too much time spent on the telephone

   b. lack of motivation

   c. poor time management skills

   d. no smoke breaks

10. Discipline, perseverance, determination, and hard work are necessary in accomplishing:

    a. short-range goals

    b. long-range goals

    c. self-actualization

    d. prevention of burnout

11. The "wear and tear" our bodies experience as we continually adjust to a changing environment is called:

    a. adaptation

    b. stress

    c. prioritizing

    d. conditioning

12. The fight-or-flight response includes all but which one of the following reactions?

    a. Respirations and heart rate increase.

    b. Digestion is activated.

    c. Hormones are released into the bloodstream.

    d. Blood supply is increased to the muscles.

13. One of the characteristics associated with burnout is that the employee does not know what is expected and how to accomplish it. This is often called:

    a. role conflict

    b. role overload

    c. role ambiguity

    d. role reversal

14. When individuals with a high need to achieve do not reach their goals, they are apt to feel:

    a. angry and frustrated

    b. tired and lonely

    c. distrustful and leery

    d. motivated and enthusiastic

15. The best way to treat burnout is to:

    a. cover it up

    b. get a prescription to help you cope

    c. prevent it

    d. encourage it

LEARNING APPLICATION

CASE STUDY

Dr. Angie Esposito is a provider at Inner City Health Care. It was her dream, even as a child, to become a physician and work in an environment where she could help people and benefit the community as well. Proud of her accomplishments, she is the first woman in her family to attend college, and she got herself through medical school with scholarships and student loans. Dr. Esposito works hard, often pulling double shifts. Liz Corbin, CMA (AAMA), has a similar dream and is working to save money to attend medical school to become a pediatrician. Dr. Esposito does her best to encourage Liz's ambitions and has taken Liz under her wing.

Late one night, Liz assists Dr. Esposito in treating three difficult emergency patients in a row. "That's it," Dr. Esposito says. "We're taking a fifteen-minute break. Ask Dr. Woo if he can cover for a short time." When Liz catches up with Dr. Esposito in the employee lounge, she finds her frustrated and in tears. "These double shifts," she says. "I'm so tired. And the patients just keep coming. I want to help them all," she sighs, and her voice trails off, "I just can't help them all. . . ."

CASE STUDY REVIEW QUESTIONS

1. Dr. Angie Esposito is experiencing burnout. What personality traits are promoting her burnout? Identify the stressors in Angie's life.

   _____

   _____

   _____

   _____

   _____

   _____

   _____

2. Liz Corbin sees her mentor breaking down under stress. Should Liz reevaluate her own long-range goals?

   _____

   _____

   _____

   _____

   _____

continues

3. Discuss the importance of keeping goals in perspective.

_____

_____

_____

_____

_____

4. What would be Liz's best therapeutic response to Dr. Esposito?

_____

_____

_____

_____

_____

CHAPTER POST-TEST

Perform this test without looking at your book. If an answer is "false," rewrite the sentence to make it true.

1. True or False? Stress is never a good thing.

_____

_____

2. True or False? Stress is something we can always prevent.

_____

_____

3. True or False? Even if you have a lot of responsibility at work, you can still avoid burnout.

_____

_____

4. True or False? Setting goals eliminates stress.

_____

_____

5. True or False? Those employees who are goal oriented are more effective than those employees who do not have a goal or future objective.

_____

_____

6. True or False? Revitalization outside the workplace is not a contributing factor to burnout.

_____

_____

7. True or False? Worry contributes to stress and does not resolve the problem that is the cause of the worry.

_____

_____

SELF-ASSESSMENT

Determining how well you now handle stress will help you to identify personal strengths and weaknesses and point you toward the skills you will need to develop to be successful on the job as a medical assistant. Complete the following stress self-test. For each question, circle the response that best describes you.

1. I exercise:
   a. three times a week
   b. less than three times a week
   c. only if I am forced to

2. When something stressful happens in my life, I:
   a. eat too much
   b. make sure I eat regular meals
   c. stop eating for days

3. If I am struggling with a problem or project, I am most likely to:
   a. consult someone who may be able to help
   b. become determined to solve the problem or finish the project on my own
   c. abandon the project or just hope the problem goes away

4. When I encounter difficult personalities, I:
   a. leave the scene and avoid the person in the future
   b. lose my temper and get into arguments
   c. practice the art of the diplomatic response

5. When offered a new challenge or responsibility that requires obtaining new skills or training, I:
   a. get tension headaches
   b. respond with enthusiasm and an open mind
   c. express concern about taking on a new duty

6. In emergency situations, I:
   a. react calmly and efficiently
   b. feel paralyzed
   c. wait for someone else to take charge

7. I feel confident and competent in group situations:
   a. only when I know everyone present
   b. most of the time
   c. hardly ever; conversations with others make me uncomfortable

8. I think meditating or taking time to be quiet and calm during a busy day is:

   a. a terrific waste of time; I always have to be doing something

   b. good for other people; I've tried it more than once, but I can't seem to get into meditation

   c. a great way to relax and refocus my mind

9. The key to handling stressful situations lies in:

   a. staying out of stressful situations

   b. examining my view of the situation from a new perspective

   c. insisting that everyone agree with my point of view

10. To accomplish my personal goals, I:

    a. am willing to get up an hour earlier each day

    b. will give up sleep altogether

    c. find myself losing sleep because I am worrying about how I am going to get everything done

11. I usually complete projects:

    a. on time

    b. at the last minute

    c. late—but only by a day

12. As I prepare for a day's activities, I:

    a. prioritize and use time management skills to budget time carefully

    b. do not prepare; I like to be spontaneous

    c. find myself overwhelmed and unable to complete anything

13. When I focus on setting a long-range goal, I:

    a. think through the short-range goals necessary to achieve it

    b. become impatient

    c. talk constantly about the goal without making plans to achieve it

14. I volunteer to take on:

    a. more tasks than any one person can easily accomplish—then amaze everyone by pulling them off

    b. only what I know I can reasonably accomplish

    c. only what is required to get the job done

15. After a stressful day, the best way to unwind is to:

    a. talk all night with family or friends about what happened

    b. rent a funny movie

    c. work late to prepare for tomorrow

16. People think of me as:

    a. a person who is unpredictable. No one knows what I will do next.

    b. someone fixed in life roles

    c. someone who is confident about who I am but who also is willing to grow and change as worthy opportunities arise

Scoring: In the "My Score" column, record the number of points earned for each of your answers. The higher your score, the less you are prone to stress. The highest possible score is 160 points. If your score is low, consider the areas you need to focus on to reduce stress in your life.

MY SCORE

1. a. 10 points b. 5 points c. 0 points
   Regular exercise reduces stress.   _____

2. a. 0 points b. 10 points c. 0 points
   Eating regular meals reduces stress.   _____

3. a. 10 points b. 5 points c. 0 points
   Problems rarely just go away; ask for help before struggling on your own.   _____

4. a. 5 points b. 0 points c. 10 points
   You will not always be able to avoid a difficult person, and argument leads to
   stress. Tact and grace are needed.   _____

5. a. 0 points b. 10 points c. 5 points
   Worrying to the point of causing physical symptoms is not productive. Closed-
   mindedness could keep you from enjoying something new and cause stressful
   reactions.   _____

6. a. 10 points b. 0 points c. 5 points
   Feelings of helplessness increase stress.   _____

7. a. 5 points b. 10 points c. 0 points
   The ability to interact comfortably with others in group situations reduces stress. _____

8. a. 0 points b. 5 points c. 10 points
   The more you can separate your sense of well-being from daily events by taking
   time to relax and refocus, the less stress you will experience.   _____

9. a. 0 points b. 10 points c. 0 points
   Stressful situations cannot always be avoided; keeping a flexible instead of a rigid
   viewpoint will reduce stress.   _____

10. a. 10 points b. 0 points c. 0 points
    Sleep is important in reducing stress. However, making time by getting up earlier
    is a good time management technique.   _____

11. a. 10 points b. 5 points c. 0 points
    Lateness causes stress for everyone.   _____

12. a. 10 points b. 0 points c. 0 points
    Unexpected things can always happen, but prioritizing and budgeting time can
    help keep a handle on the day's events and reduce stress.   _____

13. a. 10 points b. 5 points c. 0 points
    Achieving long-range goals takes perseverance and determination. Being realistic
    about goals reduces stress.   _____

14. a. 0 points b. 10 points c. 5 points
    Taking on too much responsibility leads to stress.   _____

15. a. 0 points b. 10 points c. 0 points
    Humor is an effective stress reducer—so is separating work from your home life. _____

16. a. 0 points b. 0 points c. 10 points
    Being grounded but open to new experiences reduces stress.   _____

TOTAL: _____

Areas I need to focus on to reduce stress in my life:

CHAPTER **6**

The Therapeutic Approach to the Patient with a Life-Threatening Illness

CHAPTER PRE-TEST

Perform this test without looking at your book. If an answer is "false," rewrite the sentence to make it true.

1. True or False? Patients from different cultures will view death and life-threatening illnesses in different ways.

   _____

   _____

2. True or False? The strongest influences in managing life-threatening illnesses in the life of the patient comes from the medical team.

   _____

   _____

3. True or False? Health care professionals are responsible for making sure that patients have all their legal documents in order when diagnosed with a life-threatening illness.

   _____

   _____

4. True or False? Alternative methods of treatment should be discussed with the patient, as well as no treatment at all.

   _____

   _____

5. True or False? When facing a life-threatening illness, setting goals is no longer important.

   _____

   _____

6. True or False? According to Dr. Kübler-Ross, patients go through each of the five states of grief.

_____

_____

VOCABULARY BUILDER

Misspelled Words

Find the words below that are misspelled; circle them, and correctly spell them in the space provided. Then insert the correct vocabulary terms from the list that best fit the descriptions below.

durible power of attorney for health care   living will

health care directive   sychomotor retardation

_____   _____

1. _____ allows the surrogate to make decisions related to health care when the patient is no longer able to do so.

2. A _____ allows patients to make decisions (before becoming incapacitated) of whether life-prolonging medical or surgical procedures are to continue or be withheld.

3. _____ is the slowing of mental responses, decreased alertness, and apathy.

4. A _____ is a legal document that allows a person to make choices related to treatment in a life-threatening illness.

Crossword Puzzle

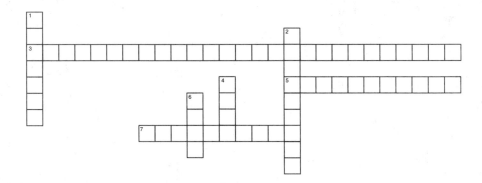

Across

3. This 1990 Act gave all patients in institutions that were Medicare or Medicaid funded certain rights.
5. Aiding health, healthful
7. This emotion is common in patients dealing with life-threatening illnesses.

Down

1. Recognition of another person's feelings by entering into those feelings
2. This type of support is vital when dealing with a life-threatening illness.
4. Late stages of HIV infection (abbreviation)
6. Abbreviation for end-stage renal disease

LEARNING REVIEW

Short Answer

1. List five issues that are appropriate to discuss with a patient facing a life-threatening illness.

_____

_____

_____

2. Discuss the pros and cons of using the words *terminal illness* or *life-threatening illness*. Which term seems more comfortable to you? Defend your rationale.

_____

_____

3. The federal government passed the Patient Self-Determination Act in _____, giving all patients receiving care in institutions that receive payments from Medicare and Medicaid written information about their right to accept or refuse medical or surgical treatment.

4. Explain what each of the letters in the acronym TEAR means as it relates to the grieving process.

T = _____

E = _____

A = _____

R = _____

5. What is the best therapeutic response to the patient with a life-threatening disease?

_____

_____

_____

_____

True or False

Mark a true statement with a T *and a false statement with an* F. *If an answer is "false," rewrite the sentence to make it true.*

____ 1. It is important for those patients who are suffering from cancer to know that the provider is willing to relieve and treat the symptoms associated with the disease.

_____

_____

____ 2. When a person is faced with a life-threatening illness, he or she will go through certain stages of grieving.

_____

_____

____ 3. It is not necessary for the health care professional to encourage patients to set goals for themselves.

_____

_____

____ 4. It is not necessary to offer nonmedical forms of assistance to patients suffering from a life-threatening illness.

_____

_____

____ 5. All patients go through the five stages of grief.

_____

_____

CERTIFICATION REVIEW

These questions are designed to mimic the certification examination. Select the best response.

1. Your patient's culture influences:

   a. his or her views about illness

   b. his or her views about treatment

   c. his or her views about death

   d. all of the above

2. Your patient has just been diagnosed with a life-threatening illness. She tells you that she would much rather die quickly than to suffer through this disease. She asks you not to say anything about her comment to the doctor. What is your best response?

   a. You have had quite a shock. Dr. King would like to talk to you about those feelings. I'll go get him for you.

   b. You, above anyone else, know what is best for your life.

   c. I know what you mean, I would feel the same way.

   d. Don't worry about that right now. Dr. King will give you medication to help with the pain.

3. The health care directive and power of attorney for health care documents are legal in how many states?

   a. 10

   b. 25

   c. 5

   d. 50

4. The slowing of physical and mental responses, decreased alertness, withdrawal, apathy, and diminished interest in work are referred to as:

   a. passive-aggressive behavior

   b. fight or flight

   c. psychomotor retardation

   d. mood swings

5. The strongest influence in managing the life-threatening illness of a patient is the:

   a. health care team

   b. family and those closest to the patient

   c. social worker

   d. hospice

6. The range of psychological suffering a patient may experience can lead to:

   a. tachycardia

   b. anorexia

   c. agitation

   d. all of the above

7. What patients fear more than anything else when facing a life-threatening illness is:

   a. pain and loss of independence

   b. dementia

   c. financial issues

   d. becoming addicted to some medications

8. In caring for individuals with life-threatening illnesses, it can be helpful to remember:

   a. that family members have the strongest influence on patients

   b. that pain must be considered within a cultural perspective

   c. that choices and decisions regarding treatment belong to the patient

   d. all of the above

9. One of the most common problems that a patient with a life-threatening illness may exhibit is:

   a. displacement

   b. denial

   c. depression

   d. assimilation

10. Referrals to community-based agencies or service groups may include:

    a. health departments

    b. social workers

    c. hospices

    d. all of the above

LEARNING APPLICATION

Role Playing Exercises

With another student, role play the following scenarios as medical assistant and patient. What is the medical assistant's appropriate therapeutic response or action?

1. The patient's husband has just found out that her husband has end-stage renal disease. She tells the medical assistant under no circumstances should her husband be informed about the prognosis.

   _____

   _____

2. The patient has been diagnosed with HIV. The medical assistant knows the patient is estranged from his or her family.

   _____

   _____

CASE STUDY 1

Jaime Carrera, a Hispanic man in his late 20s, is brought to Inner City Health Care, an urgent care center, by coworkers when he injures his head in an accident at a construction site where he is working. His head is bleeding profusely. As Jaime's coworkers watch the health care team implement Standard Precautions for infection control, one of them, his own shirt and hands covered with Jaime's blood, pulls the medical assistant aside and whispers frantically, "What are you doing? Does he have AIDS?"

CASE STUDY REVIEW QUESTIONS

1. What is the best therapeutic response of the medical assistant?

   _____

   _____

   _____

   _____

   _____

   _____

   _____

2. On what criteria do you base this response as the best therapeutic approach?

   _____

   _____

   _____

   _____

   _____

CASE STUDY 2

John Dukane, a longtime and much loved patient of the clinic, has end-stage renal disease. A kidney transplant is not appropriate due to his age, and John will not agree to receiving renal dialysis as treatment. That decision has been made clear in the provider's directive and the durable power of attorney for health care. He is healthy otherwise, and his family members feel he should try the dialysis, in hopes of extending his life by a few weeks or possibly even a few months. Discuss the arguments on both sides of the decision.

_____

_____

_____

_____

CHAPTER POST-TEST

1. True or False? Patients view death and life-threatening illnesses in different ways depending on their culture.

_____

_____

2. True or False? The strongest influences in the management of life-threatening illnesses in the life of the patient comes from the health care team.

_____

_____

3. True or False? Validating that patients have all their legal documentation in order when diagnosed with life-threatening illness is the responsibility of the health care provider.

_____

_____

4. True or False? Alternative methods of treatment, as well as the option of no treatment at all, should be discussed with the patient.

_____

_____

5. True or False? When facing a life-threatening illness, setting goals is not important.

_____

_____

6. True or False? Patients go through all five of the stages of grief as researched by Dr. Elisabeth Kübler-Ross.

_____

_____

SELF-ASSESSMENT

If you were faced with a life-threatening illness, would you choose to sustain your life regardless of the probable outcome? How far would you go with treatments? What four factors would enter into your decision? Have you discussed these issues with your family and physician?

CHAPTER **7**

Legal Considerations

CHAPTER PRE-TEST

Perform this test without looking at your book. If an answer is "false," rewrite the sentence to make it true.

1. True or False? You may discuss a person's confidential medical information as long as you do not say the patient's name.

   _____

   _____

2. True or False? Your provider does not have a contract with the patient until he or she treats the patient.

   _____

   _____

3. True or False? A provider is not obligated to care for a patient even though the patient's condition may require treatment.

   _____

   _____

4. True or False? Medical assistants do not have to worry about a "standard of care" because their employers are ultimately responsible for everything the medical assistant does under their direction.

   _____

   _____

VOCABULARY BUILDER

Misspelled Words

Find the words below that are misspelled; circle them, and correctly spell them in the spaces provided. Then insert the correct vocabulary terms from the list that best fit the descriptions below.

administrative law	expert witness	miner
agents	expressed contract	neglegance
civil law	implied consent	noncompliant
constitutional law	incompetent	plaintiffs
defendents	invation of privacy	risk management
doctrines	lible	slander
durable power of attorney for health care	litigation	statutes
	malfeasance	subpoena
emanciated minor	malpractice	tort

_____   _____   _____

_____   _____   _____

_____   _____

_____ 1. Establishes agencies that are given power to enact regulations having the force of law

_____ 2. Law that includes 27 amendments, 10 of which are the Bill of Rights

_____ 3. A 17-year-old person serving in the U.S. armed forces

_____ 4. Medical practice acts, or laws, that regulate the practice of medicine, such as licensure and standards of care

_____ 5. A patient who refuses needed care, such as a cancer patient who will not complete a series of chemotherapy treatments

_____ 6. A provider or health care professional who testifies in court to establish a reasonable and expected standard of care with respect to a specific medical situation so that jurors can understand the nature of medical information

_____ 7. The failure to exercise the standard of care that a reasonable person would exercise in similar circumstances

_____ 8. Persons who bring charges in a civil case

_____ 9. Medical assistants are _____ of their employers.

_____ 10. A patient tilts her head back and opens her eyes wide for instillation of medicated eye drops from a medical assistant without any verbal instructions to do so.

_____ 11. Professional negligence

_____ 12. *Respondeat superior* and *res ipsa loquitur*

_____ 13. Court order

_____ 14. Persons against whom charges are brought

_____ 15. A medical assistant writes in the patient's record, "Jim Marshall is a ruthless, rude man who is very full of himself. Be careful around him."

_____ 16. A patient says loudly in the reception area of Inner City Health Care, filled to capacity with waiting patients, "Dr. Reynolds should retire. I know he's not up on the latest medical techniques."

_____ 17. A 17-year-old student who lives with his or her parents

_____ 18. Actions that make the medical assistant and the employer less vulnerable to litigation

_____ 19. Lawsuit

_____ 20. Written or verbal contract that describes exactly what each party in the contract will do

Crossword Puzzle

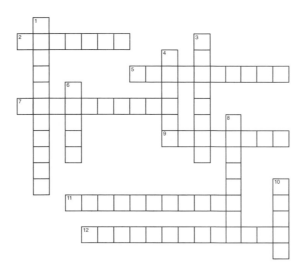

Across

2. The type of consent that is given when a patient is unconscious
5. When a doctor should have treated a patient, but did not, it can sometimes be called this.
7. Another word for lawsuit
9. Another word for laws
11. A type of lawsuit in which the doctor is accused of harming a patient
12. When a patient does not follow the doctor's orders, such as not taking medication that is prescribed

Down

1. Minors (under 18 years old) who are no longer under parental authority
3. Law that governs criminal acts
4. Person who represents another
6. Law that governs issues between persons
8. This document is a legal force with which you must comply
10. When someone harms another person's reputation by saying something untrue

LEARNING REVIEW

Identifying Civil and Criminal Law

Identify whether the following actions fall under the domain of civil law (CV) or criminal law (CM).

_____ A. A provider is siphoning off narcotics from an urgent care center's locked drug cabinet and continuing to treat patients while under the influence of the drugs.

_____ B. A woman in the advanced stages of breast cancer sues her insurer when it refuses to provide benefits for a bone marrow transplant.

_____ C. An office manager steals, or embezzles, funds from the medical practice.

Short Answer

1. List and define the four Ds of negligence.

_____

_____

_____

2. List at least 11 strategies for risk management in an ambulatory care setting that will lessen the potential for litigation.

_____

_____

_____

_____

_____

_____

_____

_____

_____

_____

_____

_____

_____

3. Before any invasive or surgical procedure is performed, patients are asked to sign consent forms, which become a permanent part of the medical record. What four things must the patient know to give informed consent?

_____

_____

_____

4. The unauthorized touching of one person by another is called _____.

5. The federal government established laws in 1968 to allow people to make a gift of all or part of their body; it is known as the _____.

6. The law mandates that the proper authorities be informed of certain harms and injuries, such as *(circle all that apply):*

   A. rape
   B. gunshot and knife wounds
   C. child abuse
   D. elder abuse

7. What term is used now in place of "domestic violence" and what does it mean? Why was this change made?

_____

_____

_____

_____

_____

8. What is the difference between an advance directive and a POLST form?

_____

_____

_____

_____

_____

_____

CERTIFICATION REVIEW

These questions are designed to mimic the certification examination. Select the best response.

1. The Patient Self-Determination Act, which includes health care directives, ensures that patients are able to:

   a. choose their own providers

   b. control their own health care decisions

   c. have guaranteed confidentiality

   d. have health care benefits

2. Which of the following covers the relationship between providers and their patients?

   a. Informed consent

   b. Locum tenens

   c. Medical ethics

   d. Criminal law

3. *Res ipsa loquitur* means:

   a. the thing speaks for itself

   b. the physician is ultimately responsible

   c. the record must be opened in court

   d. patients have a right to their records

4. The 4 Ds of negligence are:

   a. duty, derelict, danger, damage

   b. danger, duty, direct cause, disaster

   c. duty, derelict, direct cause, damage

   d. disaster, damage, direct cause, danger

5. A 17-year-old individual who is in the Navy is considered to be:

   a. *respondeat superior*

   b. an emancipated minor

   c. privileged

   d. a naval dependent

6. *Respondeat superior* is the Latin word that means

   a. providers are responsible for their employees' actions

   b. the thing speaks for itself

   c. obey your superior

   d. breach of duty of care

7. What must the inventory of controlled substances include?

   a. List of the name, addresses, and DEA registration number of the provider

   b. Date and time of inventory

   c. Signature of the individual taking inventory

   d. All of the above

8. A provider is legally bound to treat a patient until the patient:

   a. breaks an appointment

   b. does not have health insurance

   c. cannot get a referral

   d. no longer needs treatment

9. If suspicion of child abuse is aroused, the health care provider should:

   a. send the patient home

   b. treat the child's injuries

   c. inform the parents of the child's diagnosis and that it will be reported to the police and social services agency

   d. b. and c.

10. When a patient is asked to walk across the hall to the treatment room while wearing only a patient gown and is in full view of other patients, this is considered:

    a. a HIPAA violation

    b. implied consent

    c. invasion of privacy

    d. defamation of character

11. Protection of health care professionals who may provide medical care in emergencies without fear of being sued comes under:

    a. Good Samaritan laws

    b. provider's directives

    c. durable power of attorney for health care

    d. litigation

12. An order for a physician to appear in court with a medical record is:

    a. *res ipsa loquitur*

    b. *subpoena duces tecum*

    c. *respondeat superior*

    d. an interrogatory

13. When a patient reports a sore throat and the provider takes a swab for a throat culture to diagnose and treat the ailment, this act is considered:

   a. an expressed contract

   b. implied consent

   c. informed consent

   d. an implied contract

LEARNING APPLICATION

 CASE STUDY 1

On a busy afternoon at Inner City Health Care, the reception area is filled with walk-in patients, and the staff struggles to keep up with the patient load. Administrative medical assistant Liz Corbin gives the patient file for Edith Leonard to clinical medical assistant Bruce Goldman. "Dr. Reynolds wants a CBC done stat on the older adult woman in exam room 1," she tells Bruce, handing him the file. Bruce proceeds to examination room 1. Without identifying the patient, he performs a venipuncture on Cele Little, who has come to the clinic for a hearing problem. Cele asks Bruce why the procedure needs to be performed and that she does not want to have it. Bruce insists that Dr. Reynolds has ordered the procedure and performs the venipuncture anyway. The procedure frightens Cele, and she begins to fear that her hearing loss is indicative of a more serious illness.

CASE STUDY REVIEW QUESTIONS

1. What errors were made that could leave the medical assistants and provider vulnerable to litigation?

   _____

   _____

   _____

   _____

2. How might the errors leave the health care professionals open to potential lawsuits?

   _____

   _____

   _____

   _____

3. How could the errors have been avoided through effective risk management techniques?

   _____

   _____

   _____

   _____

   _____

CASE STUDY 2

Dr. Elizabeth King has just completed a routine physical examination of Abigail Johnson. Elizabeth asks Anna Preciado, RMA, to administer a flu shot to Abigail before the patient leaves the office. Abigail, an older African American woman, is accompanied by her daughter. When Anna attempts to administer the flu vaccine, Abigail says, "Is that a flu shot? They make me sick; I don't want it." Abigail's daughter says, "Yes, she does want it. Go ahead and give it to her." Abigail begins to laugh. "Okay," Anna says, "may I give you the vaccinations?" Abigail says nothing, but she rolls up her sleeve. As Anna administers the parenteral injection, the older woman looks up at her seriously and says, "I didn't want any flu shot. My daughter makes me get it every year." However, Abigail does not withdraw physically.

CASE STUDY REVIEW QUESTIONS

1. What errors were made that could leave the medical assistant and provider vulnerable to litigation?

    _____

    _____

    _____

    _____

2. How might the errors leave the health care professionals open to potential lawsuits?

    _____

    _____

    _____

    _____

3. How could the errors have been avoided through effective risk management techniques?

    _____

    _____

    _____

    _____

    _____

    _____

    _____

CASE STUDY 3

Dr. Elizabeth King is going over the daily list of scheduled patients with Ellen Armstrong, CMAS. They are standing at the front desk close to the reception area, and several patients are waiting for the first appointments of the day. Elizabeth's eyes move down the list and stops over the name Mary O'Keefe. "Mary O'Keefe," she mutters, "she's so neurotic and pestering. It's a small wonder her husband hasn't left her yet; just wait till they have that third child. . . . I don't think I have the patience for Mary today."

CASE STUDY REVIEW QUESTIONS

1. What errors were made that could leave the medical assistant and provider vulnerable to litigation?

_____

_____

_____

_____

2. How might the errors leave the health care professionals open to potential lawsuits?

_____

_____

_____

_____

3. How could the errors have been avoided through effective risk management techniques?

_____

_____

_____

_____

_____

_____

_____

CASE STUDY 4

Lydia Renzi, a deaf woman with some residual hearing, comes to Inner City Health Care and has waived her right to a certified sign language interpreter as provided under ADA. She is at the clinic today with a recurrent vaginal discharge. Lydia is diagnosed by Dr. Angie Esposito with candidiasis, a yeast infection caused by the fungus *Candida albicans*. Angie prescribes a vaginal suppository and asks Wanda Slawson, CMA (AAMA), to give Lydia instructions for using the prescription. Lydia wears a hearing aid and has trouble understanding Wanda, who is soft spoken. Wanda is also standing against a brightly lit window, and Lydia has trouble seeing her face. Lydia writes on a pad she has brought with her, "Is this a sexually transmitted illness?" In frustration, Wanda begins shouting, "You just have a yeast infection; it's not like you have herpes or anything." At that moment, another medical assistant, Bruce Goldman, is escorting a male patient past the open door of the examination room. Both men turn their heads away, though it is clear that they have overheard.

CASE STUDY REVIEW QUESTIONS

1. What errors were made that could leave the medical assistants and provider vulnerable to litigation?

   _____

   _____

   _____

   _____

2. How might the errors leave the health care professionals open to potential lawsuits?

   _____

   _____

   _____

   _____

3. How could the errors have been avoided through effective risk management techniques?

   _____

   _____

   _____

   _____

   _____

   _____

CASE STUDY 5

Construction workers Jaime Carrera and Ralph Samson are required to take a reemployment drug screening test before they can be hired to work on a new site to which they have applied. Jaime and Ralph come to Inner City Health Care, where urine specimens are collected for examination. The test comes back positive for Jaime, and his potential employer does not give him the job. Ralph tests negative. Two weeks later, Ralph returns to Inner City Health Care for a routine physical examination. "Whatever happened to Jaime Carrera?" Ralph asks Bruce Goldman, CMA (AAMA). "I haven't seen him around the site." "Oh," Bruce replies, "he tested positive for chemical substance abuse, and now he's in a rehab program that Dr. Whitney suggested."

CASE STUDY REVIEW QUESTIONS

1. What errors were made that could leave the medical assistant and provider vulnerable to litigation?

2. How might the errors leave the health care professionals open to potential lawsuits?

3. How could the errors have been avoided through effective risk management techniques?

CHAPTER POST-TEST

Perform this test without looking at your book. If an answer is "false," rewrite the sentence to make it true.

1. True or False? As long as you do not say the patient's name, you may discuss the patient's illnesses and treatments with anyone.

_____

_____

2. True or False? The patient–provider contract begins when the patient makes the appointment.

_____

_____

3. True or False? If the patient's condition should be treated, the provider is not obligated to care for the patient.

_____

_____

4. True or False? Because provider-employers are ultimately responsible for everything medical assistants do under their direction, medical assistants do not have to worry about a "standard of care."

_____

_____

SELF-ASSESSMENT

1. Have you ever been in a situation in which you were asked to disclose information about another person that might have been considered confidential? Or have you ever been told confidential information? If this has happened (or if it happens in the future), what should you have done or said? What will you do/say in the future?

_____

_____

_____

_____

_____

C H A P T E R **8**

Ethical Considerations

CHAPTER PRE-TEST

Perform this test without looking at your book. If an answer is "false," rewrite the sentence to make it true.

1. True or False? Ethics has to do with what is right and wrong.

   _____

   _____

2. True or False? Bioethics has to do with ethical issues dealing with human life.

   _____

   _____

3. True or False? When abuse is suspected, the provider and medical assistant have ethical responsibilities to report it.

   _____

   _____

4. True or False? When a patient has HIV, the provider may refuse to treat the patient.

   _____

   _____

5. True or False? A provider and a medical assistant can refuse to perform abortions.

   _____

   _____

VOCABULARY BUILDER

Misspelled Words

Find the words below that are misspelled; circle them, and correctly spell them in the spaces provided. Then insert correct vocabulary terms from the list that best fit into the descriptions below.

bioethics

code of ethics

criopreservation

genetic enginering

macroallocation

microallocation

serrogate

_____   _____   _____

_____   1. Someone who substitutes for another

_____   2. Biotechnology dealing with sophisticated medical research regarding the prevention of genetic disorders

_____   3. Medical decisions made by Congress, health systems, agencies, and insurance companies

_____   4. Set of principles and guidelines usually found in professional organizations

_____   5. Medical decisions made individually by providers and the health care team at the local level

_____   6. Applying biological systems to technological advances for disease diagnosis, production of medicine, and research

_____   7. Ethical issues dealing with life

Word Search

Find the words in the grid below. They may go in any direction.

```
S  T  R  R  E  S  O  U  R  C  E  S  I  S  V  E  T
O  Y  M  D  C  E  O  W  H  A  T  I  C  S  M  M  E
O  G  I  R  O  S  R  E  W  O  P  I  A  A  L  L  N
L  O  C  Y  D  U  A  L  W  S  T  N  C  D  G  E  G
A  L  R  T  E  B  A  R  E  E  C  R  H  N  I  C  I
C  O  O  S  S  A  O  L  N  A  O  I  I  A  L  L  N
I  N  A  P  N  N  Y  E  L  A  D  S  H  R  I  M  E
H  H  L  R  G  O  G  G  L  O  I  E  S  T  O  H  E
T  C  L  O  T  L  I  L  G  T  C  A  R  R  E  Y  R
E  E  O  T  N  N  O  S  R  R  M  A  A  S  G  Q  I
O  T  C  E  K  C  T  E  I  M  I  L  T  P  H  W  N
I  O  A  C  A  L  V  P  E  C  L  G  L  I  Y  I  G
B  I  T  T  V  D  P  L  R  Y  E  N  H  P  O  R  P
T  B  I  I  A  Z  I  Y  M  V  V  D  G  T  N  N  W
M  O  O  N  N  D  L  Y  R  E  S  E  A  R  C  H  R
N  X  N  G  E  T  A  G  O  R  R  U  S  N  K  D  D
P  C  O  N  F  I  D  E  N  T  I  A  L  I  T  Y  G
```

abuse	dilemmas	power
advertising	engineering	protecting
allocation	ethics	research
bioethical	genetics	resources
biotechnology	leadership	right
codes	macroallocation	surrogate
confidentiality	microallocation	wrong
decisions	morally	

LEARNING REVIEW

Code of Ethics Matching

The AAMA Code of Ethics presents five basic principles that medical assistants must pledge to honor as members of the medical assisting profession. For each situation presented, identify the AAMA ethical principle that applies.

A. Render service with full respect for the dignity of humanity
B. Respect confidential information
C. Uphold the honor and integrity of the profession
D. Pursue continuing education activities and improve knowledge and skills
E. Participate in community service and education

_____   1. Marilyn Johnson, CMA (AAMA), in conversation with co–office manager Shirley Brooks, CMA (AAMA), refuses to speculate about whether a diagnosis of AIDS will be confirmed for patient Maria Jover.

_____   2. Administrative medical assistant Karen Ritter joins a study group to prepare for the CMA (AAMA) certification examination as a method of securing her certification credentials, which must be updated every 5 years.

_____   3. Clinical medical assistant Anna Preciado, RMA, agrees to speak to a group of high school students who are interested in pursuing a career in the medical assisting profession.

_____   4. Liz Corbin, CMA (AAMA), politely reminds older adult patient Edith Leonard that she is a certified medical assistant, not a nurse, but assures Edith that she is qualified to perform the instillation of medicated eye drops ordered by Dr. Susan Rice.

_____   5. When patient Dottie Tate makes an appointment at Inner City Health Care for follow-up treatment of chronic back pain and a recent history of frequent falls, Bruce Goldman, CMA (AAMA), arranges for a wheelchair to accommodate Dottie's office visit.

_____   6. Karen Ritter volunteers at the local community office of Planned Parenthood on weekends.

_____   7. Jane O'Hara gently and kindly guides patient Wayne Elder, whose mild retardation often causes him to become confused in unfamiliar settings, back to the proper examination room after she finds him wandering down the hallway in search of Dr. Ray Reynolds.

_____   8. When filing a group of recent laboratory reports into the correct patient files, Ellen Armstrong, CMA (AAMA), takes care to complete the task quickly and efficiently. She performs the task at a private office station away from the general reception area and does not leave the charts open or unattended as she works.

_____   9. Audrey Jones approaches office manager Shirley Brooks, CMA (AAMA), about opportunities for obtaining advanced training to become qualified to perform a wider array of clinical procedures in the ambulatory care setting.

_____   10. Clinical medical assistant Wanda Slawson assists Dr. Mark Woo in the treatment of patient Rhoda Au, who is diagnosed with lupus erythematosus. Wendy believes the patient is foolhardy when she rejects Dr. Woo's treatment plan of Western drug therapy in favor of an approach that integrates traditional Chinese medicine. However, she respects the patient's heritage and right to choose her own health care.

Short Answer

1. According to the *Current Opinions of the Council on Ethical and Judicial Affairs of the AMA,* advertising by health care providers is considered ethical if the ad follows certain requirements. Which of the following are appropriate types of advertisements? Circle the correct responses.

   A. Testimonials from patients cured of serious illnesses or whose conditions were reversed or controlled under the care and treatment of the provider

   B. Providers' credentials and their hospital or community affiliations

   C. A description of the practice, facility hours of operation, and the types of services available to health care consumers

   D. Guarantees of cure promised within a specific time frame

2. Patient medical records are confidential legal documents. Name three instances, however, in which health professionals are allowed or required to reveal confidential patient information by law.

   _____

   _____

   _____

   _____

   _____

3. Issues of bioethics common to every medical clinic are *(circle all that apply):*

   a. allocation of scarce medical resources

   b. genetic engineering or manipulation

   c. many choices surrounding life and death

4. Individuals who are truly aware of their ethical power are able to *(circle all that apply):*

   a. not compromise any procedure or technique

   b. not put the patient at risk

   c. hide the truth regarding a possible error

5. Allocation of scarce resources may refer to *(circle all that apply):*

   a. rationing of health care

   b. denied services

   c. advertising by health care professionals

6. In the case of suspected child abuse, the medical professional should *(circle all that apply):*

   a. report the case

   b. protect and care for the abused

   c. treat the abuser, if known, as a victim also

7. List the five Ps of ethical power.

   _____

   _____

8. List the eight questions adapted from Stephen Covey's book that can be used as guidelines for making ethical decisions.

_____

_____

_____

_____

9. List three factors that constitute intimate partner violence. Does your state require that intimate partner violence be reported?

_____

_____

_____

_____

_____

_____

CERTIFICATION REVIEW

These questions are designed to mimic the certification examination. Select the best response.

1. The AAMA Code of Ethics includes all but which one of the following?

   a. We should render service with respect for the dignity of our patients.

   b. We should be paid an equitable salary/wage.

   c. We should respect confidential information.

   d. We should accept the disciplines of the profession.

   e. We should seek to improve our knowledge and skills.

2. Providers may choose who to treat but may not refuse treatment based on certain criteria. Which of the following is untrue?

   a. Providers may not refuse to treat patients based on race, color, religion, or national origin.

   b. It is unethical for a provider to refuse to treat a patient who is HIV-positive.

   c. Providers must inform a patient's family of a patient's death and not delegate that responsibility to others.

   d. Providers who know they are HIV-positive should tell their patients.

   e. Providers should report unethical behaviors committed by other providers.

3. Medical records and information in them are the property of the:

   a. patient

   b. patient and family

   c. provider and patient

   d. provider

4. Once a provider takes a case, the patient cannot be neglected or refused treatment unless:

    a. she did not pay for her last visit

    b. official notice is given from the provider to withdraw from the case

    c. the patient was a no-show

    d. the patient did not keep her last appointment

5. If a provider suspects that an HIV-seropositive patient is infecting an unsuspecting individual:

    a. every attempt should be made to protect the individual at risk

    b. the case should be reported to the CDC

    c. the patient should be dismissed from the practice

    d. the provider should notify the Department of Health

6. When a breach of ethics is about to occur, the health care provider should:

    a. rationalize her actions

    b. disregard the outcome

    c. be encouraged to step back and review his or her actions and their likely consequences

    d. not ask for help

7. Providers who know they are HIV-positive should:

    a. refrain from any activity that would risk transmission of the virus to others

    b. wear a mask

    c. inform the patients

    d. retire

8. Revealing information about patients without consent unless otherwise required to do so by law is:

    a. a breach of confidentiality

    b. bioethics

    c. a conflict of interest

    d. genetic manipulation

9. *Roe v. Wade* refers to guidelines for:

    a. artificial insemination

    b. surrogacy

    c. abortion

    d. fetal tissue transplant

LEARNING APPLICATION

 ## Critical Thinking Discussion

In small groups, explore these questions that were presented in Figure 8-1 and in the text, and present your findings to the class.

1. An increasing number of children live within dysfunctional families where one or more parent is absent, is a substance abuser, or has little time to spend with them. Many children have multiple parents or caregivers. Many spend large parts of the day in a day care environment. Child abuse is a concern. Children must be protected, but can be caught in a web of social services so overloaded and understaffed that only the most severe concerns receive attention. How do health professionals protect these children?

2. Adolescents as young as 14 to 18 years of age may seek treatment for substance abuse, birth control, even abortion without parental consent. Does this violate a parents' right to medical information regarding their children? Should the adolescent, often fearful of parental reaction, have a right to treatment?

3. Adequate and quality health care is a problem. Some adults have no health care coverage; others are part of managed care programs that keep changing as employers seek lower health care premiums. Many adults do not have an ongoing provider–patient relationship. Do medical providers have a responsibility to ensure that the needs of those without medical coverage are met? How can providers care for those without medical coverage in their communities?

4. Scientists have cloned mice, sheep, rabbits, goats, pigs, and a dog. Where does cloning stop? Will human beings be cloned if science moves forward in research with stem cells?

 # CASE STUDY

Lourdes Austen arrives at the offices of Drs. Lewis and King for her annual physical examination. It has been one year since Lourdes had surgery to remove a tumor in her breast by lumpectomy with axillary lymph node dissection, followed by a course of radiation. Lourdes's one-year mammogram and follow-up examination with her surgeon and radiologist find no evidence of a recurrence of the cancer. Lourdes is a single woman in her late 30s. As Dr. King begins the routine physical examination, assisted by Anna Preciado, RMA, Lourdes begins to cry. "I'm so happy to be alive," Lourdes says. "And so afraid of the cancer coming back. But I want to celebrate life. I've talked to my boyfriend about it and we want to get pregnant. What should I do?" Dr. King takes Lourdes's hand. "I know that living with cancer is hard. You are doing well. There are many things to consider...."

CASE STUDY REVIEW QUESTIONS

1. What bioethical dilemma exists in Lourdes's situation? In your opinion, is Lourdes's choice to become pregnant an ethical one?

   _____

   _____

   _____

   _____

continues

2. How do deeply held beliefs and attitudes about parenthood and the role of women in our society have an impact on the patient's decision? How could these beliefs have an impact on the health care team's response to Lourdes?

_____

_____

_____

_____

_____

_____

_____

_____

_____

_____

_____

_____

_____

3. What is Dr. King's best therapeutic response to Lourdes? What medical issues should the health care team consider if Lourdes becomes pregnant?

_____

_____

_____

_____

_____

_____

_____

_____

_____

_____

4. What is the role of the medical assistant in this situation?

_____

_____

_____

_____

_____

_____

_____

CHAPTER POST-TEST

Perform this test without looking at your book. If an answer is "false," rewrite the sentence to make it true.

1. True or False? Doing what is right is called ethical behavior.

_____

_____

2. True or False? Ethical issues dealing with human life are called bioethics.

_____

_____

3. True or False? The provider and medical assistant have ethical responsibilities to report suspected abuse.

_____

_____

4. True or False? A provider may refuse to treat an HIV-positive patient.

_____

_____

5. True or False? Whether to perform abortions is a choice each provider and medical assistant can make for themselves.

_____

_____

SELF-ASSESSMENT

1. Identify how you are able to demonstrate the five Ps of ethical power in your own life.

_____

_____

2. There are eight questions adapted from Stephen Covey's book that can be used as guidelines for making ethical decisions. Identify how your life fits into these guidelines and where/if you are striving to do better.

_____

_____

_____

_____

_____

CHAPTER **9**

Emergency Procedures and First Aid

CHAPTER PRE-TEST

Perform this test without looking at your book. If an answer is "false," rewrite the sentence to make it true.

1. Of the following, which is the most important in an emergency?

   a. Whether the patient has medical insurance

   b. Whether the patient is HIV-positive

   c. Whether the patient is taking any medication

   d. Whether the patient is breathing

2. The abbreviation ABC stands for:

   a. airway, biodynamics, circulation

   b. airway, bleeding, circulation

   c. airway, breathing, circulation

   d. airway, bleeding, cardiac

3. True or False? As a medical assistant, it is important to know how to respond in emergency situations.

   _____

   _____

4. True or False? A first-degree burn is the worst because it has damaged deeper tissues.

   _____

   _____

5. True or False? Whenever a person has a penetrating object embedded in his or her body, it is important that you remove it as soon as possible so you can treat the wound.

   _____

   _____

VOCABULARY BUILDER

Misspelled Words

Find the key vocabulary words below that are misspelled; circle them, and then correctly spell them in the spaces provided.

anaphalaxis	crepidation	occlusion
automated external defibillator	explicit	sprane
cardioversion	hypothermia	syncopy

_____   _____   _____

_____   _____

Word Search

Find the words in the grid below. They may go in any direction.

```
B E A W A R E E O F Y O U R O W N S A F
E T T R I A G E U Y A S S Y O U C A G Y
R E F O R O T S H C P E R S I N A S R C
N E M E R G P E N R S C Y X X M D T E N
S Y T M L I P R A Z Z E C Q L E Y R E E
Q P H V R Q P I B K K C R H T L S A N G
D C L A R C N W S G Y V O U D M H I S R
N F L I T C O R K Y N G N M Q K O N T E
E D V G N U R V K R N I M X P Q C K I M
G K V N N T V R W I M C H Q X O K T C E
A K L D H M N L S M R D O T W L U D K M
D L S F L M Z S O R J I J P A B T N L Z
N H T T Z C E C P T J A D R E E R D D L
A V G D P R C B R N T T Y Q P R R L K D
B W L R D N D F M Y R S Z T Q K R B D Z
C A R D I A C G W C P R G N I D E E L B
V G E R U T C A R F H I J L N V T Q N N
N O I S S E R P E D L F N K Z J M F M W
F A N A P H Y L A X I S W L N H B N T N
Z D T H Y P O T H E R M I A K T H B K P
```

anaphylaxis	depression	shock
bandage	dressing	spiral
bleeding	emergency	splint
breathing	first aid	sprain
cardiac	fracture	strain
comminuted	greenstick	syncope
compound	hypothermia	wounds
CPR	rescue	

LEARNING REVIEW

Matching I

Identify each of the following terms as an emergency condition (EC), an emergency or first aid procedure performed by health care professionals (EP), emergency equipment (EQ), or an emergency service provided to assist in emergency situations (ES).

____ A. First aid

____ B. Screening

____ C. Syncope

____ D. Shock

____ E. Wounds

____ F. Crash cart

____ G. Occlusion

____ H. Universal emergency medical identification symbol and card

____ I. Hypothermia

____ J. Chest Compressions

____ K. CPR

____ L. Sprain

____ M. Emergency medical service (EMS)

____ N. Fracture

____ O. Splints

____ P. Strain

____ Q. Rescue breathing

Matching II

Match each of the terms in Matching I with its definition below.

____ 1. A break in a bone. There are several types, but all are classified as open or closed.

____ 2. A tray or portable cart that contains medications and supplies needed for emergency and first aid procedures

____ 3. An injury to the soft tissue between joints that involves the tearing of muscles or tendons and occurs often in the neck, back, or thigh muscles

____ 4. A break in the skin or underlying tissues, categorized as open or closed

____ 5. Closure of a passage

____ 6. An injury to a joint, often an ankle, knee, or wrist, that involves a tearing of the ligaments. Most are minor and heal quickly; others are more severe, include swelling, and may not heal properly if the patient continues to put stress on the affected joint.

____ 7. A local network of police, fire, and medical personnel trained to respond to emergency situations. In most communities, the system is activated by calling 911.

____ 8. Identification sometimes carried by individuals to alert to any health problems they might have

____ 9. Any device used to immobilize a body part. Often used by EMS personnel

___ 10. An extremely dangerous cold-related condition that can result in death if the individual does not receive care and if the progression of the condition is not reversed. Symptoms include shivering, cold skin, and confusion.

___ 11. Fainting

___ 12. The immediate care provided to persons who are suddenly ill or injured, typically followed by more comprehensive care and treatment

___ 13. A condition in which the circulatory system is not providing enough blood to all parts of the body, causing the body's organs to fail to function properly

___ 14. The combination of rescue breathing and chest compressions performed by a trained individual on a patient experiencing cardiac arrest

___ 15. To assess patients' conditions and prioritize the need for care

___ 16. Performed on individuals in respiratory arrest, this is a mouth-to-mouth (using appropriate protective equipment) or mouth-to-nose procedure that provides oxygen to the patient until emergency personnel arrive.

___ 17. The combination of rescue breathing and this is known as CPR.

Short Answer

1. To identify the nature of the emergency and respond effectively, what five things must the medical assistant do to screen, or assess, the patient's situation?

_____

_____

_____

_____

_____

2. What five infection control measures can health care professionals follow to greatly reduce the risk for transmitting infectious disease when providing emergency care?

_____

_____

_____

_____

_____

3. For each of the patient symptoms or conditions below, identify the type of shock that is most likely.

Patient Symptom/Condition	Type of Shock
Patient suffers heart attack	_____
Patient experiences severe infection after colon surgery	_____
Patient experiences syncope after witnessing a traumatic event	_____
Patient experiences reaction to food allergy	_____
Choking patient has extreme difficulty breathing	_____
Diabetic patient lapses into a coma	_____
Patient has serious head trauma	_____
Accident victim experiences extreme loss of blood	_____

4. A common procedure for treating closed wounds is to RICE them. What do the letters of this acronym stand for?

_____

_____

5. Match each type of open wound (incision, puncture, laceration, avulsion, abrasion) to its defining characteristics.

Characteristics   **Type of Open Wound**

A wound that pierces and penetrates the skin. This wound may appear   _____
insignificant, but actually can go quite deep.

These wounds commonly occur at exposed body parts such as the fingers,   _____
toes, and nose. Tissue is torn off and wounds may bleed profusely.

A wound that results from a sharp object such as a scalpel blade.   _____

A painful wound. The epidermal layer of the skin is scraped away.   _____

A wound that results in a jagged tear of body tissues and may contain   _____
debris.

6. For each type of wound, describe proper emergency concerns, care, and treatment.

_____

_____

_____

_____

_____

_____

_____

_____

_____

_____

_____

_____

_____

_____

_____

7. Name three sources, other than heat, that can cause burns. For each, describe the proper emergency concerns, care, and treatment.

_____

_____

_____

_____

_____

_____

_____

_____

_____

_____

8. Musculoskeletal injuries, or injuries to muscles, bones, and joints, can be difficult to screen, especially for closed fractures. List five assessment techniques that health care professionals can use to determine the seriousness of musculoskeletal injuries.

_____

_____

_____

_____

9. For each set of symptoms that follows, identify the most likely emergency condition and describe emergency concerns, care, and treatment.

Symptom	Likely Emergency Condition	Emergency Concerns, Care, and Treatment
Off-color, cold skin with a waxy appearance	_____	_____
		_____
		_____
		_____
		_____
		_____
		_____
Hives, itching, lightheadedness	_____	_____
		_____
		_____
		_____
		_____
		_____
		_____

Cold, clammy skin; profuse sweating; abdominal cramps; headache; general weakness

_____ _____
_____
_____
_____
_____
_____

Lightheadedness, weakness, nausea, unsteadiness

_____ _____
_____
_____
_____
_____
_____

Moist, pale skin; drooling; lack of appetite; diplopia; full pulse

_____ _____
_____
_____
_____
_____
_____

Numbness in face, arm, and leg on one side of body; slurred speech; nausea and vomiting, loss of vision, severe headache, mental confusion, difficulty breathing and swallowing

_____ _____
_____
_____
_____
_____
_____
_____
_____

Convulsions, clenched teeth

_____ _____
_____
_____
_____
_____
_____
_____
_____
_____

Cold, clammy skin; _____ _____
rapid, weak pulse;
low blood pressure, _____ _____
shallow breathing;
dizziness, faintness, _____
thirst, restlessness,
feeling of anxiety; _____
abdomen may be stiff
and hard to the touch _____

10. Identify the method of entry into the body for each of the following poisons:

_____ 1. Carbon monoxide

_____ 2. Insect stingers

_____ 3. Chemical pesticides used in the garden

_____ 4. Spoiled food

_____ 5. Poison oak

_____ 6. Cleaning fluid fumes

CERTIFICATION REVIEW

These questions are designed to mimic the certification examination. Select the best response.

1. Which of the following is not an appropriate treatment for hypothermia?

   a. Give the victim warm liquids to drink.

   b. Remove any wet clothing.

   c. Rub the victim's skin vigorously to increase circulation.

   d. Use warm water to warm the person if possible.

2. In anaphylactic shock, the patient will:

   a. feel a constriction in the throat and chest

   b. have difficulty breathing

   c. have swelling and tingling of the lips and tongue

   d. All of the above

3. While waiting for EMS to arrive, what should be checked?

   a. Degree of responsiveness

   b. Airway, breathing

   c. Heartbeat (rate and rhythm)

   d. All of the above

4. Closed wounds that are painful and swollen require that a cold compress be applied:

   a. until the victim feels tingling

   b. for 10 minutes, then off for 40 minutes

   c. for 20 minutes, then off for 20 minutes

   d. for at least 1 hour, then off for 2 hours

5. To control nosebleeds, the patient should be seated, the patient's head elevated, and nostrils pinched for:

   a. 10 minutes

   b. 20 minutes

   c. 30 minutes

   d. 40 minutes

6. When a patient calls regarding a poisoning or suspicion of poisoning, the advice to give is to:

   a. call the poison control center

   b. give the patient charcoal

   c. tell the patient to drink milk

   d. flush the mouth with water

7. The best treatment for patients who are experiencing a seizure is to:

   a. restrain them

   b. stick a tongue depressor in their mouth

   c. protect from injury and care for them with understanding

   d. stop the seizure

8. Shock that occurs as a result of overwhelming emotional factors such as fear, anger, or grief is called:

   a. neurogenic

   b. psychogenic

   c. anaphylactic

   d. septic

9. The type of burn that may occur resulting in an entrance and exit burn wound area is:

   a. chemical

   b. electrical

   c. solar radiation

   d. explosion

10. In burn depth classifications, third-degree burns are also called:

    a. superficial

    b. full thickness

    c. partial thickness

    d. sunburns

11. The type of fracture often caused by falling on an outstretched hand that involves the distal end of the radius is called:

    a. greenstick

    b. spiral

    c. Colles

    d. implicated

12. Jaw and left shoulder pain; a rapid, weak pulse; excessive perspiration; and cold, clammy skin may be symptomatic of:

   a. seizure

   b. heart attack

   c. stroke

   d. sepsis

LEARNING APPLICATION

Screening Activity

In an urgent care setting, two or more patients may present with emergency symptoms. The order in which emergency patients will receive care depends on the health care professionals' abilities to screen patients' symptoms to determine who needs care most urgently. The following five patients present simultaneously on New Year's Eve at Inner City Health Care, an urgent care center. Office manager Walter Seals, CMA (AAMA), is working the evening shift with Dr. Mark Woo. In what order will Walter and Mark screen the priority of treatment? Number the patients 1 (most urgent) through 5 to correspond to the urgency of their conditions.

Patient	**Urgency**
Patient A presents with a gunshot wound to the leg that is bleeding severely. The patient is conscious but his pupils are dilated and he is unable to answer simple questions put to him by Walter and Dr. Woo. He cradles his right arm and will not let anyone touch it, although there is no immediate evidence of an open wound to the arm.	_____
Patient B, an elderly man, is brought in by his grandson. He describes debilitating chest pains, difficulty breathing, and nausea after eating a large family dinner. The patient's medical record indicates that he has a hiatal hernia, slipped disks, high blood pressure, and mild angina. The man is walking and speaking with moderate distress and is extremely anxious.	_____
Patient C, a young woman, presents with her boyfriend. She appears to have multiple abrasions on her right palm and knee, with damage to the right knee and ankle joints sustained after a fall while on in-line skates. Both joints are swollen and painful.	_____
Patient D, a man in his mid-30s, presents with the cotton tip of a swab stuck in his ear canal. Although the man feels a dull consistent pain in the ear, he says he has no trouble hearing. The outside of the ear appears normal, there is no bleeding evident, and the man appears annoyed but not distressed.	_____
Patient E, a young woman, presents with a group of friends, all college students, with an eye injury sustained by a champagne cork. The cork, which had a metal covering over its tip, hit the patient's eye. The young woman's eye is red and tearing and she is experiencing severe pain in the eye.	_____

CASE STUDY 1

Mary O'Keefe calls Dr. King's office in a panic. Ellen Armstrong, CMA (AAMA), answers the telephone.

Mary: "Oh my God, help me. I need Dr. King."

Ellen: "This is Ellen Armstrong. Who is this calling? What is the situation?"

Mary: "It's my baby, oh God, get Dr. King."

Ellen: "Dr. King is unavailable, but we can help you. Now, tell me your name."

Mary: "It's Mary O'Keefe. Help me, I think my baby is dead."

Ellen: "Are you at home?"

Mary: "Yes."

Ellen: "Good. Tell me what's happened."

Mary: "My son Chris pried the plug off an outlet and he's electrocuted himself!" Mary cries. "He's just lying there. I'm so scared, if I touch him, will I electrocute myself? Oh my God, my baby, my baby. What should I do?"

Ellen, who has been writing down the details on a piece of paper, motions to Joe Guerrero, another CMA (AAMA) in the office, and hands him her notes. Joe immediately accesses the O'Keefe address from the patient database and uses another telephone to call EMS with the nature of the emergency situation and directions to the O'Keefe residence. Meanwhile, Ellen remains on the line with Mary. Dr. King is on rounds at the hospital this morning and will not be in the office for at least another hour.

Ellen: "Mary, we are calling EMS, and they will be there as soon as possible. In the meantime, I'm going to need you to focus and answer my questions, okay?"

CASE STUDY REVIEW QUESTIONS

1. What steps did the medical assistant take to screen the emergency situation?

_____

_____

_____

_____

_____

_____

2. What questions should Ellen ask Mary regarding the emergency situation?

_____

_____

_____

_____

_____

continues

3. What should the medical assistant do after EMS arrives and takes over emergency care? What follow-up procedures are necessary?

_____

_____

_____

_____

_____

_____

_____

_____

_____

_____

_____

CASE STUDY 2

Lenore McDonell, a wheelchair-bound woman in her early 30s, experiences a serious laceration to the right arm sustained from a fall while performing an independent transfer from the examination table to her wheelchair. Joe Guerrero, CMA (AAMA), assists Dr. Winston Lewis in administering emergency care.

CASE STUDY REVIEW QUESTIONS

1. What Standard Precautions must the health care professionals follow before administering emergency treatment?

_____

_____

_____

2. Joe and Dr. Lewis attempt to control Lenore's bleeding by applying a dressing and pressing firmly. When the bleeding does not stop, what two actions should the health care professionals perform?

_____

_____

continues

3. In the unlikely event that bleeding continues, what piece of medical equipment will the health care team use in substitution for a tourniquet? Why is this alternative equipment effective and widely used today?

_____

_____

_____

_____

_____

4. The bleeding stops, and Joe applies a pressure bandage over the dressing. This patient is prone to fractures, and a radiograph will need to be taken. What is the next emergency procedure Dr. Lewis will perform? Why is this procedure necessary, and what equipment will the provider and medical assistant require?

_____

_____

_____

_____

_____

5. Before applying a sling, what do the health care professionals check to be sure that the medical equipment used has not been too tightly applied?

_____

_____

_____

6. What Standard Precautions will the health care team follow after the emergency treatment of the patient is successfully completed?

_____

_____

_____

7. What information will the health care team include in documenting the procedure for the patient's medical record?

_____

_____

_____

_____

_____

Research Activity

Using a medical encyclopedia or reference such as the *Physician's Desk Reference* (PDR), describe the following emergency medications and identify potential uses for each. Remember that only a provider can order medications or treatment.

Lidocaine: _____

_____

Verapamil: _____

_____

Atropine: _____

_____

_____

_____

Insulin: _____

_____

Nitroglycerin: _____

_____

Marcaine: _____

_____

Diphenhydramine: _____

_____

Diazepam: _____

_____

CHAPTER POST-TEST

Perform this test without looking at your book. If an answer is "false," rewrite the sentence to make it true.

1. Of the following, which is the most important in an emergency?

   a. Whether the patient has medical insurance

   b. Whether the patient is HIV-positive

   c. Whether the patient is taking any medication

   d. Whether the patient is breathing

2. ABC stands for:

   a. airway, biodynamics, circulation

   b. airway, bleeding, circulation

   c. airway, breathing, circulation

   d. airway, bleeding, cardiac

3. True or False? As a medical assistant, you should be prepared to respond to small-scale and large-scale emergency situations.

_____

_____

4. True or False? A first-degree burn is the worst because it has damaged deeper tissues.

_____

_____

5. True or False? Whenever a penetrating object has been embedded in a person's body, it is important that you remove it as soon as possible so you can treat the wound.

_____

_____

SELF-ASSESSMENT

1. A. On a scale of 1 to 5, rate your personal comfort in regard to the following emergency situations that medical assistants may find themselves involved with in an ambulatory or urgent care setting.

   1 = extremely uncomfortable   4 = comfortable

   2 = uncomfortable   5 = very comfortable

   3 = somewhat comfortable

   _____ Assisting in treatment of patients with injuries clearly sustained by an act of violence or abuse

   _____ Administering back blows and thrusts to a conscious infant

   _____ Performing rescue breathing on someone who has poor personal hygiene

   _____ Bandaging the open wound of an HIV-infected person

   _____ Caring for a person experiencing a seizure

   _____ Administering care to a patient who faints after venipuncture

   _____ Administering care to a patient in extreme pain

   _____ Administering care to a patient who is verbally abusive or uncooperative

2. On a scale of 1 to 5, rate your level of agreement with the statements that follow.

1 = never   4 = most of the time

2 = occasionally   5 = all of the time

3 = sometimes

_____ Life-threatening emergencies frighten me.

_____ I respond well under pressure.

_____ I am bothered by the sight of blood.

_____ I lose my temper easily, becoming openly frustrated and angry.

_____ I become frustrated and overwhelmed by feelings of helplessness in emergency situations.

_____ I remain calm and clearheaded in emergency situations.

_____ I forget about myself completely and focus on the emergency victim.

_____ I am concerned about administering care in emergency situations in which danger to myself may exist when giving such care.

_____ I am comfortable speaking to the family or friends of emergency victims.

CHAPTER **10**

Creating the Facility Environment

CHAPTER PRE-TEST

Perform this test without looking at your book. If an answer is "false," rewrite the sentence to make it true.

1. A reception area should:

    a. be comfortable and inviting

    b. be clean and uncluttered

    c. contain current reading materials for all ages

    d. All of the above

2. True or False? It is considerate, but not required, to provide at least one handicapped patient parking space.

    _____

    _____

3. Keeping the reception area clean is a responsibility of:

    a. the adminstrative medical assistant

    b. the bookkeeper

    c. the laboratory technician

    d. the office manager

    e. All of the above

4. True or False? Cultural differences will also have an impact on the amount of space necessary for the reception area.

    _____

    _____

VOCABULARY BUILDER

Misspelled Words

Find the words below that are misspelled; circle them, and correctly spell them in the spaces provided. Then insert vocabulary terms from the list that best fit into the descriptive sentences below.

accessibility   Americans with Disibilities Act   enviroment

accountibility   characteristic

_____   _____   _____

_____   1. The physical space of the reception area

_____   2. A typical or distinguishing quality

_____   3. Being ultimately responsible

_____   4. Being readily reachable

_____   5. Mandates that facilities and equipment be available to all users

Word Search

Find the words in the grid below. They may go in any direction.

```
L  S  C  I  T  A  M  R  O  F  N  I  O  O  P  E
K  E  A  T  Y  F  A  C  I  L  I  T  Y  L  S  N
O  U  L  R  R  E  C  E  P  G  T  I  A  O  C  V
N  A  R  B  E  A  A  S  N  A  A  Y  P  G  I  I
A  D  E  L  A  Y  S  I  T  C  I  T  E  N  T  R
N  T  W  O  U  T  D  L  C  D  S  V  I  I  S  O
D  E  L  W  A  A  R  E  I  I  T  .  F  T  I  N
T  E  F  I  E  A  S  O  N  K  T  K  V  I  R  M
J  J  S  R  G  S  P  O  F  G  P  B  T  V  E  E
F  N  N  I  I  H  I  I  N  M  T  Y  T  N  T  N
R  N  Z  B  G  T  T  I  H  K  O  M  O  I  C  T
L  D  L  H  P  N  M  I  Z  Z  R  C  Y  A  A  V
K  E  V  E  L  L  H  B  N  Z  N  Q  S  D  R  K
N  T  C  W  A  G  P  L  Q  G  M  Z  M  A  A  L
R  E  L  C  B  G  N  I  M  O  C  L  E  W  H  V
R  K  M  N  R  F  U  R  N  I  T  U  R  E  C  G
```

accessible   design   play

ADA   environment   reading

calming   facility   reception

characteristics   furniture   toys

comfortable   inviting   welcoming

delays   lighting

LEARNING REVIEW

Short Answer

1. What is the purpose of the ADA?

_____

_____

_____

2. When creating the facility environment, why is accessibility a major consideration?

_____

_____

_____

_____

3. Why are some medical clinics experimenting with the use of water, such as aquariums and water walls, and music in their facilities?

_____

_____

_____

_____

4. Name four ways an ambulatory care setting can accommodate the physically challenged.

_____

_____

_____

5. Identify at least four things to be done in the reception area to accommodate children.

_____

_____

_____

6. List at least five safety and evacuation considerations in the medical office.

_____

_____

_____

_____

_____

7. Create a checklist of five activities to perform on opening a medical facility for the day.

_____

_____

_____

8. Create a checklist of five activities to perform on closing a medical facility for the day.

_____

_____

_____

_____

9. Any drugs identified in the Controlled Substance Act list of narcotics and non-narcotics must be *(circle all that apply)*:

a. logged

b. in a locked and secured cabinet

c. checked when leaving the office

d. counted

10. In each of the following situations, health care professionals should strive to empower the patient with as much control and dignity as possible.

Case 1. Bill Schwartz is referred to a dermatologist by Dr. Ray Reynolds for examination of a suspicious mole on his calf. The dermatologist tells Bill that a full-body inspection will need to be done to ensure that no other areas of the skin are affected. Bill must appear disrobed in front of the dermatologist and medical assistant, who are both female.

What strategies can health care professionals use to respect the patient's dignity and lessen the sense of disproportion between health care providers and the patient?

_____

_____

_____

_____

_____

Case 2. Ellen Armstrong, CMA (AAMA), places a Holter monitor on patient Charles Williams. After the Holter monitor is in place, Charles has several questions about the patient activity diary that he would prefer to discuss with Dr. Winston Lewis.

What strategies can health care professionals use to respect the patient's dignity and lessen the sense of disproportion between health care providers and the patient?

_____

_____

_____

_____

_____

_____

Physical Office Environment Review

The physical clinic environment can contribute to the patient's sense of confidence and comfort, or it can be viewed by the patient as intimidating or anxiety producing. For each clinic area below, describe why the area could be perceived by patients as a frightening place. What can be done to make each area a more comforting and welcoming environment for patients?

A. Reception area:

_____

_____

_____

_____

_____

B. Corridors:

_____

_____

_____

_____

_____

_____

C. Examination rooms:

_____

_____

_____

_____

_____

_____

_____

Fill in the Blanks

Fill in the blanks in the sentences below, which discuss the future environment for ambulatory care.

1. Patients who are 85 years or older and who are most likely to require medical care for multiple chronic conditions is expected to increase by _____ by 2010.

2. The number of primary care providers willing to take new patients who are 65 years or older must _____.

3. _____ requires providers to have patients sign a release so the family members can be kept informed.

4. The greatest frustration of elderly patients regarding their health care experiences is the _____ _____ given by all health professionals.

5. It is important to provide clear and concise _____ instructions whenever possible in easy-to-read print.

6. The medical environment should enable all patients to _____ from one department to another with ease.

CERTIFICATION REVIEW

These questions are designed to mimic the certification examination. Select the best response.

1. HIPAA has changed the way we organize our entrance and reception areas in the following way:

    a. Patients must be able to see the receptionist at all times.

    b. Patients must have adequate parking.

    c. Patients must not be able to see or hear confidential information about other patients.

    d. The magazines must be current.

2. ADA states that:

    a. Patients must not know the names and diagnoses of other patients.

    b. Handicapped patients must have access to all patient areas with reasonable accommodations.

    c. Visually impaired patients must have adequate lighting and contrast for better viewing.

    d. An interpreter must be present with any non–English-speaking patient.

3. Patient safety within the reception area is accomplished by:

    a. providing chairs that are sturdy and in good repair

    b. containing wires and cords and keeping them out of reach

    c. attaching rugs to the flooring without loose edges

    d. containing toys within a designated play area

    e. All of the above

4. The reception area should accommodate:

    a. at least one hour's patients per provider plus a friend or relative who may accompany each patient

    b. only adult patients

    c. 2.5 seats for each examination room

    d. a. and c.

5. Before entering the exam room, health care professionals should:

    a. turn their cell phones off

    b. knock before entering

    c. wash their hands

    d. put on lab coats

6. According to the ADA, there must be one accessible entrance that should:

    a. have a padlock

    b. state that it is an exit

    c. have a doorbell

    d. be protected from the weather by a canopy or overhanging roof

7. The administrative medical assistant should be able to:

    a. perform telephone screening

    b. remember that the patient's comfort is of primary concern

    c. log data into the computer

    d. All of the above

8. A good way to check a room's readiness is to:

   a. lie on the examining table and look around

   b. place yourself in the room as a patient

   c. ask yourself how you feel about being there and what mood the surroundings create for you

   d. b. and c.

9. When closing the facility for the day, it is most important to:

   a. contact the answering service to notify them that the office is closed and who can be reached in an emergency

   b. clean all rooms

   c. lock the doors

   d. turn off the lights

10. Making facilities and equipment available to all users is called:

    a. maintenance

    b. accessibility

    c. promotion

    d. standardization

11. HIPAA requires that clinic facilities:

    a. have adequate corridors and bathrooms to accommodate wheelchair patients

    b. place an administrative medical assistant in an area seen and heard by all patients

    c. protect the confidentiality of patients checking in at the reception desk

    d. provide space for children in the clinic

12. The primary goal of maintaining a comfortable environment in which patient care is given is to:

    a. feed anxiety

    b. aggravate illness

    c. promote health

    d. stimulate the senses

13. Space planners suggest:

    a. that the reception area accommodate at least two hours' patients per provider

    b. that the reception area accommodate a friend or relative who might accompany each patient

    c. that there be 2.5 seats in the reception area for each examination room

    d. only b. and c.

14. Any drugs kept in the office that are identified as controlled substances must always be kept:

    a. in the refrigerator

    b. in a locked, secure cabinet

    c. in the provider's desk drawer

    d. in the administrative medical assistant's desk drawer

LEARNING APPLICATION

Lydia Renzi, a near-deaf woman with some residual hearing, is a patient of Dr. Angie Esposito's at Inner City Health Care. Lydia is fluent in American Sign Language (ASL) and usually wears a hearing aid when she is away from home. Lydia calls to make her appointment at Inner City Health Care using a telecommunications device for the deaf (TDD) and the services of a government-funded relay operator. Although Lydia often chooses not to be accompanied by an interpreter, Inner City Health Care always provides the option to supply the services of a qualified professional sign language interpreter in compliance with the ADA. When Lydia arrives at Inner City Health Care with a high fever and a suspected case of the flu, the staff accommodates Lydia's special needs in several simple ways. Remembering that people who are hearing impaired rely on visual images to receive and to convey messages, Liz Corbin, CMA (AAMA), always faces Lydia directly so that the patient can see her facial expressions and lip movements. Liz holds eye contact with Lydia and does not break it until she is sure that Lydia understands her message and has time to think and respond. Special care is taken to provide Lydia with written instructions for prescriptions and for following through on home care.

CASE STUDY REVIEW QUESTIONS

1. What are the special communication needs of the hearing-impaired patient in the ambulatory care setting?

2. How can the medical assistant's actions make a direct impact on the quality of care given to hearing-impaired patients?

continues

3. Suppose that Lydia is an elderly woman who is embarrassed and sensitive about her hearing loss and will not admit that she has trouble hearing others. How might the medical assistant accommodate the special needs of this patient?

_____

_____

_____

_____

_____

_____

_____

Role-Play Exercises

The administrative medical assistant is the person who sets the social climate for the interchange between the patient and the health care team. A friendly, reassuring demeanor and an ability to screen situations are essential skills. With another student, role-play as a patient and an administrative medical assistant. Have the "patient" say each of the phrases below. When you are finished role-playing, write what you have said and done in response to each statement below.

1. A patient with intense stomach pain doubles over and then bolts up to the reception desk, saying, "I'm going to throw up."

_____

_____

_____

_____

_____

_____

_____

2. When presented with a bill, the patient exclaims, "I can't pay for all of this now! Every time I come here it seems like the doctor bill goes up a hundred dollars."

_____

_____

_____

_____

_____

_____

3. A patient is looking for the correct exit from the examination area to the waiting area and makes a wrong turn into the administrative medical assistant's area. He asks, "Where do I go?"

_____

_____

_____

_____

4. A patient new to an HMO plan does not realize that a separate referral form is needed for a follow-up visit with the gastroenterologist one week after a colonoscopy test has been performed. She says, "I drove an hour to get to this appointment. No one told me I needed another form."

_____

_____

_____

_____

_____

_____

_____

_____

CHAPTER POST-TEST

Perform this test without looking at your book. If an answer is "false," rewrite the sentence to make it true.

1. A reception area should:

   a. be comfortable, clean, and uncluttered

   b. contain current reading materials for all ages

   c. have adequate lighting for reading

   d. contain accommodations for patients with disabilities

   e. All of the above

2. True or False? It is required to provide one handicapped patient parking space.

   _____

   _____

3. Keeping the reception area clean is a responsibility of:

   a. the administrative medical assistant

   b. the bookkeeper

   c. the laboratory technician

   d. the office manager

   e. all employees

4. True or False? Cultural differences do have an effect regarding the amount of space necessary for the reception area.

   _____

   _____

SELF-ASSESSMENT

1. Visualize your last visit to a medical facility. Was the reception area clean, tidy, welcoming, and comfortable? What would you do to improve it?

_____

_____

_____

2. List at least three things you would add to any reception area to make it even more accommodating. Think of items not mentioned in the textbook.

_____

_____

_____

_____

_____

_____

CHAPTER **11**

Computers in the Ambulatory Care Setting

CHAPTER PRE-TEST

Perform this test without looking at your book. If an answer is "false," rewrite the sentence to make it true.

1. The keyboard and the mouse are considered to be:

   a. the most common types of input device

   b. the most common types of output device

   c. portable memory storage devices

   d. read-write devices

2. To ensure that your work in the computer is safe from hackers, you should:

   a. store all work on data storage devices

   b. defragment frequently

   c. use firewalls

   d. backup frequently

3. Circle each of the following tasks that are performed by a computer as part of a total practice management system:

   a. Keeping track of appointments

   b. Writing and forwarding prescriptions to the patient's pharmacy

   c. Creating patient statements

   d. Processing insurance claims

   e. Reading directions on how to download a software program

4. The "brain" of the computer is called the:

   a. motherboard

   b. modem

   c. video card

   d. central processing unit (CPU)

5. To prevent unauthorized use of your clinic computers, you should:

   a. keep the computer in a locked cabinet at all times

   b. keep the computer in a locked cabinet at night

   c. assign every employee a password

   d. have only one person on the computer at a time

VOCABULARY BUILDER

Misspelled Words

Find the words below that are misspelled; circle them, and correctly spell them in the spaces provided. Then insert the correct vocabulary terms from the list that best fit the descriptions below.

electronic medical records	hardware	RAM
erganomics	Internet	total practice management
fishing	modom	system

_____   _____   _____

_____ 1. A device used by a computer to communicate to a remote computer through phone lines

_____ 2. Maximizing the user's safety when setting up a workstation that involves preventing back, neck, and eye strain

_____ 3. Acronym for *random access memory*, a type of computer memory that can be written to and read from

_____ 4. The physical equipment used by the computer system to process data

_____ 5. The practice of attempting to acquire sensitive information (such as passwords or bank account numbers) by masquerading as a trusted source through email communication

_____ 6. Electronic patient records from a single medical practice, hospital, or pharmacy

_____ 7. A worldwide computer network available via modem

_____ 8. A category of software that deals with the day-to-day operations of a medical practice

Crossword Puzzle

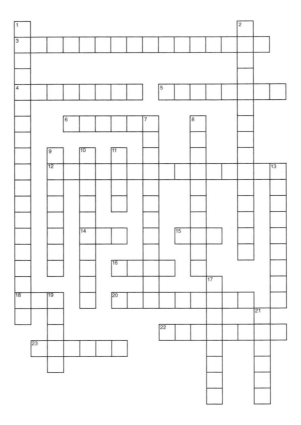

Across

3. Also known as a microcomputer
4. A worldwide computer network available via modem
5. Components of a computer system that you can touch, see, or hear
6. A unit composed of a number of parts that function together to perform a particular task
12. Software that provides instructions to the computer hardware and also runs computer programs
15. Acronym for *read only memory*
16. Amount of memory needed to store one character
18. Stores in-progress data and is the acronym for *random access memory*
20. Nonportable storage device that is read-write with permanent memory
22. Hardware connections that are made using a crossover cable between computers that have an installed network interface controller
23. Storage device for workstations

Down

1. Software that performs a specific data processing function
2. Removes blank spaces left from deleted files
7. Processes data in health care facilities such as patient account processing, insurance claim processing, and statistical analysis of research data
8. A readily transportable data storage device that moves data between computers that are not connected on a network
9. Frequently referred to as a computer program
10. Electronic or optical connection of computers and peripheral equipment for the purpose of sharing information and resources
11. The raw material and collection of characters and numbers entered into a computer
13. A large computer system used for large volumes of repetitive calculations and for governmental provider service programs such as Medicare and Medicaid
17. Allows site access to your computer
19. An input or output device which alters digital data from the computer and transmits it over telephone lines
21. Data storage device capacity

LEARNING REVIEW

Short Answer

1. List the tasks that should be performed by members of the health care team when maintaining the computer.

_____

_____

_____

2. What precautions must be taken to ensure that data are not lost during a power outage?

_____

_____

_____

3. What are the three most common networks encountered in the medical office?

_____

_____

_____

4. Name several hardware connections to a network.

_____

_____

_____

5. Name several wireless connections to a network.

_____

_____

_____

6. Name the two different techniques used by antivirus software to scan files to identify and eliminate computer viruses and malware.

_____

_____

_____

_____

7. List at least six of the defenses that should be used in protecting the health care facility's computer system.

_____

_____

_____

_____

8. The four fundamental elements of all computer systems are:

_____

_____

9. List the HIPAA compliance measures to be taken that will ensure that all PHI data are accurate and not altered, lost, or destroyed.

_____

_____

_____

_____

_____

10. The identifying characteristics of a secure site are *(circle all that apply)*:

    a. small padlock icon in the Web browser window

    b. site address: https://

    c. an "S" in the upper left corner of the screen

    d. site address: http://

11. What is meant by "electronic medical record" and "electronic health record"? Distinguish between the terms.

    _____

    _____

    _____

    _____

CERTIFICATION REVIEW

These questions are designed to mimic the certification examination. Select the best response.

1. A flash drive is a:

    a. memory device

    b. type of software device

    c. DVD drive

    d. safety warning

2. What step(s) should be followed when selecting software?

    a. Choose a knowledgeable vendor.

    b. Determine what tasks will be computerized.

    c. Software available for each task should be identified and evaluated on a trial basis.

    d. All of the above

3. A personal digital assistant is classified as a:

    a. supercomputer

    b. mainframe computer

    c. minicomputer

    d. microcomputer

4. Computers in the medical office or clinic are used to perform:

    a. routine office tasks

    b. maintenance of electronic medical records and management of the clinic or practice

    c. clinical laboratory applications

    d. a. and b. only

    e. a., b., and c.

5. Defragmenting gets rid of:

   a. fragments of information that you do not need anymore

   b. old information no longer needed

   c. empty spaces on the hard drive

   d. removal of software that you do not use

6. The fastest, most complex, and most expensive computer that is also used in medical research is the:

   a. mainframe

   b. supercomputer

   c. minicomputer

   d. personal digital assistant

7. The smallest but most widely used type of computer in today's heath care facility is the:

   a. microcomputer

   b. supercomputer

   c. mainframe computer

   d. minicomputer

8. Examples of output devices would be:

   a. printers, fax machines, monitors

   b. keyboard, mouse

   c. scanners, electronic tablets

   d. touch screens, digital cameras

9. What step(s) should be taken in the changeover to a computer system?

   a. Schedule during a down period, such as a long holiday or vacation period.

   b. Introduce the new system while continuing to use the old system.

   c. Transfer files and data and when the staff is comfortable with the system and their computer skills, then make the changeover.

   d. All of the above

10. Manuals and documents that define how programs operate are called:

   a. the operating system

   b. system software

   c. computer system documentation

   d. application software

11. Compact disks and digital video versatile disks are two types of

   a. hard drives

   b. optical drives

   c. flash drives

   d. tape drives

12. Data storage device capacity is often referred to as

    a. hardware

    b. the operating system

    c. memory

    d. algorithms

13. Portable memory storage devices from which the storage media can be readily removed and transported are called:

    a. flash drives

    b. ROM

    c. RAM

    d. optical drives

LEARNING APPLICATION

 CASE STUDY

Due to an influx of patient volume, the practice of Drs. Lewis and King will have to hire more administrative staff and expand their office space. Three more computers have been installed, with updated software programs. Shirley Brooks, CMA (AAMA), practice manager, is trying to avoid any future safety issues in the workplace.

CASE STUDY REVIEW QUESTION

1. What factors should she take into consideration when setting up each workstation to be "ergonomically correct"?

    _____

    _____

    _____

    _____

    _____

    _____

    _____

    _____

    _____

    _____

    _____

    _____

CHAPTER POST-TEST

Perform this test without looking at your book. If an answer is "false," rewrite the sentence to make it true.

1. The most common type of input device is the:

   a. USB port

   b. flash drive

   c. monitor

   d. keyboard

2. To ensure that your computer information is safe from unauthorized viewing within the office:

   a. use firewalls

   b. defragment frequently

   c. use passwords

   d. back up frequently

3. Which of the following is *not* a function of a total practice management system?

   a. Keeping track of appointments

   b. Keeping track of accounts receivable

   c. Keeping track of accounts payable

   d. Processing insurance claims

   e. Reading directions on how to download software

4. Part of the system that carries out instructions defined by the program software or the data input then sends the results to the selected output devices is called the:

   a. motherboard

   b. modem

   c. video card

   d. CPU

5. To prevent unauthorized use of your clinic's computers, you should:

   a. establish only one person who has access to the computer

   b. keep the computer in a locked cabinet at night

   c. assign every employee a password

   d. have only one person on the computer at a time

SELF-ASSESSMENT

How comfortable are you with moving a computer from one area to another and hooking up all the cords, connections, and wires? What do you think you could do to become more comfortable with computer hardware connections? Look at the connections of your computer and its accessory hardware. Is it color coded or marked in some way?

_____

_____

_____

_____

CHAPTER **12**

Telecommunications

CHAPTER PRE-TEST

Perform this test without looking at your book. If an answer is "false," rewrite the sentence to make it true.

1. True or False? When transferring a call, it is not necessary to obtain the patient's name and phone number.

_____

_____

2. True or False? Some patients need to be handled with a firm voice on the phone.

_____

_____

3. True or False? It is not necessary to ask permission prior to putting a patient on hold.

_____

_____

4. True or False? When taking a message, be as brief as possible. The patient's name and phone number is enough information.

_____

_____

5. True or False? Patients cannot expect confidentiality on their home answering machines.

_____

_____

6. True or False? All angry calls should be immediately forwarded to the provider.

_____

_____

VOCABULARY BUILDER

Misspelled Words

Find the words below that are misspelled; circle them, and correctly spell them in the spaces provided. Then fill in the blanks in the following paragraph with the appropriate terms. (Hint: not all terms will be used.)

answering services	etiguette	jargon
articulate	faximile	modulated
buffer words	fluant	obfucation
clincial email	Good Samaritan laws	pagers
enunciate	handheld devices	pronounciation

_____   _____   _____

_____   _____   _____

When speaking on the telephone, medical assistants must use proper telephone _____, which means being courteous and professional to others. To ensure that listeners understand what is said, it is important to _____, or say the words clearly. Simple terms rather than medical _____ promote mutual understanding rather than confusion or _____. The use of slang words and expressions is considered unprofessional and disrespectful. When speaking with a caller who is not _____ in English, it is helpful to speak slowly and use short sentences. Proper _____ of all words in a carefully _____ voice will also help people understand what you are saying, especially non–English-speaking people. Good communication skills are of real benefit to a medical assistant when using the telephone and when speaking directly to patients.

Matching

Match the following devices or services listed in Column A with corresponding descriptions in Column B.

_____ 1. pager

_____ 2. answering service

_____ 3. cellular phone

_____ 4. automated routing unit

_____ 5. fax

_____ 6. email

A. Takes calls when the office is closed

B. Sends a message via phone lines to an electronic mailbox located in another person's computer

C. A one-way communication device used to contact staff when away from the office

D. A portable telephone

E. A document sent over telephone lines from one facsimile machine or modem to another

F. A system that allows callers to reach specific people or departments by pressing a specified number on a touch-tone telephone

LEARNING REVIEW

Short Answer

1. Name four reasons why a potential patient will contact an ambulatory care facility by telephone.

   _____

   _____

   _____

   _____

2. Many providers and health care professionals use paging systems. Paging systems allow the medical assistant to alert a provider or other health care professional who is not on-site to call in for an important message. Name and describe four paging system options.

   _____

   _____

   _____

   _____

   _____

   _____

   _____

   _____

3. Many hospitals and ambulatory care settings have telephone systems to manage heavy telephone traffic; these are called _____ .

4. No call should be left unattended for more than _____ seconds.

5. What is the difference between enunciation and pronunciation?

   _____

   _____

6. Name the three different types of Voice-over-Internet Protocol (VoIP) services in use.

   _____

   _____

7. List three advantages of email and three disadvantages of email.

   Advantages:

   _____

   _____

   _____

   Disadvantages:

   _____

   _____

   _____

8. Explain the difference between email and clinical email.

_____

_____

_____

_____

9. Why is it important for email to be encrypted?

_____

_____

Scope of Practice Review

Indicate the calls described below that fall within the scope of practice for a medical assistant (MA) to respond to and the calls that should be directed to the provider (P).

Type of Call	Who Should Handle
Insurance questions	_____
Scheduling patient testing and office appointments	_____
Medical advice	_____
Requests for prescription refills	_____
Provider's family members	_____
General information about the practice	_____
Poor progress reports from a patient	_____
Requests for medications other than prescription refills	_____
Other providers	_____
Salespeople	_____
STAT reports	_____

Patient Confidentiality Activity

Because medical assistants must observe laws regarding both patient confidentiality and the patient's right to privacy, it is crucial for the medical assistant to understand and comply with legal and ethical principles and the restrictions governing the issues of patient confidentiality. Indicate by checking off the appropriate box whether the medical assistant may discuss a patient's medical condition or reveal details from the medical record.

	Yes	No	Yes, with signed release
Patient's spouse or family member			
Patient's employer			
Patient's attorney			
Another health care provider			
Patient's insurance carrier			
Referring provider's office			
Credit bureau or collection agency			
Member of the office staff, as necessary for patient care			
Other patient			
People outside the office (friend, family acquaintance)			
Patient's parent or legal guardian, except concerning issues of birth control, abortion, or STDs			

CERTIFICATION REVIEW

These questions are designed to mimic the certification examination. Select the best response.

1. Telephone calls that may be handled by the medical assistant include all but which one of the following?

    a. Billing questions

    b. Appointment changes

    c. Requests for prescription refills

    d. Calls from other physicians

2. When a medical assistant is talking to a patient on the telephone and another line rings, what should the medical assistant do?

    a. Ask permission from the first caller to put her on hold, answer the second call and then ask permission from that caller to put him on hold, and go back to the first caller to finish up.

    b. Put the first call on hold, answer the second call and handle that issue, then go back to the first caller.

    c. Let the second line ring; it will be picked up by an answering system.

    d. Finish with the first caller, then answer the second line.

3. Which of the following is *not* a good idea in a medical office?

    a. Using a speaker phone to listen to voice messages

    b. Speaking quietly on the telephone so other patients cannot hear

    c. Using a privacy screen to reduce the chance of being overheard on the telephone

    d. Using only email so you will not be overheard

4. After-hours telephone messages are usually directed to:

    a. the provider's home

    b. the medical manager's home

    c. a voice mail system or answering service/machine

    d. an email system

5. When talking to older adult patients on the phone:

    a. if the patient is hearing impaired, speak slower, clearer, and a little louder

    b. assume that they are senile or at least forgetful and repeat all the information several times

    c. if the person has difficulty understanding, simplify the information, ask if there are any questions, and try to explain patiently in simple terms

    d. All of the above

    e. a. and c. only

6. Guidelines of the Health Insurance Portability and Accountability Act (HIPAA) for telephone communication include:

    a. Determine if patients have specific instructions on who has been granted privilege to their private medical information.

    b. Determine if patients have a particular number they want called for confidential communications.

    c. Ask if it is acceptable to leave a message if patients are not at the number provided.

    d. All of the above

7. The best solution for handling a caller who refuses to give information after gentle prodding is:

    a. tell the patient to call back when he is ready to cooperate

    b. hang up on the caller

    c. take a message and then give it to the provider

    d. argue with the patient, telling him that he is being unreasonable and that you need the information

8. The administrative medical assistant should always try to answer a call:

    a. by the end of the first ring if possible but definitely within three rings

    b. after five rings

    c. after two rings and before five rings

    d. within a minute

9. Before transferring a call to the appropriate party, a guideline to follow is:

    a. Put the caller on hold, then transfer the call.

    b. Put the caller on hold and contact the person to whom the call is going, to see if the person can speak to the caller.

    c. Transfer the call immediately.

    d. Get the caller's name, number, and any pertinent information.

10. If a call is a medical emergency, what protocol should be followed in handling that type of situation?

   a. Tell the patient to go to the emergency room.

   b. Keep the caller on the line and call 911 on another line.

   c. Put the caller on hold and try to get the provider on the phone.

   d. Tell the patient that you will call 911 for her and then call her back.

11. To ensure sensible risk management when making calls, you should protect the patient's privacy at all times; this is referred to as:

   a. confidentiality

   b. jargon

   c. elaboration

   d. screening

LEARNING APPLICATION

 # CASE STUDY

As Inner City Health Care, an urgent care center, continues to grow, increasing both patient load and staff, the existing telephone system, consisting of a simple intercom and four telephone lines, is no longer sufficient to handle the call volume and allow for full, immediate accessibility for all staff members. Callers are frustrated by the length of time it takes to get through and by long amounts of time spent on hold. Messages are often late in getting properly routed. Administrative medical assistant Karen Ritter suggests to office manager Jane O'Hara that an automated routing unit (ARU) might be more efficient for the growing clinic's needs. At the next regularly scheduled staff meeting, the provider-employers give the go-ahead to research an ARU.

CASE STUDY REVIEW QUESTIONS

1. ARU systems provide several options for callers that identify specific departments or services that callers can be connected with directly. What kinds of caller options might be appropriate for Inner City Health Care?

   _____

   _____

   _____

   _____

   _____

2. What can be done so the patient with an emergency or the hearing-impaired patient can speak automatically to a "live" operator?

   _____

   _____

   _____

   _____

continues

3. How can an ARU help staff members receive their calls more efficiently?

_____

_____

_____

4. How can the office manager and medical assistant implement the ARU system with a minimum of disruption to provider(s), staff, and patients?

_____

_____

_____

_____

_____

_____

_____

Role-Play Exercises

Effective telephone communication requires prompt and professional responses from medical assistants. With another student, role-play as patient and medical assistant. When you are finished role-playing, write what you have said as the "medical assistant" below.

1. Patient Nora Fowler calls with a question about medication prescribed for her rheumatoid arthritis and insists on a call back from Dr. Elizabeth King. Dr. King is presently on rounds at the hospital and will not be available until 4:30 PM. Nora's tone of voice indicates that she is upset, and she states that her medication is not helping her discomfort. It is clear from the conversation that Nora has discontinued taking her medication.

_____

_____

_____

_____

_____

_____

2. While speaking on telephone line 1 with patient Bill Schwartz, who is calling to schedule a physical examination, medical assistant Wanda Slawson receives another call on line 2 from a laboratory with a summary of emergency test results for another patient. Wanda knows that Dr. Susan Rice is waiting for the test results.

_____

_____

_____

3. Medical assistant Bruce Goldman takes a call from patient Juanita Hansen. Juanita is inquiring about a bill and indicating that her insurance carrier, Blue Cross, did not pay the entire fee for her son's last examination, which left her with a balance owed to Inner City Health Care. Office manager Walter Seals is responsible for managing insurance claims and inquiries.

_____

_____

_____

_____

Hands-on Activities

1. Each morning, medical assistant Ellen Armstrong is responsible for transcribing messages left on the medical practice's answering machine the evening before. Using the message pad slips below, transcribe each message completely and appropriately. In the space for "Attachments," list any records, files, or documents that should be attached to the message slip for the recipient's review.

A. "Ellen, this is Anna Preciado. Can you tell Marilyn Johnson, the office manager, that I won't be in tomorrow for the afternoon shift? I have a 101-degree temperature and bad flu symptoms. Check with Joe Guerrero to see if he can come in to sub for me as the clinical medical assistant. Yesterday he told me he would be available if I wasn't feeling well enough to come in. I know Dr. Lewis has several patients scheduled for clinical testing in the afternoon. I can be reached at 555-6622."

B. "This is Charles Williams. Dr. Lewis put me on a Holter monitor today. It's about 11:00 PM and one of the leads came off. I put it back on, but I am worried about whether I will have to do this test again. Can you call me tomorrow at home before 8:00 AM at 555-6124 or at the office after 9:00 AM at 555-8125? Thanks."

To: _____ Date: _____

From: _____ Time: _____

Telephone #: _____

Message: _____

_____

_____

_____

                        Initials: _____

Attachments: _____

_____

To: _____ Date: _____

From: _____ Time: _____

Telephone #: _____

Message: _____

_____

_____

_____

                        Initials: _____

Attachments: _____

_____

CHAPTER POST-TEST

Perform this test without looking at your book. If an answer is "false," rewrite the sentence to make it true.

1. True or False? When transferring a call, it is important to obtain the patient's name and phone number.

_____

_____

2. True or False? Some patients will become defensive when a firm voice is used on the phone.

_____

_____

3. True or False? The patient should always be asked if she can be put on hold.

_____

_____

4. True or False? When taking a message, be brief but thorough. The patient's name, phone number, questions, best time for a callback, and any other pertinent information that is useful should be noted.

_____

_____

5. True or False? Patients should expect confidentiality at all times, even on their home answering machines.

_____

_____

6. True or False? The provider should be alerted to any angry calls regarding patient care and treatment.

_____

_____

SELF-ASSESSMENT

1. Discuss the following questions with another classmate or in a small group. During the discussion, consider how different people react in different ways, depending on their personalities, their patience, and their confidence levels. After the discussion, spend a moment in self-reflection to think of ways you can improve your telephone communication skills.

   (1) Have you ever conversed with someone on the telephone whom you could not understand?

   _____

   _____

   (2) Was it the language of the individual, their accent, enunciation, or volume?

   _____

   _____

   (3) Would it have been easier to understand the individual if you were face to face with that person?

   _____

   _____

(4) How did you handle the situation? Did you ask the person to speak louder, slower, or more clearly?

_____

_____

(5) How do you think most people would handle a situation in which they could not hear the speaker clearly? What if the speaker were an older adult? a non–English speaker? A person in pain or very ill?

_____

_____

2. Of the following telecommunication devices and methods, with which are you most familiar and which will you need to learn more about? What do you think is the best way to become more familiar with the following devices and methods?
   • Email
   • Pagers
   • Multiline phones
   • Cell phones
   • Fax machines
   • Answering services

_____

_____

_____

_____

CHAPTER **13**

Patient Scheduling

CHAPTER PRE-TEST

Perform this test without looking at your book. If an answer is "false," rewrite the sentence to make it true.

1. Circle the letter that lists correct types of scheduling systems:

   a. wave, modified wave, double booking, mile-a-minute

   b. open hours, wave, clustering, stream, double booking

   c. first-come, first-served; open hours; clustering

2. Below are guidelines to scheduling. Which one is correct?

   a. Urgent calls should be sent to the hospital, which is better equipped to handle them.

   b. Urgent calls should be assessed before determining the best course of action.

   c. Referrals by other physicians need to be seen immediately.

   d. Appointments for pharmaceutical and medical supply representatives should be referred to the physician.

3. Information that should be obtained from all new patients includes all but which one of the following?

   a. The patient's full legal name

   b. The patient's birth date

   c. The patient's address and telephone numbers

   d. The reason for the visit

   e. The patient's insurance information

   f. The patient's family health history

4. True or False? All medical offices are changing to electronic appointment scheduling.

   _____

   _____

5. True or False? When providing a sign-in sheet for patients, it is permissible to request the reason for the visit.

   _____

   _____

6. True or False? It is not necessary to note cancellations or no-shows in the patient's chart.

_____

_____

VOCABULARY BUILDER

Misspelled Words

Find the words below that are misspelled; circle them, and correctly spell them in the spaces provided. Then replace the highlighted words in the following paragraph with the correct vocabulary terms from the list.

clustering	modified wave scheduling	screaning
double booking	no-show	stream scheduling
encription technology	open hours	wave scheduling
matrics	practice based	

_____ _____ _____

_____ 1. Inner City Health Care reserves 9 AM to 12 PM on Thursday mornings for walk-in patients who are seen on a first-come, first-served basis within that time frame.

_____ 2. At the offices of Drs. Lewis and King, Ellen Armstrong, CMA (AAMA), schedules Mary O'Keefe for a 1:00 PM appointment for some blood work and Martin Gordon for a 1:00 PM appointment for a blood pressure check so Dr. King can assess whether his medication is at the proper level.

_____ 3. Lenny Taylor, an older adult patient with mild dementia, forgets his third appointment with Dr. James Whitney.

_____ 4. At Inner City Health Care, vaccinations are scheduled every 10 minutes from 10 AM to 12:20 PM on Mondays; Tuesday office hours are reserved for new patients only.

_____ 5. Three patients are scheduled to receive treatments in the first half hour of every hour.

_____ 6. Dr. Elizabeth King prefers to see patients for regular gynecologic examinations in consecutive appointments scheduled from 8:30 AM to 11:30 AM and obstetric patients from 1:00 PM to 3:30 PM.

_____ 7. When patient Herb Fowler calls to set up an appointment with Dr. Winston Lewis for his chronic cough, Ellen Armstrong, CMA (AAMA), asks Herb a series of questions to ascertain the nature, extent, and urgency of his condition.

_____ 8. Dr. Winston Lewis prefers that each patient be assigned a specific time, scheduling at 30- or 60-minute intervals on a continuous basis throughout the day.

_____ 9. An ophthalmologist schedules three patients at the beginning of each hour for comprehensive examinations, followed by single appointments every 10 to 20 minutes during the rest of the hour for quick, follow-up procedures such as removing eye patches or instilling eye drops.

_____ 10. On the 15th day of each month, office manager Walter Seals, who is responsible for efficient patient flow at Inner City Health Care, asks each of the urgent care center's five providers to confirm their scheduling commitments for the upcoming month to block off unavailable times in the appointment book.

_____ 11. The medical assistant uses software to protect patients' confidentiality in electronic format.

LEARNING REVIEW

Short Answer

1. Appointment books are legal documents recording patient flow. For a manual appointment system, where pencil is used for ease in rescheduling, what can the medical assistant do to ensure that a permanent record is secured?

_____

_____

_____

2. For a computerized appointment system, what can a medical assistant do to ensure that a permanent record of patient flow is secured?

_____

_____

_____

_____

3. Name two primary goals in determining the best method for scheduling patient appointments.

_____

_____

_____

4. What is the typical scheduling time for each of the following types of office visits for an internal medicine practice?

(1) Patient consultation: _____

(2) Established patient routine follow-up: _____

(3) New patient: _____

(4) Complete physical examination: _____

(5) Cold/flu symptoms: _____

(6) Vaccination: _____

5. What are six variables involved in the process of scheduling appointments for patients and other visitors to the ambulatory care setting?

_____

_____

_____

_____

6. Patient flow analysis sheets help medical practices determine the effectiveness of patient scheduling and devise plans for improving a smooth patient flow through the ambulatory care setting. What kinds of issues can a study of these data reveal?

_____

_____

_____

_____

7. What are the five steps of scheduling a specific appointment time for a patient?

_____

_____

_____

_____

_____

_____

8. Two ways of reminding patients of upcoming appointments are to give the appointment card personally to the patient and to mail the card to the patient. Identify a third reminder system. What procedures must be observed to protect patient confidentiality when using this third method?

_____

_____

_____

_____

9. Identify seven scheduling styles.

_____

_____

10. Identify the best scheduling system for the examples below, and explain the reasoning behind your choice.
   (1) Hospital emergency room:

   _____

   _____

   _____

   _____

   (2) Laboratory for blood testing:

   _____

   _____

   _____

   _____

   (3) Two or more patients are given a particular appointment time:

   _____

   _____

   (4) Best-known and widely used scheduling system:

   _____

   _____

   _____

11. Patient Mark Johnson is a no-show for his appointment. Other than marking the no-show appropriately on the appointment schedule, what other action must be taken to document Mr. Johnson's no-show status? Why is it important to accurately and completely document patient no-shows and cancellations?

_____

_____

_____

_____

_____

_____

_____

True or False

Mark a true statement with a T *and a false statement with an* F. *If an answer is "false," rewrite the sentence to make it true.*

____ 1. In scheduling, double booking means to keep two appointment books going for the same doctor.

_____

_____

____ 2. One major purpose of screening when scheduling appointments is to determine if the patient has an emergency or urgent situation/illness.

_____

_____

____ 3. If a patient routinely cancels or misses three consecutive appointments, the provider may decide to terminate services.

_____

_____

____ 4. The appointment book/record may be subpoenaed, and therefore is considered a legal document.

_____

_____

____ 5. Providing patients with appointment cards is an effective way to prevent missed appointments.

_____

_____

____ 6. It is important to provide an appointment to a referral patient as soon as possible.

_____

_____

____ 7. There is an unexpected delay in the schedule caused by an office emergency. It is not necessary for the medical assistant to provide the patient with an estimate of how long the delay will be.

_____

_____

____ 8. A hurried, disinterested manner toward patients is just as often the basis for legal action as is a negligent act.

_____

_____

___ 9. A permanent record or daily appointment sheet does not have to indicate any changes such as cancellations, walk-ins, urgent care needs, and no-shows.

_____

_____

___ 10. If at the same time when scheduling an appointment for a patient in the office, the phone rings, the medical assistant should first excuse herself and take the call.

_____

_____

CERTIFICATION REVIEW

These questions are designed to mimic the certification examination. Select the best response.

1. Scheduling outpatient procedures:

   a. is done at the end of each day

   b. is best done with the patient present

   c. will be easier with a calendar for visualization of days discussed

   d. b. and c.

2. One principle above all else in scheduling for the office is:

   a. flexibility

   b. neatness

   c. accountability

   d. estimation

3. The type of scheduling that requires visits to be set up around patients with specific chronic ailments such as diabetes and hypertension is called:

   a. screening

   b. referral appointments

   c. group scheduling

   d. stream appointments

4. The general rule for no-shows and cancellations is that after _____ consecutive missed appointments, the provider will review the patient's record and could terminate care.

   a. five

   b. three

   c. two

   d. ten

5. What, more than anything else, determines the success of a day in the ambulatory care setting?

   a. Patient care

   b. Efficient patient flow

   c. Operational functions

   d. Interpersonal skills

LEARNING APPLICATION

When patient Lenore McDonell falls from the examination table and lacerates her arm while attempting an independent transfer from the table to her wheelchair, clinical medical assistant Joe Guerrero alerts Dr. Winston Lewis, and the two begin to implement emergency procedures to control Lenore's bleeding and assess damage to the arm. Lenore's fall occurred at the end of her appointment, a routine checkup with Dr. Lewis.

Administrative medial assistant Ellen Armstrong must adjust Dr. Lewis's schedule to accommodate the emergency situation. Martin Gordon, a man in his mid-60s, diagnosed with prostate cancer, waits in the reception area for Dr. Lewis's next appointment. Mr. Gordon's appointment, a 6-month follow-up, is expected to take 30 minutes. Mr. Gordon is also being rated for depression related to his cancer diagnosis. Hope Smith, a new patient in good general health, is scheduled for a complete examination; she is due to arrive at the office of Drs. Lewis and King at the Northborough Family Medical Group within 20 minutes. Jim Marshall, an impatient and aggressive businessman, is scheduled for the first afternoon appointment after Dr. Lewis's lunch commitment. Mr. Marshall's appointment for a physical examination and ECG to investigate chest pains he has experienced recently is expected to take 45 minutes. Dr. Lewis's schedule is completely booked for the rest of the day.

CASE STUDY REVIEW QUESTIONS

1. What scheduling alternatives will Ellen offer Mr. Gordon, who is already waiting in the reception area? What special considerations regarding Mr. Gordon should Ellen take into account and why?

_____

_____

_____

_____

_____

_____

_____

2. What is Ellen's first action regarding Ms. Smith, Dr. Lewis's next patient due to arrive? What scheduling alternatives should Ellen offer her?

_____

_____

_____

_____

_____

_____

continues

3. What scheduling alternatives, if any, should Ellen present to Mr. Marshall? Explain your logic.

_____

_____

_____

_____

_____

4. How is screening important to Ellen's rescheduling of Dr. Lewis's patients? What important administrative and communication skills will Ellen use to handle this emergency situation efficiently and professionally?

_____

_____

_____

_____

_____

_____

_____

_____

_____

_____

_____

Hands-on Activity

Patient Martin Gordon has a 30-minute appointment scheduled with Dr. Lewis on Wednesday, February 7, 20XX for routine follow-up for prostate cancer. He calls the office on January 30 and would like to reschedule his appointment for two weeks later at 3:00 PM the same time. You mark through his name on the appointment schedule with a single line in red pen, and document the change in the patient's chart. Now, complete the appointment card below to be mailed to Mr. Gordon as a reminder of his new appointment time.

LEWIS & KING, MD
L&K
2501 CENTER STREET
NORTHBOROUGH, OH 12345

M _____

has an appointment on

Mon. _____   at _____

Tues. _____   at _____

Wed. _____   at _____

Thurs. _____   at _____

Fri. _____   at _____

If unable to keep appointment, kindly give 24 hours' notice.

MOSS Activities

Using Medical Office Simulation Software and the skills learned in Procedure 13-4, schedule the following appointments:

1. A 30-minute appointment for Edward Gormann on July 10, 2009, for an earache.

2. A 15-minute appointment for Megan Caldwell on July 15, 2009, to check for strep throat.

CHAPTER POST-TEST

Perform this test without looking at your book. If an answer is "false," rewrite the sentence to make it true.

1. Circle the letter that lists correct types of scheduling systems.

   a. Modified wave, wave, clustering, and mile-a-minute

   b. Stream, open hours, wave, grouping, separating

   c. First-come, first-served; open hours; clustering

   d. Open hours, wave, clustering, stream, double booking

2. Below are guidelines to scheduling. Which one is correct?

   a. Urgent calls should be scheduled for the next available appointment time.

   b. Urgent calls should be sent to the hospital, which is better equipped to handle them.

   c. If a referral patient calls, it is best to obtain information from the referring provider's office to determine the urgency of the appointment.

   d. Appointments for pharmaceutical and medical supply representatives should be referred to the physician.

3. Information that should be obtained from all new patients includes all but which one of the following?

   a. The patient's full legal name

   b. The patient's birth date

   c. The patient's address and telephone numbers

   d. Family health history

   e. Reason for the visit

   f. The patient's insurance information

4. True or False? Many medical offices are changing to electronic appointment scheduling.

   _____

   _____

5. True or False? When a patient cancels or is a no-show, it must always be documented in the patient chart.

   _____

   _____

SELF-ASSESSMENT

1. When you call a provider's office, do any of the following aggravate you? Do you think other people are aggravated by these?

   a. Being put on hold right away or too often

   b. The administrative medical assistant asking too many questions

   c. Not enough appointment time choices; that is, you have to wait too long for an appointment

   d. Not getting a real person; that is, having to listen to electronic choices and make selections

   e. Other (add your own idea) _____

2. Now go to each of the situations in Question 1 and determine an action that could alleviate all or some of the aggravation. Keep in mind that the situation might still exist (e.g., the receptionist might still have to ask a lot of questions), but how might he or she make the experience more pleasant?

   _____
   _____
   _____
   _____

3. When you visit a provider's office, do any of the following aggravate you?

   a. The administrative medical assistant does not acknowledge you right away.

   b. The wait is too long.

   c. The waiting room is noisy, messy, or uncomfortable.

   d. There are no magazines of interest to you.

   e. Other (add your own idea) _____

4. Similar to the instructions in Question 2, go to each of the situations in Question 3 and determine solutions that could alleviate all or some of the causes of aggravation. Keep in mind that the solutions in this case are obvious and doable.

   _____
   _____
   _____
   _____

5. Think of your most pleasant interaction with a provider's office as a patient making an appointment, scheduling a procedure, changing an appointment, or even canceling an appointment. What made the experience more pleasant? Was it the voice of the administrative medical assistant? his or her tone? actual words? the overall options? or something else?

   _____
   _____
   _____
   _____

6. As you enter your career as a medical assistant, try to remember how the patient feels. Try to recall situations that bother you when you are a patient. Try to keep these issues in mind and see if you can eliminate or alleviate them to make your patients as comfortable as possible. Maybe you are just the person who will help to make the experience of seeing a doctor more pleasant for your patients. Try to be like the person you thought of for Question 5. This is not an easy thing to do when you are busy and stressed. Can you think of ways you can remind yourself every day of these lessons?

_____

_____

_____

_____

CHAPTER **14**

Medical Records Management

CHAPTER PRE-TEST

Perform this test without looking at your book. If an answer is "false," rewrite the sentence to make it true.

1. True or False? Out-guides indicate when patient charts are out of order.

   _____

   _____

2. Which of the following is *not* an important skill to have when filing?

   a. You should know the alphabet.

   b. You should know the basic rules of filing.

   c. You should pay attention to details.

   d. You should be good at math.

3. True or False? Medical records are important for many reasons. They provide information for medical care, legal protection, and research purposes.

   _____

   _____

4. True or False? It is acceptable to release medical information to family members as long as they can show proper picture identification.

   _____

   _____

5. True or False? The standard in court is that if there is no record of information related to the appointment, including care and treatment of that patient, then it did not happen.

   _____

   _____

6. True or False? All medical filing systems use the alphabetic filing system.

   _____

   _____

VOCABULARY BUILDER

Misspelled Words

Find the words below that are misspelled; underline them, and correctly spell them in the space provided. Then, fill in the blanks in the following sentences with the appropriate terms. (Hint: not all words will be used.)

accession record	key unit	SOAP
captions	out-gide	source-orientated medical record
coding	perging	tickler file
cross-reference	problem-orientated medical record	unit

_____   _____   _____

_____

1. To remember to check with the reference laboratory on Friday to obtain patient Martin Gordon's test results, Ellen Armstrong, CMA (AAMA), places a note in her _____.

2. Every six months, Marilyn Johnson follows office policy and procedures for _____ inactive files to remove and archive those not in active use.

3. The organized method of identifying and separating items to be filed into small subunits is accomplished with the use of _____ units.

4. When Liz Corbin, CMA (AAMA), retrieves Annette Samuels's chart for Dr. Woo, she places an _____ in the filing cabinet to show that the file has been removed from storage.

5. The _____ is a journal (or computer listing) where numbers in a numeric filing system are pre-assigned. The log sequentially lists numbers to be used to assign to numeric records.

6. The file for Kent Memorial Hospital contains three indexing _____ to be considered when preparing the filing label.

7. If a _____ card is required in the alphabetic card file of a numeric filing system, such as when making note of an established patient's married name, a card is prepared that includes an **X** next to the file number to indicate that this card does not designate the primary location card for the file.

8. In the _____ system of recordkeeping, patient problems are identified by a number that corresponds to the charting relevant to that problem number; that is, asthma #1; dermatitis #2; and so on.

9. When a filing system other than alphabetic is being used, the proper _____ must be determined for the chart or file so it can be retrieved.

10. _____ are used to identify major sections of file folders by more manageable subunits, such as GA-GE, or Miscellaneous. Captions are marked on the tabs of the guides.

11. Inner City Health Care uses the _____ method of recordkeeping, which groups information according to its origin; for example, laboratories, examinations, provider notes, consulting providers, and other types of information.

12. Some medical facilities have added two additional letters, "E" and "R," to the _____ approach, which stand for "education for patient" and "response of patient to education and care given."

LEARNING REVIEW

Short Answer

1. Why is accurate, up-to-date, complete documentation in patient medical records essential in the ambulatory care setting?

_____

_____

_____

_____

_____

2. Why is the POMR system commonly used by family practice offices?

_____

_____

_____

3. Why is a color-coding system effective in the ambulatory care setting?

_____

_____

4. How important is an effective, easy-to-use, and easy-to-access filing system to the efficiency of the ambulatory care setting?

_____

_____

_____

_____

_____

_____

5. List at least four advantages of EMRs.

_____

_____

_____

_____

6. What does the acronym SOAPER stand for?

_____

_____

_____

7. List three numeric filing systems that are used in medical facilities.

_____

_____

_____

8. List at least five standards required by the HIPAA Security Rule for electronic medical records.

_____

_____

_____

_____

_____

_____

_____

Indexing Units Exercise

Assign the correct units to the following items to be filed using the rule for filing patient records that is listed for each.

1. Names that are hyphenated are considered one unit.

   A. Jackson Hugh Levine-Dwyer

   unit 1 _____   unit 2 _____   unit 3 _____

   B. Leslie Jane Poole-Petit

   unit 1 _____   unit 2 _____   unit 3 _____

2. Seniority units are indexed as the last indexing unit.

   A. Keith Wildasin Sr.

   unit 1 _____   unit 2 _____   unit 3 _____

   B. Gerald Maggart III

   unit 1 _____   unit 2 _____   unit 3 _____

3. Titles are considered as separate indexing units. If the title appears with first and last names, the title is considered the last indexing unit.

   A. Dr. Louise Udolf

   unit 1 _____   unit 2 _____   unit 3 _____

   B. Prof. Valerie Rajah

   unit 1 _____   unit 2 _____   unit 3 _____

4. The names of individuals are assigned indexing units respectively: last name, first name, middle, and succeeding names.

   A. Lindsay Adair Martin

   unit 1 _____   unit 2 _____   unit 3 _____

   B. Abigail Sue Johnson

   unit 1 _____   unit 2 _____   unit 3 _____

5. When indexing names of married women, the name is indexed by the legal name.

   A. Mary Jane O'Keefe (Mrs. John)

   unit 1 _____   unit 2 _____   unit 3 _____   unit 4 _____

   B. Nora Patrice Fowler (Mrs. Herb)

   unit 1 _____   unit 2 _____   unit 3 _____   unit 4 _____

6. Foreign language units are indexed as one unit with the unit that follows. Spacing, punctuation, and capitalization are ignored.

A. Joseph Jack de la Hoya

unit 1 _____ unit 2 _____ unit 3 _____

B. Maurice John van de Veer

unit 1 _____ unit 2 _____ unit 3 _____

Multiple Choice

Circle the right answer(s) from the choices below.

1. The most important reason for using numeric filing is that:
   a. it preserves patient confidentiality
   b. a larger number of records can be easily filed
   c. a computer can more readily read numeric filing labels

2. Walter Seals, CMA (AAMA), is filing using a terminal digit filing system. For the patient file labeled 67 84 30, what is unit 1?
   a. 67
   b. 30
   c. 80

3. Outgoing correspondence is:
   a. friendly correspondence
   b. correspondence sent out of the medical office
   c. correspondence to be thrown away

4. Karen Ritter, CMA (AAMA), is filing patient files using a numeric filing system. She comes across a file for a patient who has not yet been assigned a number. Karen should put the file:
   a. in the miscellaneous numeric file section
   b. in a pending filing bin until the provider can assign a number
   c. directly behind the rest of the files

5. An out-guide in paper or manual records should contain:
   a. a record of when the chart was removed
   b. the signature of the patient's physician
   c. a record of when the file is expected to be returned

6. State statutes have ruled that medical records are the property of the:
   a. state medical society
   b. ones who create them
   c. patient only

7. Any information to be released from the medical record:
   a. goes to medical insurance
   b. requires a provider's signature
   c. requires patient notification and approval
   d. requires a subpoena

8. Filing equipment:

   a. should have a locking capability

   b. is available in vertical or lateral styles

   c. is to be stored in an area accessible only to authorized personnel

   d. All of the above

9. EMR stands for:

   a. emergency room

   b. a popular color-coding system's trade name

   c. electronic medical records

   d. emergency medical rules

10. Release marks include:

    a. date stamp and initials

    b. out-guides

    c. tabs

    d. SOAP/SOAPER

CERTIFICATION REVIEW

These questions are designed to mimic the certification examination. Select the best response.

1. The POMR is also known as:

   a. a source-oriented medical record

   b. a SOAP/SOAPER system

   c. a traditional method

   d. a problem-oriented medical record

   e. none of the above

2. The SOAP/SOAPER format is:

   a. a way to sanitize instruments

   b. a form of patient electronic records

   c. a type of filing system

   d. a specific charting system

   e. none of the above

3. If a patient needs to return for another examination in six months, you might use a reminder system. What is the name of that system?

   a. Reminder system

   b. Recall system

   c. Phone log

   d. Tickler system

   e. Out-guide

4. The most common method of filing in today's medical office is:

  a. alphabetically

  b. numerically

  c. by insurance

  d. by subject

  e. color coding

5. If a medical document is filed in multiple places, you might use a(n):

  a. index

  b. out-guide

  c. cross-reference

  d. multiple reference

  e. cross-filed card

6. The best method to use for making a correction in a paper medical record is:

  a. use a "white out" product

  b. scribble over the error with a magic marker

  c. put "x's" through the error

  d. draw a single line through the error, make the correction, write "CORR" or "CORRECTION" above the area corrected, and add your initials and date.

7. Identifiable patient information that should *not* appear on the outside of the chart would include:

  a. patient's address

  b. patient's social security number

  c. patient's birth date

  d. patient's phone number

  e. all of the above

8. Closed files are usually kept:

  a. 3 to 6 years beyond the statute of limitations

  b. 2 to 5 years

  c. indefinitely

  d. 10 years

9. The three types of cabinets used in medical clinics are:

  a. vertical, lateral, and movable

  b. metal, hanging, and color coded

  c. horizontal, lateral, and movable

  d. open, locked, and movable

10. Captions are used:

  a. to separate file folders

  b. to identify major sections of file folders

  c. in vertical and lateral systems

  d. a. and c. only

LEARNING APPLICATION

Filing Order Review

Using the numbers 1, 2, and 3, label the patient names in each group according to the correct filing order of names in an alphabetic filing system.

____ L. Sanders

____ Larry Paul Samuels

____ Lawrence P. Sanders

____ James Edward Reed Sr.

____ James Edward Reed

____ James Edward Reed Jr.

____ Lynn Elaine Brenner

____ Lynn Ellen Brenner

____ Lynn Eloise Brenner

____ Patrick Sam Saint

____ Patrick Sam St. Bartz

____ Paul Sam Saint

MOSS Activities

Using Medical Office Simulation Software and the skills learned in Procedure 14-7, register the following new patients, to establish a new record for each.

1. Ms. Julia E. Martin, a new patient of Dr. Schwartz. (Hint: Dr. Schwartz is a participating provider of Julia's insurance plan, ConsumerOne HRA, and accepts assignment.)

Home contact information	13 Cobble Stone Ave Douglasville, NY 01234 (123) 457-1212
Marital Status	Single
Social Security Number	999-76-1234
Date of Birth	December 1, 1980
Employer	Clear Lake Elementary 5526 Gravel Way, Douglasville, NY 01234 (123) 528-1132
Primary Insurance Information	ConsumerOne HRA ID Number: 999761234-01 Group Number: CLE5610 Policyholder: Self

2. Mr. Adair Smith, a new patient of Dr. Heath, who was referred by Dr. Samantha Green. (Hint: Dr. Heath is a participating provider of Adair's insurance plan, Medicare, and accepts assignment.)

Home contact information	159 Broad Street Douglasville, NY 01234 (123) 528-4092
Marital Status	Married to Mackenzie Smith
Social Security Number	999-54-3579
Date of Birth	April 26, 1938
Employer	Retired
Primary Insurance Information	Medicare ID Number: 999543579A

3. Remi Beaufort, a new patient of Dr. Heath, who is brought to the office by his father, Joseph Beaufort. (Hint: Dr. Heath is a participating provider of the insurance plan, and accepts assignment.)

Home contact information	43 Clay Lane Douglasville, NY 01234 (123) 457-3393
Marital Status	Single
Social Security Number	999-23-8989
Date of Birth	June 8, 1991
Employer	Full-time student at Clear Lake Elementary
Guarantor information	Joseph Beaufort Social Security Number: 999-44-8754 Date of Birth: August 17, 1964 Employer: The Rockwell Group
Primary Insurance Information	Signal HMO Policyholder: Joseph Beaufort ID Number: 999448754-03 Group Number: TRG01 Office co-pay: $10.00

CHAPTER POST-TEST

Perform this test without looking at your book. If an answer is "false," rewrite the sentence to make it true.

1. True or False? When patient charts are out of order, we use out-guides to help us see the error better.

_____

_____

2. When filing, you need to be skilled in all but which one of the following?

   a. Knowing the alphabet

   b. Knowing the basic rules of filing

   c. Being able to pay attention to details

   d. Being good at math

3. True or False? Medical records are important for many reasons. Their most important purpose is for legal protection.

   _____

   _____

4. True or False? It is acceptable to release medical information to a family member as long as you have written authorization from the patient.

   _____

   _____

5. True or False? Proper documentation in a patient's chart is the standard in court because if there is no record of treatment, then it did not happen.

   _____

   _____

6. True or False? Medical filing systems may be based on the alphabet, a numeric system, or by subject.

   _____

   _____

SELF-ASSESSMENT

To perform this self-assessment, you must first perform an exercise: Go to your spice drawer, a stack of magazines, a bunch of bills/statements, or even your clothes closet, drawers, or the shelves you keep your towels on. (Maybe organize something in your medical assisting classroom or laboratory area!)

1. Think of the best way to organize them. Is it by size, color, or both? Alphabetically? By date? Frequency of use?

   _____

   _____

   _____

   _____

2. Perform the organization. What was the most difficult part: planning how to best accomplish it, or actually doing it? Did you have to take everything out and place it back in order, or were you able to just move things around? Was this a time-consuming exercise? Is the order now a useful tool? Did you have any decisions to make, such as do you file red pepper under red or pepper? Should your pants be organized with their matching tops, or should all the pants be together and all the tops together? Should the medications be organized in alphabetic order, or by classification (type of action)?

   _____

   _____

   _____

   _____

3. Now choose another item to organize in a different way. How did this second exercise differ? (For example, towels might have been organized by size or by color, whereas your spices would be organized alphabetically.) Do you think another person would have chosen a different method?

_____

_____

_____

_____

4. Who do you think decides in an office how a particular area is to be organized? Do you think there might be different ways?

_____

_____

_____

_____

5. Pretend that your provider's office has its patients' charts filed alphabetically, but now they are moving to more computerized records and want to change their files to a numeric system. Make a list of the supplies the staff will need, calculate the time it might take, and make up a plan on how to accomplish this (remember the files are still being used every day). Does this seem like a major undertaking? Could any files be purged (pulled out of circulation) during this reorganization?

_____

_____

_____

_____

CHAPTER **15**

Written Communications

CHAPTER PRE-TEST

Perform this test without looking at your book. If an answer is "false," rewrite the sentence to make it true.

1. The four major letter styles are *(circle four of the following):*

   a. full block

   b. modified block, standard

   c. facilitated block

   d. simplified block

   e. simplified

   f. modified block, indented

2. The part of a letter that includes a specially designed logo with the address and phone numbers is called the:

   a. salutation

   b. inside address

   c. letterhead

   d. reference heading

   e. enclosure

3. True or False? Whenever documents are to be included in a mailed letter, the word *enclosure* should be written out completely and placed one or two lines below the reference initials.

   _____

   _____

4. True or False? Envelopes should be addressed using block (uppercase) letters and no punctuation.

   _____

   _____

5. A computerized feature that allows you to send the same letter, although personalized, to many different people using a database is called:

a. word processing letters

b. mail merge

c. database letters

d. merge correspondence

6. True or False? All letters in the complimentary closure are uppercase.

_____

_____

VOCABULARY BUILDER

Misspelled Words

Find the words below that are misspelled; underline them, and correctly spell them in the space provided. Then, fill in the blanks in the passage below with the correct vocabulary terms. (Hint: not all terms will be used.)

bond paper	mail merge	proofread
form letters	modified block letter	simplified letter
full block letter	optical character reader	watermarque
keed	portfoleo	ZIP+4

_____   _____   _____

There are four major types of letter styles in which medical assistants commonly write. Of these, the _____ _____ style is the most time-efficient, because it does not use excessive tab indentations for the address, complimentary closure, or keyed signature. In the _____ style, all lines begin at the left margin with the exception of the date line, complimentary closure, and keyed signature. Medical assistants may choose to use the _____ style, which is the style of letter recommended by the Administrative Management Society. In this style, all lines are _____, or input by keystroke, flush with the left margin. When selecting paper supplies, the medical assistant should choose _____ _____ with a _____, or image imprinted during the papermaking process that is visible when a sheet is held up to the light. When preparing letters for outgoing shipments, it is important for the medical assistant to pay attention to several factors, including addresses. Medical assistants should machine-print addresses (including the _____ code) with a uniform left-hand margin so that the addresses can be read by the U.S. Postal Service's _____ (abbreviated OCR). One creative approach to letter composition is to create a _____ or database of frequently used _____.

LEARNING REVIEW

Abbreviations Exercise

Write what each abbreviation stands for.

1. Enc. _____
2. c _____
3. P.S. _____
4. OCR _____
5. CAP _____
6. ROM _____
7. LC _____
8. WF _____

Matching

Match the common proofreader's mark in Column I to its meaning in Column II.

____ 1. #   A. "Let it stand"
____ 2. ^   B. Paragraph indent
____ 3. BF   C. Insert space
____ 4. STET   D. Move left
____ 5.]   E. Italic type
____ 6. [F. Align type horizontally
____ 7. :| G. Insert
____ 8. =   H. Boldface type
____ 9. ITAL   I. Move right
____ 10. ¶   J. Insert colon

True or False

Mark true statement with a T *and false statements with an* F. *If an answer is "false," rewrite the sentence to make it true.*

____ 1. Modified block, standard, is the most efficient letter style for the ambulatory care setting.

_____

_____

____ 2. Paper for written communications in the office should be of good quality, contain a watermark, and be at least 20-pound stock.

_____

_____

____ 3. A written record of what transpires during a meeting is called the agenda.

_____

_____

____ 4. Business correspondence should be clear, concise, and accurate.

_____

_____

____ 5. First class mail is divided into two mail subclasses.

_____

_____

Processing Mail Exercise

For each type of mail below, list the action the medical assistant should take or to what department or person the medical assistant should forward the mail.

Type of Mail	Action Taken
Invoices for supplies and equipment	
Magazines for reception area	
Insurance forms	
Patient payments	
Medical journals	
Personal or confidential letters	

CERTIFICATION REVIEW

These questions are designed to mimic the certification examination. Select the best response.

1. The "salutation" of a letter is the:

   a. signature

   b. greeting

   c. return address

   d. closing remark (such as: "Sincerely")

   e. the recipient's name, title, and address

2. When addressing an envelope, the proper way to list the state is:

   a. to write it out completely

   b. to abbreviate it using at least the first four letters

   c. to capitalize it using the official two-letter abbreviation

   d. any of the above as long as it is in uppercase letters and is written clearly

3. Which of the below would be incoming mail to a provider's office?

   a. email

   b. insurance forms

   c. medical journals

   d. letters from patients

   e. all of the above

4. The medical assistant may, with the provider's permission, sign certain letters such as:

   a. the ordering of supplies or subscriptions

   b. notification of collection procedures and reminder of payments

   c. dismissal letters

   d. a. and b.

5. When addressing an envelope:

   a. the address should be machine printed with a uniform left margin

   b. all punctuation should be eliminated

   c. use dark ink on a light background using uppercase letters

   d. All of the above

6. The types of envelopes most often used are:

   a. number 7

   b. number 6 ¾

   c. number 10

   d. b. and c.

7. Periodical is the new term for:

   a. second class mail

   b. third class mail

   c. priority mail

   d. parcel post mail

8. Before presenting any correspondence to the provider for signature, the document should be:

   a. date stamped

   b. checked for accuracy

   c. folded and put in an envelope

   d. typed on plain white paper

9. The most secure service the USPS offers is:

   a. priority mail

   b. express mail

   c. registered mail

   d. certified mail

LEARNING APPLICATION

Ellen Armstrong, CMA (AAMA), enjoys working on correspondence for Drs. Lewis and King and takes pride in her written communication skills. As an ongoing project, office manager Marilyn Johnson asks Ellen to make suggestions for updating and revising the style manual used in the medical office for written communication guidelines. Ellen suggests the addition of a section in the style manual to discuss bias in language. Bias-free language is sensitive in applying labels to individuals or groups and uses sex-specific words and pronouns appropriately. For example, "dementia" is used instead of "crazy" or "senile." Instead of using "layman," consider using "layperson." Apply "he or she" only in sex-specific usage. Marilyn and the provider-employer ask Ellen to implement the addition to the style manual.

CASE STUDY REVIEW QUESTIONS

1. Why is bias-free language an important consideration in written communication for the ambulatory care setting?

   _____

   _____

   _____

   _____

   _____

2. List other examples of biased language and give suggestions for bias-free alternatives.

   _____

   _____

   _____

   _____

   _____

   _____

Proofreading Exercise

Proofread the letter below, correcting all errors by inserting the proper proofreader's marks directly onto the text. (Consult your textbook for a list of common proofreader's marks and refer to a medical dictionary, if necessary.)

JAMES CARTER, MD, NEUROLOGY
Metropolitan University Medical Center, 8280 Wright Avenue, Northborough, OH 12382

February 2, 20XX

Elizabeth Kind, M.D
Northborough Medical Family Group
The offices of Lewis & King, MD
2501 Center Street
Nrothborough, OH 12345

RE: MARGARET THOMAS

Dear Dr. King:

Thank you for refering Margaret Thomas to my neurological practice. Margaret come to you recently as a new patient for a comprehensive physical examination to evaluate troubling symptoms she had been experiencing for several months. Margaret notices symtoms of tremor, difficulty walking, defective judgement, and hot flushes; she is not able to poinpoint the exac ttime symptoms began. Your physical examination suggested the possible diagnoisis of parkingson's Disease. Margaret presented today for a complete nuerological evaluation.

MEDICAL/SURGICAL HISTORY. The patient is posiitive for the usual childhood diseases and the births of three children, following normal pregnancies. Her surgical history includes an Appendectomy performed 10 years ago. She has a food allergy to shellfish, but no known allergies to medications. She takes Pepto-Bismol and Metamusil for frequent stomach upset and constipation. She is a widow with two children, ages twenty three, twenty-five, and 29,and is a retired homemaker. She does not smoke and has an occassional glass of wine. Her family history is positive for colon cancer in her mother and parenteral grandfather and for lung cancer in her father.

PYHSICALEXAMINATION. VITAL SIGNS: The patient has normal vital signs for a 52-year old Caucasian female. HEENT: The patient had a normacephalic and atraumatic exam. There is mild bobing of the head and facial expressions appear fixed. Pupils equal, round, regular, react to light and acommodation. The fundi were benign. There was normal cup to disc ratio of 0.3. Tympanic Membranes were both clear and mobile. Her nose was clear. the oropharynz ws clear without any evidence of lezions. There was not cervical adenopathy, no thyromegely, or other masses. NECK: Musles of the neck are quite rigid and stiff. CHEST: Cear to percussion and auscultation. HEART: Regular rate and rhythm without murmurs or gallops. there was no jugular venous distention, no peripheral edema, no carotid buits. Pulses were 2+ and symetrical. Abdomen. Some what obese, but benigh. There was not organomegaly or masses. Bowel tones were normal. There was no rebound tenderness. BACK: Examination reveals loss of posturalreflexe and patient stands with head bent forward and wals as if in danger of falling forward. There is difficulty in pivoting and loss of balance. GENITOURINARY: Normal. EXTREMITIES: Thre is moderate bradykinesia. Chracteristic slow, turning motion (pronation-supination) of, the forearm and the hand and a motion of the thumb against the fingers as if rolling a pill between the fingers is noted. This condition seems to worsen when the patient is concentrating or feeling anxious.

continues

(continued)

NEUROLOGICAL. The patient was cooperative and answered all questions. There is no history past of mental disorders or cardiovascular disease. There is muscle weakness and rigidity in all four extremities. Intellect remains intact;

LABORATORY DATA: Urinanalysis reveals low levels of dopamin. Cat scan reveals degeneration of nerve cells occuring in the base1 ganglia.

ASSESSMENT. Based on the patient history and neurologic examination, it appears most likely that the patient has mild to moderate Parkinsons Disease.

PLAN. 1. Recommend physical therapy focussed on learning how to manage diffi-cult movements such as descneding stairs safely.
2. Exercises to maintain flexibility, motility, and mental well-being.
3. Levadopa to increase dopamine levels in the brain to control symptoms. Please advise the patient that alchohol consumption shoudl be limited because it acts antegonistically to levodopa.
4. Relaxation and stress management counseling.

PROGNOSIS. Parkinson's disease progresses slowly. Patient should be follow on a regular basis and observed for any signs of damentia which may result in about 1-third of cases.

Sincerely,

James Carter, MD

DD: February 2, 20XX
DT: February 3, 20XX
JC/bl

MOSS Activity

Using Medical Office Simulation Software, follow the steps below to generate a letter to a patient. Use the scenario information to compose the body of the letter in full block letter style. When you have finished, print the letter, then fold and insert the letter properly into a correctly addressed envelope.

1. Open MOSS and log in.

2. From the top menu, select Billing, then Patient Ledger.

3. Click on the magnifying glass button next to the Patient Account field.

4. Search for patient Megan Caldwell, and click View.

5. Click on the Correspondence button below the patient ledger.

6. A dialog box will open. Save the file output a location of your choosing which is easily accessible to you, and click OK. Now, a letter template will generate.

7. Compose a letter in full block style, based on the following scenario information. (Hint: Select the text "Type Message Here…." and delete it. Now you are ready to type your letter.)

   • Megan Caldwell's PAP test results were abnormal and Dr. Schwartz would like her to schedule a colposcopy with biopsy in the next few weeks so he can determine the cause of the abnormal results. Please refer to the enclosed brochure for information on this procedure.

8. Proofread the letter for errors, and when you are satisfied that it is complete, save and print the letter.

9. Properly address an envelope to the patient Megan Caldwell.

10. Fold and insert the letter properly into the envelope and turn it in to your instructor.

CHAPTER POST-TEST

Perform this test without looking at your book. If an answer is "false," rewrite the sentence to make it true.

1. The most commonly used of the four major letter styles in the ambulatory care setting is:

   a. full block

   b. modified block, standard

   c. facilitated block, indented

   d. simplified

2. The part of a letter that includes the return address and perhaps a logo is the:

   a. salutation

   b. inside address

   c. letterhead

   d. reference heading

   e. enclosure

3. Whenever documents are to be included in a mailed letter, the word *enclosure* should be indicated by:

   a. Enclosures

   b. Enc.

   c. 1 Enc.

   d. 2 Enclosures

   e. Enclosures (2)

   f. any of the above

4. True or False? Envelopes should be addressed using a combination of uppercase and lowercase letters and with the proper punctuation.

   _____

   _____

5. When it is desirable to send the same letter, although personalized, to many different people, a computerized feature that can be used is called:

   a. word processing letters

   b. mail merge

   c. database letters

   d. merge correspondence

6. True or False? Only the first letter of the first word in the complimentary closing is uppercase.

   _____

   _____

SELF-ASSESSMENT

In your written communications, are you able to express yourself accurately and concisely? Able to communicate ideas effectively? Capable of proofreading and editing for content? Use this simple self-assessment to gauge your comfort and proficiency in written communications by identifying strengths and pinpointing any weak areas that could use improvement. For each statement below, circle the corresponding letter to the response that best describes you.

1. When writing a letter, I generally feel:

    a. confident. I communicate effectively on the page and enjoy writing letters.

    b. at ease. My written communication skills are acceptable.

    c. uncomfortable. I would rather communicate verbally than through writing.

2. As far as content goes, when I am given the required information and asked to compose a letter, I:

    a. almost always understand exactly what I am being asked to communicate and am able to convey it precisely in letter form

    b. generally understand what I am being asked to communicate, but sometimes have to fine-tune my letters

    c. often have trouble understanding what I am being asked to communicate and usually have to go back and ask questions about the letter's content

3. In general, when choosing words for written correspondence, I feel:

    a. secure about my ability to select appropriate language and use medical terminology accurately

    b. pretty confident, although my general vocabulary and knowledge of medical terminology could use some improvement

    c. frustrated; I always seem to confuse words and medical terms no matter how hard I try not to

4. As far as spelling goes, I am:

    a. a top-notch speller; I always keep both a standard and medical dictionary on hand for the words I am not sure of

    b. an adequate speller; sometimes I confuse a word here or there; I always have to proofread carefully for spelling errors

    c. a below-par speller; my letters are always littered with misspellings and someone else has to proofread my work

5. Grammatically speaking, I am:

    a. above average; I routinely find mistakes in my colleagues' work

    b. passable; I make minor mistakes but usually catch them while proofreading

    c. hopeless; people find mistakes in my work even after I have checked it twice

6. Regarding proofreader's marks, I am:

    a. highly capable of proofreading my work; if colleagues need someone to proof their work, I am first on their list

    b. an okay proofreader; I occasionally overlook a mistake, but nobody's perfect

    c. frightened; proofreading marks are just a bunch of meaningless squiggles to me

7. How would you describe your formatting skills?

   a. Exemplary. I understand all basic letter forms, and all of my letters are rigorously formatted according to correct specifications.

   b. Satisfactory. Every so often, I confuse styles or forget an annotation; but in general, all my letters are formatted correctly.

   c. Fair to nonexistent. I have trouble understanding why every letter has to be so formally constructed.

8. When adhering to office style guidelines, I:

   a. always follow the guidelines

   b. usually have no problem sticking to style guidelines; when I make a mistake, it is a rare event

   c. need improvement; my letters are frequently littered with style inconsistencies, and I do not understand the need for an office style as long as each letter is written with accurate information

9. Overall, I think of writing letters in the health care environment as:

   a. one of my strong suits

   b. a task that I am able to accomplish, just not one I particularly enjoy

   c. a necessary evil

Scoring: If your answers were mostly A responses, you have strong written communications skills and enjoy writing letters. If your responses were mostly Bs, your written communications skills are good but could stand some improvement. Try reviewing pertinent information in this chapter to strengthen areas that need it. If your answers were mostly Cs, you need to work on your written communication skills. Volunteer to take on as many written correspondence assignments as you can—practice may help you overcome your apprehension about writing letters and will almost certainly raise the quality of your work.

_____
_____
_____
_____
_____
_____
_____
_____
_____
_____

C H A P T E R **16**

Medical Documents

CHAPTER PRE-TEST

Perform this test without looking at your book. If an answer is "false," rewrite the sentence to make it true.

1. True or False? Outsourcing is rapidly eliminating the need for the traditional transcriptionists in medical facilities.

   _____

   _____

2. True or False? Anyone who has computer abilities and can spell well can perform medical transcription well.

   _____

   _____

3. True or False? Medical documents are only for the clinic and provider who generated them, so they are called "internal documents."

   _____

   _____

4. True or False? Medical transcription is a profession that has not really undergone many changes in the last decade or so.

   _____

   _____

5. True or False? If a medical transcriptionist encounters a term that cannot be interpreted or something new that cannot be referenced, that section of the document should be flagged.

   _____

   _____

6. True or False? Medical transcriptionists do not need to be concerned with HIPAA regulations.

   _____

   _____

VOCABULARY BUILDER

Find the words below that are misspelled; circle them, and correctly spell them in the spaces provided. Then insert the correct vocabulary terms from the list that best fit the descriptions below.

athentication	discharge summery	priveliged
autapsy report	editor	progress notes
chart notes	electronic health records	proofreading
chief complaint	gross examination	quality assurence
confidentilty	history and physical	review of symptems
consultation reports	medical transcriptionist	risk management
correspondence	outsourcing	turnaround time
currant	patholigy	voice recognition software

_____   _____   _____

_____   _____   _____

_____   _____   _____

1. Today, the _____ may be more involved with quality assurance than actually transcribing medical records, notes, letters, and documents.

2. The part of the pathology report that describes the size and shape of a biopsy is called a _____ .

3. The part of patients' hospital records that describe their entire hospital stay, progress, and condition on release is called a _____ .

4. The part of the patient's medical record that contains information related to the main reason for the encounter, as well as a synopsis of the patient's previous medical information, is called the _____ .

5. Reports such as history and physicals that should be completed within 24 hours are called _____ reports.

6. A type of signature that may use various computer key entries as identification is referred to as _____ .

7. Software that translates spoken sounds into written words is called _____ .

8. A medical report generated to describe the examinations of tissues or cells obtained through a surgery or medical procedure is the _____ report.

9. The practice of contracting transcription with a service outside of the clinic or hospital to a company where it can be done at a lower cost and with a faster turnaround time is called _____ .

Definitions

Define the following terms.

1. Joint Commission:

_____

_____

_____

2. Consultation report:

_____

_____

_____

_____

3. Editing:

_____

_____

4. Flag:

_____

_____

_____

5. Turnaround time:

_____

_____

_____

_____

LEARNING REVIEW

Short Answer

1. List five personal attributes of the medical transcriptionist.

_____

_____

_____

_____

_____

2. Give two examples of each type of turnaround time report and the time of the turnaround.

STAT _____ _____

Current _____ _____

Old _____ _____

3. List at least four advantages of outsourcing.

_____

_____

_____

_____

_____

4. Offices using electronic medical records may delegate much of the medical transcriptionist's responsibility to other medical personnel. Identify the items below that may be entered into an electronic medical record by the medical assistant by writing (MA) next to the entry, and those items that may be entered by the provider (P).

Reason for the patient's visit   _____

Entering chart notes   _____

Entering vital signs   _____

Entering and transmitting prescription to a pharmacy   _____

Transmitting the medical record to another provider   _____

Entering current medications   _____

Entering the chief complaint   _____

Abbreviations Exercise

Write what each abbreviation stands for.

1. EHR   _____

2. MT   _____

3. TAT   _____

4. QA   _____

5. VRS   _____

6. CMT   _____

7. CC   _____

8. ROS   _____

9. H&P   _____

10. DS   _____

11. OR   _____

12. HIPAA   _____

True or False

Mark a true statement with a T *and a false statement with an* F. *If an answer is "false," rewrite the sentence to make it true.*

_____ 1. Medical records are documents governed by laws and may be subpoenaed for review by various courts.

_____

_____

_____ 2. The medical report may play a major role in substantiating injury or a malpractice claim.

_____

_____

_____ 3. The Joint Commission allows 36 hours from admission for a history and physical report to be dictated, transcribed, and filed into the patient's medical record.

_____

_____

____ 4. When transcribing radiology or imaging reports, the date of service should be used rather than the date of dictation.

_____

_____

____ 5. Electronic signatures on medical documents are allowed by both Medicare and the Joint Commission.

_____

_____

____ 6. When editing the transcribed document, it may be necessary to change the dictator's style or meaning.

_____

_____

____ 7. Once a job has been accepted, the transcriptionist or transcription service is legally bound to meet the schedule, short of "an act of nature."

_____

_____

____ 8. Meeting deadlines is irrelevant and there is not stringent adherence to turnaround time.

_____

_____

____ 9. Risk management personnel should be consulted first before divulging files to an attorney or insurance representative.

_____

_____

____ 10. Provider-directors or office managers should not be responsible for the wrongful acts of medical transcriptionists working under their supervision.

_____

_____

CERTIFICATION REVIEW

These questions are designed to mimic the certification examination. Select the best response.

1. Association for Healthcare Documentation Integrity (AHDI) credentials _____.

   a. MTs

   b. CMTs

   c. CMTs and RMTs

   d. CMAs and RMAs

2. A digital dictation system allows you to measure to:

    a. the 30th or 90th of a minute

    b. 60 seconds

    c. the 10th or 100th of a minute

    d. 30–40 seconds

3. The medical report must be:

    a. dated correctly

    b. signed or initialed by the dictator

    c. legible

    d. all of the above

4. The specific time period in which a document is expected to be completed from the time it is received by the transcriptionist until it is returned to the provider and made part of the permanent medical record is called:

    a. filing time

    b. turnaround time

    c. completion time

    d. return time

5. Radiology, pathology, and laboratory reports are usually termed as _____ to indicate the need for immediate turnaround.

    a. ASAP

    b. current

    c. old

    d. STAT

LEARNING APPLICATION

CASE STUDY

You are transcribing a report when you notice it is a report about your neighbor. The report states that the test run for multiple sclerosis is positive. You had just spoken to your neighbor yesterday and she was concerned that she hadn't heard from her provider and was wondering about the results of her tests.

CASE STUDY REVIEW QUESTIONS

1. What should you do?

    _____

    _____

    _____

    _____

    _____

Proofreading Exercise

Correct the following paragraph.

```
her past medical history is postivie for the usual childhood diseases and the births of to
children following normal pregnancies she has a negative pasts urgical history. she has
no allergies To medications and takes tylenol for occasional headashes She is married
and has to children, ages 3 and 12 months. She does not smoke or drink
```

CHAPTER POST-TEST

Perform this test without looking at your book. If an answer is "false," rewrite the sentence to make it true.

1. True or False? The need for the traditional medical transcriptionist in a medical facility today is declining due to outsourcing.

   _____

   _____

2. True or False? Medical transcription is a job for people with good computer abilities and word processing speed; who have excellent spelling, grammar, and punctuation skills; and who care enough to do the best job possible.

   _____

   _____

3. True or False? Medical documents are not only for the clinic and provider who generated them, they are also legal documents used by many professionals.

   _____

   _____

4. True or False? Medical transcription is a profession that has undergone numerous changes in the last decade or so.

   _____

   _____

5. True or False? If a medical transcriptionist cannot interpret a portion of the sentence or cannot make reference, then that portion of the document should be flagged.

   _____

   _____

6. True or False? Because medical transcriptionists work within the medical field with medical information, they need to be concerned with HIPAA regulations.

   _____

   _____

SELF-ASSESSMENT

1. Do you think you would enjoy working as a transcriptionist? What is it about the profession that appeals to you? What is it about the profession that does not appeal to you?

_____

_____

_____

_____

_____

Name _____   Date _____   Score _____

Medical Insurance

CHAPTER PRE-TEST

Perform this test without looking at your book. If an answer is "false," rewrite the sentence to make it true.

1. True or False? Managed care has simplified the patient's responsibility for payment.

_____

_____

2. True or False? With managed care options, there is less emphasis on the medical assistant needing to be accurate and timely when filing insurance claims.

_____

_____

3. True or False? Preexisting conditions usually require a waiting period.

_____

_____

4. True or False? "Coordination of benefits" means that the insurance companies will take care of the paperwork.

_____

_____

5. True or False? Co-payment is the amount the insurance will cost the patient each month.

_____

_____

VOCABULARY BUILDER

Misspelled Words

Find the words below that are misspelled; circle them, and correctly spell them in the spaces provided. Then, insert the correct vocabulary terms from the list that best fit the descriptions below.

ajustment	preautherization	referral
benefit period	prefered provider organization	resourse-based relative value scale
Medicare Part D	primary care provider	self-insurance
point-of-service plan	proof of eligibility	usual, customarry, and reasonable

_____   _____   _____

_____   _____   _____

1. The _____ is a doctor chosen by the patient who is the first doctor the patient sees and is responsible for making referrals for further treatment by a specialist or for hospitalization.

2. A _____ allows the enrollee to have the freedom to obtain medical care from an HMO provider or to self-refer to a non-HMO provider at a greater cost.

3. The _____ was developed using values for each medical and surgical procedure based on work, practice, and malpractice costs and factoring in the regional differences.

4. _____ means that prior notice and approval needs to be obtained before services will be covered.

5. A _____ is an organization of providers who network together to offer discounts to purchasers of health care insurance.

6. The _____ is the specified time during which benefits will be paid under certain types of health insurance coverages.

7. The amount a provider writes off the patient's account is known as an _____.

8. _____ is prescription drug coverage by Medicare.

Abbreviations Exercise

List what each of the following acronyms stands for.

1. CMS _____

2. COB _____

3. DEERS _____

4. EPO _____

5. HMO _____

6. IDS _____

7. MCO _____

8. POS _____

9. PPO _____

10. UCR _____

LEARNING REVIEW

Short Answer

1. What questions should the medical assistant ask when screening for medical insurance coverage?

_____

_____

_____

2. What measures do managed care organizations employ to ensure cost-effective services?

_____

_____

_____

3. What are the six models of managed care organizations in use?

_____

_____

_____

4. List seven pieces of information that should be maintained in a log regarding preauthorization, precertification, or referral procedures for various insurance carriers.

_____

_____

_____

_____

_____

5. Identify the three common elements involved in computing a provider's fee schedule.

_____

_____

_____

6. The insurance carrier generates an EOB and an RA. Explain what these are and who they are sent to.

_____

_____

_____

_____

7. List three examples of insurance fraud, and three examples of insurance abuse.

A. Fraud:

_____

_____

_____

_____

B: Abuse:

_____

_____

_____

_____

Matching

Match the statements below to the appropriate Medicare Part.

_____ 1. Covers outpatient expenses including providers' fees, lab tests, and radiologic studies

_____ 2. Covers hospital admission and stays

_____ 3. Offers prescription drug coverage for everyone covered by Medicare

_____ 4. Referred to as Medicare advantage plans

_____ 5. Does not require a monthly premium

_____ 6. Has a "donut hole" or coverage gap

_____ 7. Will start paying for services after a $131 deductible has been met

_____ 8. Requires a monthly premium

_____ 9. Covers hospice care

_____ 10. Covers charges for durable medical equipment

A. Medicare Part A

B. Medicare Part B

C. Medicare Part C

D. Medicare Part D

CERTIFICATION REVIEW

These questions are designed to mimic the certification examination. Select the best response.

1. The portion of the medical fees that the patient needs to pay at the time of services is called:

a. co-pay

b. fee for service

c. out-of-pocket expenses

d. premium

2. The largest medical insurance program in the United States is:

   a. Blue Cross/Blue Shield

   b. Medicaid

   c. Medicare

   d. TRICARE

3. The cost that patients must pay each month (sometimes provided by their employers) is called the:

   a. out-of-pocket expense

   b. co-pay

   c. premium

   d. relative value scale

4. Which of the following describes HIPAA?

   a. It is about confidentiality, patient privacy, and security of personal health information.

   b. It protects health insurance coverage for workers and their families when they change or lose their jobs.

   c. It includes national standards for electronic health care transactions.

   d. It establishes rules for national identifiers for providers, health plans, and employers.

   e. a. and c. only

5. Noncovered services are also known as:

   a. nonallowed services

   b. exclusions

   c. out-of-pocket services

   d. expensive services

6. A statement summarizing how the insurance carrier determined reimbursement for services received by the patient is called a(n):

   a. EOB

   b. RA

   c. day sheet

   d. personal financial statement

7. The medical insurance that covers medical care for certain qualifying low-income individuals is:

   a. Medicare

   b. CHAMPUS

   c. TRICARE

   d. Medicaid

8. To ensure that there is a successful flow of adequate income in the clinic or office, the medical assistant should:

   a. bill the insurance carrier or patient as needed

   b. complete forms properly

   c. keep track of aging accounts

   d. All of the above

9. Improper billing practices are considered:

   a. fraud

   b. nonproductive

   c. abuse

   d. risky

10. Which of the following is a problem with work-related health insurance coverage?

    a. Part-time employees are usually not eligible.

    b. Medical benefits may not transfer equally.

    c. Insurance companies often refuse to provide coverage for some procedures, including experimental treatments.

    d. All of the above

11. The person covered under the terms of an insurance policy is called the:

    a. primary

    b. secondary

    c. beneficiary

    d. elector

12. When more than one policy covers the individual, the _____ determines which of the policies will pay first.

    a. deductible

    b. exclusion

    c. coinsurance

    d. coordination of benefits

13. Where does one find the address to which insurance claims are to be sent?

    a. The telephone book

    b. On the back of the insurance card

    c. In the insurance provider manual

    d. None of the above

14. Blue Cross and Blue Shield are examples of:

    a. MCOs

    b. HMOs

    c. PPOs

    d. traditional insurance organizations

LEARNING APPLICATION

CASE STUDY

Lourdes Austen, a one-year survivor of breast cancer, is covered by an HMO. Lourdes's primary care provider, Dr. King, recommends that Lourdes receive a colonoscopy because she has a family history that is positive for colon cancer, and medical studies have demonstrated a link between colon and breast cancers in families. Lourdes's HMO requires preauthorization before a specialist's care can be provided. Dr. King supplies the referral to a gastroenterologist who will perform the colon screening test and gives Lourdes the necessary completed referral form to take with her to her scheduled appointment. During the colonoscopy procedure, one benign polyp is removed, and the gastroenterologist requests that Lourdes return for a follow-up examination in one week.

Lourdes makes an appointment with the specialist's administrative medical assistant. When she returns one week later, the medical assistant informs Lourdes that she must have a new referral form for the office visit or the HMO will not approve payment; Lourdes will have to pay for the examination herself. "But we drove 40 minutes to get here, and no one ever told me I'd need another form for this. I thought it was all covered under the colonoscopy," Lourdes says.

CASE STUDY REVIEW QUESTIONS

1. Lourdes's HMO policy requires preauthorization. Is there anything that can be done to secure a proper referral without having to schedule another appointment for the patient or force the patient to pay for the office visit?

_____

_____

_____

_____

_____

_____

2. What is the role of the specialist's administrative medical assistant in this situation? Could the situation have been prevented?

_____

_____

_____

_____

_____

_____

CHAPTER POST-TEST

Perform this test without looking at your book. If an answer is "false," rewrite the sentence to make it true.

1. True or False? Managed care has made the patient's responsibility for payment more complex.

_____

_____

2. True or False? With managed care options, there is more emphasis on the medical assistant needing to be accurate and timely when filing insurance claims.

_____

_____

3. True or False? Preexisting conditions always require a waiting period.

_____

_____

4. True or False? "Coordination of benefits" means that the insurance companies will handle all the paperwork necessary for payment.

_____

_____

5. True or False? Co-payment is the amount the insurance will cost the patient's employer each month.

_____

_____

SELF-ASSESSMENT

1. Take a close look at your insurance coverage. If you do not have medical insurance coverage, take a look at the coverage of a close friend or relative or choose a policy you would like to have.

   A. Does it require a co-pay?

   B. How much is the co-pay for a doctor's visit?

   C. How much is the co-pay or a hospital stay? surgery?

   D. How much is the co-pay for medication?

   E. Does prescribed medication have to be from a formulary list?

   F. How much is the total amount you would have to pay for any given year?

2. Some people advocate doing away with health insurance for office visits and medications and just having insurance for big expenses such as catastrophic coverage. Discuss this idea with a group of at least three people. These people may be your classmates or friends/family. Write up a list of the advantages and disadvantages.

_____

_____

_____

_____

3. Some people advocate a "socialistic" method of health insurance such as Canada has. Look online for information about Canada's health care system and make a list of the advantages and disadvantages. Which way would you vote if you had a choice?

_____

_____

_____

_____

C H A P T E R **18**

Medical Insurance Coding

CHAPTER PRE-TEST

Perform this test without looking at your book. If an answer is "false," rewrite the sentence to make it true.

1. True or False? Medical insurance coding is a way of keeping track of the doctor's financial records.

   _____

   _____

2. CPT stands for:

   a. Comprehensive Patient Treatments

   b. Current Procedural Terminology

   c. Curative Procedures Tried

   d. Curative Patient Treatments

3. ICD stands for:

   a. Incidental Codes of Diagnosis

   b. Internal Codes for Decisions

   c. International Codes for Diagnosis

   d. International Classification of Diseases

4. True or False? Third party usually means the insurance company.

   _____

   _____

5. True or False? Insurance claim forms and submissions are fairly straightforward; therefore, most anyone can perform these duties with some basic training.

   _____

   _____

VOCABULARY BUILDER

Misspelled Words

Find the words below that are misspelled; circle them, and then correctly spell them in the spaces provided.

bundeled codes

claim register

Current Procedural Terminoligy

E Codes

encounter form

explanation of benifts

Healthcare Common Procedure Coding
System

International Classification of Deseases

modifyers

point-of-service device

Uniform Bill (UB-04)

V Codes

_____

_____

_____

_____

_____

Abbreviations Review

Write what the following abbreviations and acronyms stand for.

1. EOB _____

2. HCPCS _____

3. ICD _____

4. POS _____

5. CPT _____

Definitions

Write the definition of the following terms or phrases.

1. Bundled codes _____

_____

_____

2. Claim register _____

_____

_____

3. Current Procedural
   Terminology _____

_____

_____

4. E Codes _____

_____

_____

5. Encounter form

_____

_____

_____

_____

_____

6. Explanation of
   benefits

_____

_____

_____

_____

_____

7. Healthcare Common
   Procedure Coding
   System

_____

_____

_____

8. *International
   Classification of
   Diseases*, 9th Revision,
   Clinical Modifications
   (ICD-9-CM)

_____

_____

_____

9. Point-of-service device

_____

_____

_____

_____

10. Uniform Bill (UB-04)

_____

_____

_____

11. V Codes

_____

_____

_____

12. Modifiers

_____

_____

_____

LEARNING REVIEW

Short Answer

1. CPT is updated annually and published by the American Medical Association. It is divided into seven sections. Name them.

   _____

   _____

   _____

2. Codes for diagnoses are found in the ICD-9-CM. The ICD-9-CM is divided into three volumes. Specify what information each volume contains.

   (1) Volume I:

   _____

   _____

   _____

   (2) Volume II:

   _____

   _____

   _____

   (3) Volume III:

   _____

   _____

   _____

3. In which volume of the ICD would a medical assistant first look to find the diagnosis code for osteomyelitis? What is the diagnosis code for unspecified osteomyelitis of the ankle or foot?

   _____

   _____

4. Injury codes cannot stand alone but must be accompanied by E Codes. What does the "E" stand for?

   _____

   _____

5. V Codes are the last main section of Volumes I and II. What are V Codes?

   _____

   _____

6. Errors in coding insurance claims can have far-reaching effects for both the patient and the provider. Name three effects.

   _____

   _____

   _____

   _____

7. Differentiate between bundled and unbundled codes.

_____

_____

_____

_____

8. List five common errors that may occur when completing insurance claim forms.

_____

_____

_____

_____

_____

9. Identify seven basic elements necessary to have documented in a compliance program.

_____

_____

_____

_____

_____

_____

_____

Diagnosis and Procedure Identification

For each entry in the following table, insert a "D" for diagnosis or a "P" for procedure on the first line. Then, enter the appropriate diagnosis or procedure code, referencing the textbook, the current revision of the ICD, or the current edition of the CPT.

Diagnosis/Procedure	Entry	Code
_____	1. Services requested after hours in addition to basic services	_____
_____	2. Medicine given or taken in error	_____
_____	3. Anorexia nervosa	_____
_____	4. Pneumonocentesis, puncture of lung for aspiration	_____
_____	5. Diabetic ketoacidosis	_____
_____	6. Urinalysis; qualitative or semi-qualitative, except immunoassays, microscopic only	_____
_____	7. Bruxism	_____
_____	8. *Pneumocystis carinii* pneumonia	_____
_____	9. Amniocentesis	_____
_____	10. Epstein-Barr virus infection	_____

_____   11. Gait training (includes stair climbing)   _____

_____   12. Medical testimony   _____

_____   13. Therapeutic or diagnostic injection (specify material injected);   _____
subcutaneous or intramuscular

_____   14. Narcotics affecting fetus or newborn via placenta or breast milk   _____

CERTIFICATION REVIEW

These questions are designed to mimic the certification examination. Select the best response.

1. What is the name of the coding system that includes codes for services provided to **Medicare or Medicaid** patients?

    a. HCFA

    b. CPT

    c. ICD-9

    d. HCPCS

    e. WHO

2. A diagnosis code of 670.51 has been entered on the claim form. **What system is used to assign that code?**

    a. CPT

    b. ICD-9

    c. ICD-10

    d. HCPCS

    e. RVS

3. In the CPT manual, the description of the level of E&M codes includes which of the following?

    a. Complexity of the medical decision making

    b. Level of history taken

    c. Number of systems examined and documented

    d. New versus established patient

    e. All of the above

4. Which of the following is a description of Volume II of the ICD-9?

    a. Known as the Tabular Index, lists all diagnostic codes in numeric order

    b. An alphabetic listing of all known diagnoses, including symptoms and accidents and their causes

    c. Lists procedures in tabular form

    d. All of the above

5. Deliberately billing a higher rate than what was performed to obtain greater reimbursement is called:

    a. encoding

    b. downcoding

    c. upcoding

    d. exploding

6. One way to prevent a breach of confidentiality when processing insurance claim forms is to:

    a. ask the patient, parent, or guardian to sign an Authorization to Release Medical Information form before the claim is completed

    b. ask the patient for verbal approval before sending in the claim

    c. have the patient write a letter requesting that the information be forwarded

    d. have the insurance carrier contact the patient

7. When coding, it is imperative:

    a. to be as precise as possible

    b. not to guess

    c. not to code what is not there

    d. All of the above

8. Submitting claims electronically:

    a. can improve cash flow

    b. ensures consistency

    c. will reduce the amount of supplies required

    d. All of the above

9. Using an electronic device for direct communication between medical offices and a health care plan's computer is called:

    a. subrogation

    b. point of service

    c. diagnosis-related groups

    d. prospective payment

10. The most common claim form for the ambulatory setting is the:

    a. CMS-1450

    b. HCFA-1000

    c. CMS-1500

    d. CPT-1500

11. The codes showing that a patient has been seen for reasons other than sickness or injury are:

    a. S Codes

    b. D Codes

    c. V Codes

    d. X Codes

12. The insurance claims processor will confirm that:

    a. there are no exclusions or restrictions for payment of that diagnosis

    b. the claim was received within seven days of the appointment

    c. the procedure relating to the diagnosis is medically necessary

    d. a. and c.

13. A provider's fee profile is:

    a. based on an average of all the practice's fees

    b. a continuous record of usual charges made for specific services

    c. an average of fees charged over a period of three months

    d. the amount paid by insurance carriers

LEARNING APPLICATION

CASE STUDY

Lourdes's colonoscopy required the following diagnoses and procedures. Give the correct coding for processing the insurance claim for this patient.

CASE STUDY REVIEW QUESTION

Colonoscopy with biopsy, single or multiple   _____

Benign neoplasm of the colon   _____

Family history of malignant neoplasm of the gastrointestinal tract   _____

Personal history of malignant neoplasm of the breast   _____

Low-complexity office visit   _____

CPT Review

For each procedure listed, give the correct procedure code and name the CPT section in which the code can be found.

Procedure	Code	Section
Chemotherapy administration, intravenous infusion technique, up to 1 hour	_____	_____
Hepatitis B surface antibody (HBsAb)	_____	_____
Simple repair of superficial wounds of scalp, neck, axillae, external genitalia, trunk or extremities (including hands and feet) 7.6 to 12.5 cm	_____	_____
Electrocardiogram, routine ECG with 12 leads; with interpretation and reports	_____	_____
Hepatic venography, wedged or free, with hemodynamic evaluation, radiologic supervision, and interpretation	_____	_____
Hepatitis Be antigen (HBeAg)	_____	_____
Anesthesia for arthroscopic procedures of hip joint	_____	_____

CHAPTER POST-TEST

Perform this test without looking at your book. If an answer is "false," rewrite the sentence to make it true.

1. True or False? Medical insurance coding is a way of putting procedures and treatments into numeric form.

_____

_____

2. CPT stands for:

   a. Comprehensive Procedural Terminology

   b. Current Procedural Terminology

   c. Complete Procedural Terminology

   d. Curative Procedural Terminology

3. ICD stands for:

   a. International Codes for Diagnosis

   b. Internal Codes for Diagnosis

   c. International Codes for Diseases

   d. International Classification of Diseases

4. True or False? A third party is one that is involved with reimbursement procedures.

_____

_____

5. True or False? Insurance coding, claim forms, and submissions are complex enough that medical coders and billers need extended training and experience to do it well.

_____

_____

SELF-ASSESSMENT

1. Have you considered whether you would like to be an insurance coder and biller? Think about the following questions.

   A. What qualities do you possess that would make you a good candidate for a career in medical billing and coding?

   _____

   _____

   _____

   B. What qualities do you not possess but could obtain?

   _____

   _____

   _____

C. What do you think you would like best about a position in medical coding and billing?

_____

_____

_____

D. What would be your least favorite part of the job?

_____

_____

2. Explore the profession of medical coding. Look on the Internet for coding organizations offering certification examinations. Differentiate among the various credentials available to coders.

_____

_____

_____

_____

_____

_____

_____

_____

_____

_____

_____

_____

_____

_____

_____

_____

_____

_____

_____

C H A P T E R **19**

Daily Financial Practices

CHAPTER PRE-TEST

Perform this test without looking at your book. If an answer is "false," rewrite the sentence to make it true.

1. True or False? The management of the business details of a practice usually becomes the responsibility of the medical assisting staff.

   _____

   _____

2. True or False? Every patient, regardless of insurance coverage, should be charged the same fee for the same service.

   _____

   _____

3. True or False? You should discourage the use of credit/debit cards for making payments for services rendered.

   _____

   _____

4. True or False? Purchase orders are to be written up when the purchase arrives.

   _____

   _____

5. True or False? Petty cash is available for authorized use when the purchase is minor or unexpected and when a check is not necessary.

   _____

   _____

VOCABULARY BUILDER

Misspelled Words

Find the words below that are misspelled; circle them, and correctly spell them in the spaces provided. Then insert correct vocabulary terms from the list that best fit into the descriptive sentence below.

accounts payible	debit	payee
accounts recievable	dispursements	pegboard system
adjustments	encounter form	petty cash
balance	guaranter	posting
cashier's check	leadger	traveler's check
certified check	money market account	voucher check
credit	National Provider Identifier	
day sheet	notary	

_____   _____   _____

_____   _____

_____ 1. A record of daily patient transactions used in conjunction with pegboard systems

_____ 2. Small cash sum kept on hand in the office for minor or unexpected expenses

_____ 3. Decreases the balance due

_____ 4. Replaces all other identifiers used by providers for reimbursement and other transactions with private payers and the government

_____ 5. As a noun, this term denotes "the amount owed"; as a verb, the term means "to verify posting accuracy"

_____ 6. Accounting function that describes the act of recording financial transactions into bookkeeping or accounting systems

_____ 7. Increases or decreases to a patient account not due to charges incurred or payments received

_____ 8. Sum owed by a business for services or goods received

_____ 9. Sum owed to a business for services or goods supplied

LEARNING REVIEW

Short Answer

1. Identify two work guidelines essential to creating and maintaining accurate financial records.

_____

_____

2. Identify six habits essential to creating and maintaining accurate paper financial records.

_____

_____

_____

_____

_____

3. Identify seven of the nine features that may be a part of the checking account.

_____

_____

_____

_____

_____

_____

4. What are five rules to ensure that checks are properly written and recorded?

_____

_____

_____

_____

_____

5. Give three reasons why it is important to ensure that proper control is utilized when purchasing supplies and equipment.

_____

_____

_____

6. When office supplies arrive, what should be done to verify that the correct items and quantities have been received? What should be done to prepare the invoice for payment?

_____

_____

_____

_____

_____

_____

_____

7. Describe the following types of checks, which are different from checks issued from a standard business checking account.

   (1) Cashier's check:

   _____

   _____

   _____

   (2) Certified check:

   _____

   _____

   _____

   (3) Money order:

   _____

   _____

   _____

   (4) Voucher check:

   _____

   _____

   _____

   _____

   (5) Traveler's check:

   _____

   _____

8. Adjustments are entries made to a patient's account that do not represent charges or payments. Name three reasons why adjustments may sometimes be made to a patient's account.

_____

_____

_____

9. Deposits are generally made daily. All checks to be deposited must be endorsed. Define endorsement. Identify the best method of endorsing checks in the ambulatory care setting and describe the benefits of using this method.

_____

_____

_____

_____

_____

10. Checks received from patients and others must be inspected before preparing the checks for deposit. What guidelines should medical assistants follow in accepting and inspecting checks?

_____

_____

_____

11. If a check is returned to the ambulatory care setting for insufficient funds, what procedures should be followed?

_____

_____

_____

12. It is crucial to balance all financial information for each day and for the month's end. Month-end figures on the day sheet must agree with the patient ledgers. Why is it important to go through this time-consuming accounting process?

_____

_____

_____

_____

_____

_____

_____

CERTIFICATION REVIEW

These questions are designed to mimic the certification examination. Select the best response.

1. The pegboard system of bookkeeping is sometimes called the:

   a. write-it-once system

   b. ledger system

   c. double-entry system

   d. duplicated page system

2. NSF stands for:

   a. nonsufficient funds

   b. not sufficient funds

   c. not satisfactory funding

   d. negligent status of funding

3. A restrictive endorsement stamp is used to:

   a. stamp on the ledger to signify that payment has been made

   b. stamp the doctor's signature on insurance forms and other documents

   c. stamp on the statement to signify that you have sent a check

   d. stamp on the back of a check to signify "for deposit only"

4. When reconciling a bank statement:

   a. the reconciling should be done every month

   b. the checkbook entries should be checked against the bank statement

   c. the reconciling should be done daily by computer

   d. all reconciling should be done in ink to avoid any unauthorized entries

   e. a. and b.

5. If a check has been deposited and is now returned due to insufficient funds, it will be necessary to:

   a. redeposit the check

   b. call the bank that returned it and verify availability of funds so the check can then be redeposited

   c. call the patient who wrote the check

   d. discard the check and credit the amount back to the patient's account

6. The most common method(s) of tracking a patient's balance is (are):

   a. the pegboard system

   b. computerized financial systems

   c. the ledger card

   d. a. and b.

7. The pegboard system consists of:

   a. day sheets

   b. ledger cards

   c. encounter forms

   d. receipt forms

   e. All of the above

8. In cases of divorced parents where one parent has physical custody of the child and is considered the one responsible for payment if the child is not insured with a contracted insurance carrier, the parent is called:

   a. the payee

   b. the guarantor

   c. the subscriber

   d. none of the above

9. The number required by the Centers for Medicare & Medicaid Services (CMS) on claims for clinical diagnosis services is called the:

   a. insurance registration number

   b. client number

   c. National Provider Identifier

   d. contract number

10. The Advanced Beneficiary Notification form is used primarily for:

    a. Medicaid patients

    b. HMO patients

    c. Medicare patients for the purpose of collecting payments that are not allowed

    d. CHAMPUS patients

11. A patient encounter form:

    a. is also called a charge slip

    b. is also called a superbill

    c. is also called a pegboard form

    d. both a. and b.

12. In most practices there is a need to have cash available on a daily basis to:

    a. make change for a patient paying cash for services

    b. make funds available for all office personnel

    c. pay for minor and incidental expenses

    d. provide funds for weekly lunches for all employees

13. When a check must be guaranteed for the amount in which it is written, a _____ is issued.

    a. cashier's check

    b. certified check

    c. voucher check

    d. traveler's check

14. Restricting the use of a check should it be lost or stolen may be done through:

    a. reconciling

    b. balancing

    c. special endorsement

    d. blank endorsement

LEARNING APPLICATION

Hands-on Activities

1. Administrative medical assistant Karen Ritter is responsible for assisting the office manager and accountant in performing accounts payable activities for Inner City Health Care. On September 4, she receives a $323.45 bill from RJ Medical Supply Company for blood pressure equipment the office received on August 30. Noting that the company demands payment within 30 days of billing, Karen writes a check disbursing funds to the company on September 15. The balance in the office's checking account before this check is written is $26,100.00. Using this information, write out the check and stub below. Karen will submit the check to Susan Rice, M.D., for her signature.

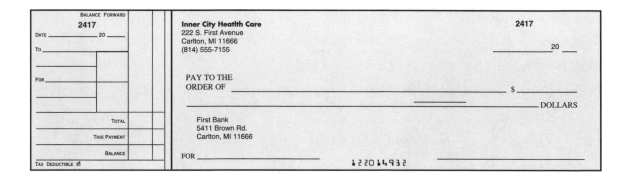

2. Office manager Walter Seals, CMA (AAMA), is responsible for purchasing office supplies for Inner City Health Care. On September 10, Walter completes purchase order #1742 to Mayflower Supply, requested by administrative medical assistant Karen Ritter. The items are taxed at 8%, and the shipping fee is prepaid. The items are billed and shipped to Inner City Health Care; the terms are net due 30 days. Complete the purchase order form below.

PURCHASE ORDER   NO. 1742

Bill To:	Ship To:	Vendor:

REQ BY	BUYER	TERMS

QTY	ITEM	UNITS	DESCRIPTION	UNIT PR	TOTAL
				SUBTOTAL	
				TAX	
				FREIGHT	
				BAL DUE	

Inner City Health Care   Mayflower Supply, Inc.

222 S. First Avenue   642 East 65th Street

Carlton, MI 11666   Carlton, MI 11623

(814) 555-7155   (814) 555-9999

2 boxes of fax paper, #62145, at $8.99 a box

5 day-view desk calendars, #24598, at $4.25 each

4 cases of copier paper, #72148, at $20.00 a case

5 boxes of highlighter pens, 12 to a box, #26773, at $3.98 a box

4 computer printer cartridges, #96187, at $49.99 each

MOSS Activities

1. Using Medical Office Simulation Software and the skills learned in Procedure 19-3, post procedure charges for the following patients. If a patient has a co-payment due, post the co-payment at the time of procedure posting.

   A. Edward Gormann was seen in the office on July 10, 2009, complaining of an earache.

Reference Number	1010
Office Visit Type	Established patient, expanded problem-focused (99213)
Diagnosis Codes	Otitis media (382.9)
Co-payment	The patient pays his $20.00 with a check, #751, at the time of service.

   B. Julia Martin was seen in the office on July 10, 2009, complaining of heartburn.

Reference Number	1011
Office Visit Type	New patient, problem-focused (99203)
Diagnosis Codes	Gastroesophageal reflux (530.81)

   C. Megan Caldwell was seen in the office on July 15, 2009 to check for strep throat.

Reference Number	1035
Office Visit Type	Established patient, problem-focused (99212)
Procedures	Rapid strep test (87880)
Diagnosis	Strep throat (034.0)
Co-payment	The patient pays her $20.00 with cash at the time of service.

   D. Remi Beaufort was seen in the office on July 15, 2009 for a mono screen.

Reference Number	1036
Office Visit Type	New patient, expanded problem focused (99202)
Procedure Codes	Mono screen (86308)
Diagnosis Codes	Mononucleosis (075)
Co-payment	The patient's father pays the $20.00 with a check, #1056, at the time of service.

2. Using Medical Office Simulation Software and the skills learned in Procedure 19-4, perform insurance billing for the procedures posted in the first exercise, for patients Gormann, Martin, Caldwell, and Beaufort.

   A. Choose Electronic for the Transmit Type.

   B. Print or save the prebilling worksheet for each patient to be turned in to your instructor.

   C. Print or save the resulting transmission report to be turned in to your instructor.

3. Using Medical Office Simulation Software and the skills learned in Procedure 19-5, post insurance payments for the same group of payments.

   A. The office receives an EOB from Flexihealth PPO InNetwork on July 30, 2009:

   • For patient Edward Gormann, the plan allowable was $98.24 less the patient's $20 co-pay. The net amount the plan paid for the visit was $78.24 (post an insurance adjustment of $12.76).

   • For patient Megan Caldwell, for the 99212 charge, the plan allowable was $70.80 less the patient's $20 co-pay. The net amount the plan paid for this charge was $50.80 (post an insurance adjustment of $9.20). For the rapid strep test, the plan allowable was $40.71 (post an insurance adjustment of $5.29).

   B. The office receives an EOB from ConsumerOne HRA on July 24, 2009, for Julia Martin's charge. The plan allowable was $177. Write off the remaining amount as an insurance adjustment.

   C. The office receives a RA from Signal HRA on July 31, 2009, for Remi Beaufort's charges. For the 99202 charge, the plan allowable was $130, less the patient's $10 co-pay. The net amount the plan paid for this charge was $110 (post an insurance adjustment of $27). For the mono screen, the plan allowable was $15.05 (post an insurance adjustment of $1.95).

CHAPTER POST-TEST

Perform this test without looking at your book. If an answer is "false," rewrite the sentence to make it true.

1. True or False? The management of the business details of a practice usually becomes the responsibility of the medical assisting staff.

   _____

   _____

2. True or False? The same fees for services should be charged to every patient, regardless of whether they have insurance coverage.

   _____

   _____

3. True or False? You should encourage the use of credit/debit cards for medical bills.

   _____

   _____

4. True or False? Purchase orders are to be written up before the purchase is made.

   _____

   _____

5. True or False? Petty cash is available for authorized use when employees need cash for minor, routine, or small unexpected expenses.

   _____

   _____

SELF-ASSESSMENT

1. In your personal checkbook or banking system at home, how often do you reconcile?

_____

_____

_____

_____

2. When you do reconcile, do you balance? How much time will you spend on the reconciliation to balance? If you reconcile your bank statements on a regular basis and balance each month, congratulations! If you do not reconcile on a regular basis, start today. Gather your last bank statement. If you do not have one, call the bank and have them send you one or download one from the Internet if your bank offers Internet banking. Accept the beginning balance on the bank statement. Gather the check stubs/copies that you have written within the bank statement's beginning and end dates. Check off all the checks that have gone through the bank and are listed on the statement.

Add up the outstanding checks (i.e., the ones that have not gone through yet). Subtract them from the ending balance. Add in any interest you have earned for the month. Subtract any fees you have been charged. Does your amount match the bank statement? If not, go back over your math to make sure you added and subtracted correctly and fix any errors. If you still cannot balance, call the bank and ask to sit down with a representative/clerk so they can help you balance. After you balance once, the next month will be much easier. If your bank offers Internet or online banking, and you are not using that option, consider it. Why are you not using it? Talk to a representative to be sure the online service is secure and your information is protected. If you are satisfied that it is a safe and secure service, consider taking advantage of the online option. Reconciling the monthly statements online is easy to do because the math is done for you by the computer! If you are using online banking, do you think it saves you time? Does it save you money? Is it easier than reconciling manually?

_____

_____

_____

_____

_____

C H A P T E R **2 0**

Billing and Collections

CHAPTER PRE-TEST

Perform this test without looking at your book. If an answer is "false," rewrite the sentence to make it true.

1. The Truth-in-Lending Act states:

   a. Providers cannot charge more than 10% interest on their patient accounts.

   b. Providers must charge interest if the account is more than four months past due.

   c. Providers must notify patients in writing if interest is to be charged on their accounts.

   d. If the provider and patient agree to an installment plan of more than four payments, the installment charge must be stated in writing.

2. True or False? The best opportunity for collection is at the time of services.

   _____

   _____

3. True or False? Large clinics with numerous statements to send out each month will find the monthly billing cycle method to be the most efficient.

   _____

   _____

4. True or False? A collection ratio of 80% is considered a good ratio.

   _____

   _____

VOCABULARY BUILDER

Misspelled Words

Find the words below that are misspelled; circle them, and correctly spell them in the spaces provided. Then match the correct vocabulary term to its definition below.

accounts recievable ratio   collection ratio   statute of limatations

collection agency   probate court   Truth-in-Lending Act

_____   _____

_____   1. Also known as the Consumer Protection Act of 1967; an act requiring providers of installment credits to state the charges in writing and to express the interest as an annual rate

_____   2. An outside establishment that collects outstanding debt

_____   3. Defines the period of time in which legal action can take place

_____   4. Shows the status of collections and the possible losses in a medical facility

_____   5. A measure of how effective collections are and an indication of how quickly outstanding accounts are paid

LEARNING REVIEW

Short Answer

1. A billing efficiency report allows for careful monitoring of follow-up bills; that is, whether they were paid, if the insurance has paid, and an assessment of the patient's responsibility for payment. What five pieces of data are included in these reports from which production efficiency is calculated?

_____

_____

_____

2. Identify and explain the five most common reasons some patient accounts become past due.

_____

_____

_____

_____

_____

3. In the pegboard system, what method is used to identify the age of accounts?

_____

_____

_____

_____

_____

4. Name five criteria according to which computer programs can age accounts.

_____

_____

_____

5. The computer can also generate accounts receivable reports. Name three pieces of information included on a computer-generated accounts receivable report.

_____

_____

6. Collection agencies generally provide two services to an ambulatory care facility. Name and describe each type of service.

_____

_____

_____

_____

_____

7. Collection of fees when a patient has died is directed to the executor of the estate. Place an X next to each action below that represents a responsible action in collecting past due accounts from deceased patients' estates.

_____ If there is no known administrator, address the statement to "Estate of [insert patient's name]" and mail to the patient's last known address.

_____ Send an invoice via certified mail with a complete breakdown of all monies owed by the deceased patient's spouse or closest relative, noting that the survivor is responsible for making payment in full.

_____ Mail the account information via certified mail, return receipt, to the administrator of the estate, whose name can be obtained from the probate department of superior court.

_____ If unsure how to proceed, contact the office's attorney or the probate court for advice.

8. With regard to collections, the statute of limitations is usually defined by the class of the overdue account. Name the three classes of accounts.

_____

_____

_____

9. There are certain legal rules and ethical guidelines to follow when placing collection calls. Circle all that apply.

(1) Callers must identify themselves and validate that the person they are talking to is the responsible party.

(2) Threaten to turn the call over to a collection agency.

(3) Do not call the patient's place of employment.

(4) Do not make repeated calls to the debtor's friends or family.

True or False?

Mark a true statement with a T *and a false statement with an* F. *If an answer is "false," rewrite the sentence to make it true.*

____ 1. Most states regulate the time frame when collection calls can be placed, which is usually between the hours of 8 AM and 8 PM.

_____

_____

____ 2. Emancipated minors are responsible for their own accounts.

_____

_____

____ 3. The expense of hiring an outside collection agency may not always justify the amount of fees to be collected.

_____

_____

____ 4. Not all accounts can be collected, so it is best to identify them early, write them off, and save the practice time and money.

_____

_____

____ 5. An account assigned to a collection agency can be filed in small claims court.

_____

_____

CERTIFICATION REVIEW

These questions are designed to mimic the certification examination. Select the best response.

1. Patients who owe money but have moved and left no forwarding address are referred to as:

   a. deadbeats

   b. skips

   c. nonpayers

   d. dead accounts

2. Statutes of limitations vary from state to state but should be investigated if an unpaid account is more than:

   a. 3 years old

   b. 5 years old

   c. 10 years old

   d. without a time limit if the account is more than a certain amount

3. Lack of payment from a patient may not be considered serious until after:

   a. 30 days

   b. 60 days

   c. 90 days

   d. 120 days

4. For an insurance claim pending more than 45 days, the medical assistant should:

   a. call the carrier and find out if the claim was received

   b. rebill the insurance company

   c. check on the processing status of the claim with the carrier

   d. a. and c.

5. The most appropriate time to discuss fees for financial concerns of the patient is:

   a. when services are rendered

   b. when scheduling an appointment

   c. by mail after services are rendered

   d. when the insurance company does not pay the fee

6. The Truth-in-Lending Act is also known as the:

   a. Consumer Protection Act of 1967

   b. Fair Debt Collection Practice Act

   c. Patient Bankruptcy Protection Act

   d. Accurate Billing and Collection Act

7. The charge slip is also known as the:

   a. ledger

   b. encounter form

   c. day sheet

   d. CMS-1500

8. When a patient files for bankruptcy:

   a. there is little likelihood that the debt can be collected

   b. it is best to close the account and identify the loss

   c. file a proof-of-claim form and provide a copy of the patient's outstanding account to the bankruptcy court

   d. take the account to small claims court

9. In determining how aggressive to be in debt collections, you should consider:

   a. the previous month's billing backlog

   b. production efficiency

   c. the terms of the insured's policy

   d. the value of the dollar owed

LEARNING APPLICATION

Hands-on Activity

Complete the charge slip for Charles Williams' office visit, based on the information below.

Charles Williams, 62 years old, is a new patient of Dr. Winston Lewis at the offices of Drs. Lewis and King. On July 1, 20XX, five days before the patient's birthday, Charles comes to see Dr. Lewis for an appointment with a chief complaint of intermittent, irregular heartbeats or palpitations, dizziness, and chest pain. Dr. Lewis performs a comprehensive physical examination and orders several tests, including an ECG, complete blood count (CBC), and urinalysis with microscopy. The total fee for the office visit and tests is $345—$200 for the physical examination, $75 for the ECG, $25 for the urinalysis, $25 for venipuncture, and $20 for the CBC, which Charles pays for by check at the time of service. Charles is insured by a private carrier, All-American Insurance Company, group #333210, ID number 112-45-9980, which he receives through his employer, High Tech Computer Group. Dr. Lewis asks Ellen Armstrong, CMA (AAMA), to schedule a return appointment in exactly one week to go over the results of Charles's tests. Ellen schedules the appointment and prepares a charge slip for Charles's visit. She refers to his patient information sheet for the correct personal information. Charles Williams lives at 123 Greenside Street, Northborough, OH, 12346.

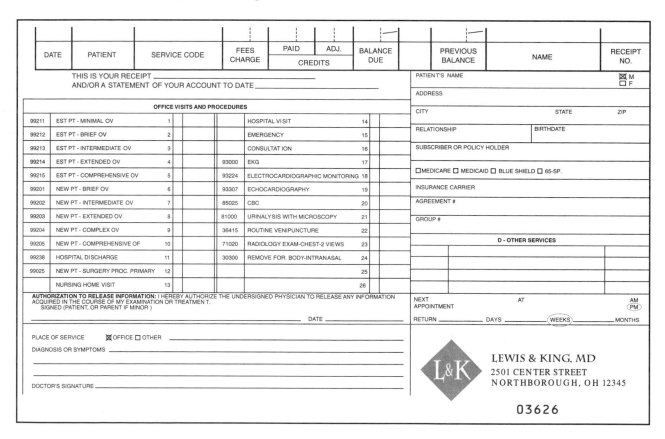

Role Play Activity

In groups of three, role play a collection call using the information in Figure 20-6 in your text. One student should role play the medical assistant, one should be the Patient O'Keefe, and the third person should observe and critique. At the conclusion of the role play, the "medical assistant" and "patient" should each discuss how it felt to be the person in that role.

CHAPTER POST-TEST

Perform this test without looking at your book. If an answer is "false," rewrite the sentence to make it true.

1. The Truth-in-Lending Act states:

   a. Providers can charge more than 10% interest on their patient accounts.

   b. Providers can charge interest only if the account is more than four months overdue.

   c. Providers must notify patients in person if interest is to be charged on their accounts.

   d. If the provider and patient agree to an installment plan of more than four payments, the installment charge must be stated in writing.

2. True or False? The best opportunity for collection is within 30 days of the time of service.

3. True or False? Large clinics with numerous statements to send out each month will find the cycle billing method to be the most efficient.

4. True or False? A collection ratio of 90% is considered a good ratio.

SELF-ASSESSMENT

Think about a time or times when you paid a bill late or did not paid it until the following month. Without disclosing too much personal information, answer the following:

1. What was your reason(s)?

2. Did you receive an overdue notice or a phone call?

3. Which do you think would be more difficult to receive, the notice or the phone call?

4. Are you likely to become defensive if the caller or notice has a threatening tone or a more understanding tone? Justify your response.

_____

_____

_____

_____

5. Could the tone of the notice/call leave you feeling good/bad about the event? Explain.

_____

_____

_____

_____

6. Identify ways the situation could have been handled better.

_____

_____

_____

_____

7. Will your experience affect the way you treat people who owe your clinic money?

_____

_____

_____

_____

C H A P T E R **2 1**

Accounting Practices

CHAPTER PRE-TEST

Perform this test without looking at your book. If an answer is "false," rewrite the sentence to make it true.

1. True or False? Accounts receivable is the amount the provider is owed by patients.

_____

_____

2. The purpose of cost analysis is to determine the:

   a. costs of each service

   b. fixed costs

   c. variable costs

   d. total of all of the above

3. True or False? Income statements should show both profits and expenses.

_____

_____

4. True or False? The W-4 form shows the employee's withholding allowance.

_____

_____

VOCABULARY BUILDER

Misspelled Words

Find the words below that are misspelled; circle them, and correctly spell them in the spaces provided. Then match the vocabulary words to the appropriate definition below.

accounting   cash bases   income statement
accounts payible   check register   libilities
accounts recievable ratio   collection ratio   owner's equity
accrual basis   cost analisys   trial balance
assets   cost ratio   utilazation review
balance sheet   fixed costs   varieble costs

_____   _____   _____

_____   _____   _____

_____

_____ 1. Financial statement showing net profit or loss

_____ 2. Costs that vary in direct proportion to patient volume

_____ 3. Categorizes and records all checks written

_____ 4. Formula that measures the speed in which outstanding accounts are paid

_____ 5. The purpose of this is to determine the cost of each service

_____ 6. An itemized statement of assets, liabilities, financial condition, and owner's equity

_____ 7. System of reporting income where income is recognized at the time the money is collected

_____ 8. Costs that do not vary in total as the number of patients varies

_____ 9. System of monitoring the financial status of a facility and the financial results of its activities, providing information for decision making

_____ 10. Debts and other financial obligations for which one is responsible

_____ 11. Formula that shows the percentage of outstanding debt collected

_____ 12. Properties of value that are owned by a business entity

_____ 13. Created by totaling debit balances and credit balances to make sure that total debits equal total credits

_____ 14. The amount by which a business's assets exceed the business's liabilities

_____ 15. Formula that shows the cost of a procedure or service and helps determine the financial value of maintaining certain services

_____ 16. System of reporting income where income is reported at the time charges are generated

_____ 17. A review of medical services before they can be performed

LEARNING REVIEW

Short Answer

1. There are a variety of methods used for financial management in the ambulatory care setting. Name three bookkeeping systems that are appropriate for use in a medical office.

_____

_____

2. Medical software packages have the ability to code information obtained in the ambulatory care setting for use in a database. When completing insurance claim forms or generating reports, the software has the capability to include the most common procedural and diagnostic codes. What other kinds of codes can a computerized accounting system generate that will facilitate the billing?

_____

_____

_____

3. The computer can also be used in the preparation of financial documents. Name four financial documents.

_____

_____

4. Name three ways computer service bureaus handle accounts from medical facilities.

_____

_____

_____

_____

_____

5. Identify at least four steps to take to reduce the chance of embezzlement.

_____

_____

_____

_____

_____

6. To protect the practice from financial loss, providers can purchase fidelity bonds. Name and describe the three kinds of bonds. Place an X in front of the one that offers the most assurance.

   1. _____   _____

   2. _____   _____

   3. _____   _____

7. How might the office manager use data from the budget sheet?

_____

_____

_____

8. Why is it important to implement and track budgets for specific categories of income and expense in the ambulatory care setting?

_____

_____

_____

Matching I

Match the appropriate noncomputerized bookkeeping system to the following duties performed by the medical assistant.

A. Single-entry

B. Pegboard

C. Double-entry

_____ 1. Office manager Walter Seals was responsible for implementing a computer system at Inner City Health Care. Before the computerized accounting program was put into effect, the urgent care center relied on a manual system of checks and balances that allowed the provider-employers to keep a firm hold on the relation between the facility's assets and the sum of liabilities and net worth.

_____ 2. During a temporary one-week down period in the computer system at the offices of Drs. Lewis and King while a system upgrade is installed, administrative medical assistant Ellen Armstrong completes each day's financial transactions in a daily journal, then transfers this information to the ledger through the posting process. The information will be entered into the computer once the system is up and running again.

_____ 3. When the patient returns the charge slip to the reception desk after an examination, medical assistant Karen Ritter carefully replaces and lines up the charge slip with the patient's name on the day sheet, then correctly inserts the ledger card under the last page of the charge slip. She proceeds to enter the total charges due and any patient payments.

Fixed and Variable Costs Exercise

Fixed costs are expenses that do not vary in total as the number of patients seen by the medical practice grows or shrinks. Variable costs are expenses that are directly affected by patient volume. From the list below, identify expenses that qualify as fixed costs (FC) and those that are variable costs (VC).

_____ 1. Interpreting laboratory test results

_____ 2. Annual depreciation of the cost of an automatic electrocardiograph (ECG) machine

_____ 3. Medical benefits for the office staff

_____ 4. Purchase of reagent test strips for urinalysis

_____ 5. Magazine subscriptions for the facility reception area

_____ 6. Monthly telephone expenses

_____ 7. Medical journal subscriptions for the providers

_____ 8. Purchase of a HemoCue blood glucose system

_____ 9. Printing cost of a patient education brochure

_____ 10. Purchase of open-shelf lateral files

_____ 11. Adding a new position, such as a clinical medical assistant, to the office staff

_____ 12. Property taxes on the medical facility building and grounds

_____ 13. The monthly cost of janitorial services

_____ 14. Purchase of disposable needle-syringe units

_____ 15. Disposable paper gowns for patient examinations

CERTIFICATION REVIEW

These questions are designed to mimic the certification examination. Select the best response.

1. The system that is based on the accounting principle that assets equal liabilities plus owner's equity is the:

    a. single-entry system

    b. double-entry system

    c. standard of billing services bureaus

    d. accounts receivable accounting principles

2. Of the following statements, which is false?

    a. Double-entry bookkeeping is expensive.

    b. Double-entry bookkeeping is accurate.

    c. Double-entry bookkeeping is more time consuming.

    d. Double-entry bookkeeping has checks and balances in place.

3. Owner's equity is *not* the same as:

    a. net worth

    b. proprietorship

    c. capital

    d. accounts payable

4. Bonds may be purchased to protect the practice from:

    a. embezzlement

    b. financial loss

    c. malpractice suits

    d. a. and b.

    e. all of the above

5. A total practice management system has the ability to:

    a. process insurance claims electronically

    b. manage payroll and purchases

    c. generate financial records

    d. All of the above

6. Computerization of medical facilities has increased because of:

    a. emphasis being placed on the accurate documentation of medical records

    b. patient load

    c. increase in managed care plans

    d. a. and c.

7. The trial balance is created by:

   a. collecting data from the current year and previous year and converting them into a ratio

   b. totaling debit balances and credit balances to confirm that total debits equal total credits

   c. reporting outside revenue sources and overhead expenses

   d. recording two sets of entries, such as increase in assets and increase in liabilities

8. Providers should purchase fidelity bonds because they:

   a. are worth the price

   b. provide a sense of security

   c. lessen the chances of embezzlement

   d. will reimburse the practice for any monetary loss caused by the practice's employees

9. A proper contract should be negotiated and signed with any computer and billing service bureau because it:

   a. is considered a legal document

   b. ensures confidentiality and strict privacy of patient information

   c. is in compliance with HIPAA

   d. b. and c.

10. Financial records should provide the following at all times:

    a. salaries earned by providers and staff

    b. amount earned, owed, and collected within a given period

    c. where expenses were incurred in a given period

    d. b. and c.

11. A hospital cost report for Medicare is a part of:

    a. financial accounting

    b. managerial accounting

    c. cost accounting

    d. cost analysis

12. Examples of variable costs include all of the following *except:*

    a. clinical supplies

    b. equipment costs

    c. depreciation

    d. laboratory procedures

13. The accounts receivable trial balance:

    a. tells you how much the practice owes to creditors

    b. shows any problems between the daily journal and the ledger

    c. tracks all disbursements and compares the total with the purchases

    d. uses an NCR transfer strip to copy pertinent information

14. Calculating and reviewing costs provide ambulatory care settings with:

   a. data to set fees

   b. monitoring of the practice's performance

   c. offline batch processing

   d. a. and b.

LEARNING APPLICATION

CASE STUDY 1

When the offices of Drs. Lewis and King agreed to accept individuals covered by a large managed care organization, the decision of the provider-owners was based on a complete financial analysis and projection of the expected effects the new patient load would have on the medical practice. As a result, the group practice added a second office manager and a new clinical medical assistant to the existing staff.

CASE STUDY REVIEW QUESTIONS

1. As Drs. Lewis and King absorb the new managed care patients into the practice, what can the provider-owners do to determine whether their financial analysis and projection were accurate?

   _____

   _____

   _____

2. Once the practice has assembled financial data on the effects of the new patient load, how will these data be used?

   _____

   _____

   _____

   _____

   _____

3. What beneficial effects might the addition of a clinical medical assistant have on the medical practice?

   _____

   _____

   _____

   _____

   _____

CASE STUDY 2

A group practice of radiologists charges $225 for a routine mammogram. Total expenses related to the mammogram procedure equal $30,000 per month, and the practice performs a monthly average of 200 mammograms.

CASE STUDY REVIEW QUESTIONS

1. What is the average cost ratio for the mammogram procedure? Show your calculations in the space provided.

   _____

   _____

2. Given the cost to patients for the mammogram procedure, is the group practice making a profit or loss on performing mammograms? What amount is the profit or loss per procedure? What amount is the profit or loss for the entire month?

   _____

   _____

   _____

Hands-on Activities

1. At the offices of Drs. Lewis and King, the total accounts receivable at the end of May is $100,000 and the monthly receipts total is $75,000; the total accounts receivable at the end of June is $82,000 and the monthly receipts total is $31,000; the total accounts receivable at the end of July is $86,000 and the monthly receipts total is $20,000; the total accounts receivable at the end of August is $93,000 and the monthly receipts total is $45,000. What is the accounts receivable ratio for each month? Show your calculations in the space provided. Which month has the healthiest accounts receivable ratio? Why?

   May: _____   July: _____

   June: _____   August: _____

   _____

   _____

   _____

2. For the month of September, receipts at the offices of Drs. Lewis and King totaled $35,000. The Medicare/Medicaid adjustment for the month was $1,750, and the managed care adjustment was $4,500. Total charges for the month of September equaled $53,000. What is the collection ratio for the month of September? Show your calculation in the space provided.

   _____

   _____

3. For the month of October, receipts at the offices of Drs. Lewis and King totaled $41,000. The Medicare/Medicaid adjustment for the month was $2,000, the Worker's Compensation adjustment was $750, and the managed care adjustment was $4,700. Total charges for October equaled $55,000. What is the collection ratio for the month of October? Show your calculation in the space provided.

---

4. Income statements reveal the cumulative profit and total expenses for each month.Monthly income and expenses are then added to arrive at year-to-date totals, which are compared with the annual budget for particular income and expense categories. Use the following information to complete the expense analysis table for the first quarter office expense costs of the offices of Drs. Lewis and King. The total office expense budget for the year is $20,000 divided evenly per quarter.

Telephone expenses	January $323.46
	February $425.93
	March $393.87
Postage and mail expenses	January $725.45
	February $550.90
	March $601.33
Office supply expenses	January $1,200.62
	February $325.45
	March $446.26
Yearly budget	Telephone expenses $4,000
	Postage and mail expenses $8,000
	Office supply expenses $8,000

Office Expenses	January	February	March	Year to Date	Budget for Year
Telephone	_____	_____	_____	_____	_____
Postage	_____	_____	_____	_____	_____
Office supplies	_____	_____	_____	_____	_____
TOTALS	_____	_____	_____	_____	_____

CHAPTER POST-TEST

Perform this test without looking at your book. If an answer is "false," rewrite the sentence to make it true.

1. True or False? Accounts payable is the amount the provider is owed by patients.

---

2. The purpose of cost analysis is to:

   a. determine the costs of each service

   b. determine the fixed costs

   c. determine the variable costs

   d. determine the total of all of the above

3. True or False? Both profits and expenses should be shown on income statements.

_____

_____

4. True or False? Employees' withholding allowance is recorded on the W-4 form.

_____

_____

SELF-ASSESSMENT

Personal finances, as well as the finances of businesses such as ambulatory care settings, require careful planning, management, and budgeting. You can use the systems of business financial management to gain insights into your personal spending patterns and to help develop and fine-tune smart financial habits and attitudes. For each statement, circle the response that best describes you.

1. I think saving money is:

    a. important; I make every effort to put away a sum of money as savings on a regular basis.

    b. great if you can find a way; I would like to save, but I have trouble finding ways to do it.

    c. not important right now; I have too many expenses—what I really need is a loan!

2. When planning a large purchase, such as a computer or a car, I:

    a. set a limit for spending and affordable installment payments and stick to it.

    b. have a rough idea of what I can afford, but do not do any advance planning.

    c. try to buy what I want and think about paying for it later.

3. When considering monthly personal income and expenses, I:

    a. know exactly how much money is coming in and how much is going out to pay bills.

    b. know I can cover my bills but do not keep track of exactly how much I make or spend.

    c. hope for the best, and if I fall short—charge it!

4. When I have extra money, I:

    a. save one-third, use one-third to pay off debts, and use the last third on a special purchase.

    b. save half or use it to pay off debts and spend the other half on a special purchase.

    c. spend it all on a special purchase.

5. My checkbook is:

    a. always balanced.

    b. sometimes balanced.

    c. rarely balanced.

6. When choosing a bank for my savings or checking, I:

    a. research interest rates, features, funds, and services carefully to find the best deal.

    b. choose the bank that pays the highest interest rate.

    c. just pick whatever is most convenient; banks are all the same.

7. I think planning for retirement is:

   a. a priority now; the sooner you start saving, the more your money grows!

   b. important but not the most essential financial responsibility I have right now.

   c. not something I think about now—that is too far away; who can predict the future?

8. People think of me as someone who:

   a. pays attention to detail and is neat and organized.

   b. always manages to get the job done at the last minute.

   c. struggles to keep up with routine or repetitive tasks.

9. I think analyzing financial data is:

   a. a smart way to assess current spending patterns and guide future spending.

   b. a great thing to do if you have enough time and willpower.

   c. a waste of time; besides, I just do not want to know.

10. I am the kind of person who:

    a. sets short- and long-term financial goals for income and spending and works toward implementing them in a responsible way.

    b. has short- and long-term financial goals but cannot get around to planning for them.

    c. makes financial decisions on a day-to-day basis; it is enough to deal with one day at a time.

Scoring: If your answers were mostly A responses, congratulations! You have developed a financially responsible outlook and good record-keeping habits. If your responses were mostly Bs, you are thinking about financial realities and recognize the importance of a strong financial awareness. Focus on specifics where you can improve your financial skills. If your responses were mostly Cs, you need to work on achieving good personal financial habits. Start working on your record-keeping skills by taking the plunge and keeping a weekly journal of expenses to see where your money goes!

CHAPTER **22**

Infection Control and Medical Asepsis

CHAPTER PRE-TEST

Perform this test without looking at your book. If an answer is "false," rewrite the sentence to make it true.

1. The single most important action you can take to avoid acquiring communicable diseases is to:

    a. not mingle with people in crowded areas

    b. wear a mask when in public

    c. wear gloves at all times

    d. wash hands frequently

2. To sanitize something means literally to:

    a. wash and rinse well

    b. sterilize it

    c. disinfect it

    d. wipe it off

3. True or False? The difference between sterilizing and disinfecting is that sterilization gets rid of all microbes and their spores, whereas disinfection gets rid of surface microbes, but not their spores.

   _____

   _____

4. Epidemiology is the study of:

    a. communicable diseases only

    b. diseases and other conditions and their patterns

    c. *epi-*, or surfaces

    d. bugs

5. The word *pathogen* means:

    a. all "germs" or microorganisms

    b. bacteria and viruses only

    c. only those microorganisms that cause diseases

    d. all of the above

VOCABULARY BUILDER

Misspelled Words

Find the words below that are misspelled; circle them, and correctly spell them in the spaces provided. Then insert one of the correct vocabulary terms into the sentences below. Each word will be used once.

contaminated	infection control	sanitization
ecoriated	medical asepsis	transmision
epidemology	microorganisms	

_____   _____   _____

1. _____ is the study of the history, cause, and patterns of infectious diseases.

2. Microscopic living creatures, also known as _____, that are capable of causing disease are called pathogens. The spread of infectious diseases can occur through direct contact, indirect contact, inhalation, ingestion, or bloodborne contact.

3. _____ refers to various methods, including the CDC's Standard Precautions, that health care professionals use to eliminate or reduce the risk of spreading disease.

4. Spreading disease is another way of describing the _____ of infectious microorganisms from one person to another.

5. _____ involves specific techniques that are designed to destroy pathogens after they leave the body and to decrease the risk for spreading infection to others.

6. To reduce the risk that any item, including equipment, surgical trays, and instruments, could be _____ or exposed to microorganisms or infectious material, various sterilization techniques are used.

7. Before instruments or other fomites are disinfected or sterilized, they must be scrubbed or cleaned and rinsed to remove tissue, debris, or other impurities that may harbor pathogens, a process called _____ .

8. Medically aseptic hand washing techniques should be performed on a regular basis to ensure the reduction of pathogens spread by the hands. To reduce the risk for chapped, _____ skin, medical assistants can apply water-based antibacterial lotion to the hands after washing.

Matching

Match the following terms with the correct definitions.

amoebic dysentery	infectious agent	pathogen
bloodborne pathogen	malaria	scabies
fomites	palliative	trichomoniasis

_____ 1. Infection with a *Trichomonas* parasite, which can be transmitted through sexual intercourse

_____ 2. Infectious skin disease caused by the itch mite, *Sarcoptes scabiei,* which is transmitted by direct contact with infected persons

_____ 3. An agent that relieves only symptoms of the disease instead of curing the infection

_____ 4. A pathogen responsible for a specific infectious disease

_____ 5. Infectious intestinal disease characterized by inflammation of the mucous membrane of the colon and diarrhea

_____ 6. Any microorganism capable of causing disease found in blood or components of blood

_____ 7. Infectious disease caused by protozoan parasites within red blood cells; transmitted to humans by female mosquitoes

_____ 8. Substances that absorb and transmit infectious material, that is, contaminated items such as equipment

_____ 9. Any disease-producing microorganism

Definitions

Write a brief definition for each correct vocabulary term.

1. Resistance:

_____

_____

2. Vaccine:

_____

_____

3. Antibody:

_____

_____

4. Immunoglobulins:

_____

_____

5. Immunity:

_____

_____

6. Disinfection:

_____

_____

7. Antigen:

_____

_____

Word Search

Find the words in the grid below. They may go in any direction.

```
H  P  B  F  H  X  V  L  N  O  I  T  A  Z  I  T  I  N  A  S  S  P
V  A  L  N  V  C  H  N  P  K  D  C  K  D  R  B  N  L  F  W  T  R
T  N  I  D  I  S  I  N  F  E  C  T  I  O  N  L  M  M  P  J  E  E
J  T  N  D  D  G  T  K  F  L  L  P  Q  P  N  Y  Y  V  K  M  R  V
N  I  F  E  N  R  O  B  D  O  O  L  B  G  O  S  A  L  X  M  I  E
O  B  L  T  J  T  K  L  D  I  S  E  A  S  E  C  P  H  M  D  L  N
I  I  A  A  P  A  T  H  O  G  E  N  J  T  C  K  S  R  G  L  I  T
T  O  M  N  T  C  O  N  T  R  O  L  B  I  L  M  Y  O  E  K  Z  I
C  T  M  I  A  Y  S  U  R  I  V  M  N  M  K  H  H  N  R  A  E  O
E  I  A  M  Y  I  R  R  T  J  K  E  I  V  A  P  O  L  V  C  D  N
T  C  T  A  C  T  R  V  Y  C  S  C  B  N  N  I  K  S  N  L  I  W
O  S  I  T  T  V  T  E  I  G  R  Y  D  Q  S  G  S  U  O  N  M  M
R  H  O  N  T  X  Q  T  T  O  O  W  D  S  L  N  Y  R  I  J  M  S
P  L  N  O  M  A  P  A  O  C  A  L  I  N  O  L  S  G  T  H  U  U
X  Z  H  C  T  E  S  R  U  S  A  M  O  I  X  R  Z  I  C  K  N  G
B  P  G  N  S  T  G  E  H  T  S  B  T  I  E  L  X  C  E  B  I  N
R  X  X  I  P  A  R  I  P  N  O  U  H  I  M  R  T  A  F  R  Z  U
L  K  T  J  N  G  N  P  A  S  A  C  R  L  D  E  M  L  N  J  A  F
T  N  Z  I  P  G  Q  R  Q  C  I  R  L  R  W  H  D  W  I  K  T  F
A  P  S  J  M  H  T  H  E  L  A  S  M  A  X  M  Z  I  D  M  I  Y
B  M  L  Y  N  H  F  R  N  B  R  L  Z  B  V  V  M  T  P  D  O  K
S  T  X  R  H  G  P  Y  Q  K  L  G  L  M  X  E  H  V  M  E  N  Z
```

antibiotics	disinfection	precautions
antiseptic	epidemiology	prevention
asepsis	fungus	protection
autoclave	hand washing	sanitization
bacteria	immunization	spread
barriers	infection	sterilize
bloodborne	inflammation	transmission
contaminated	microorganisms	vaccines
control	microscopic	virus
disease	pathogen	

LEARNING REVIEW

Fill in the Blanks

Immunity is defined as the ability of the body to resist disease. Identify the correct terms or the specific form of immunity that may occur in response to specific antigens.

1. The immune response that involves T cells and B cells to attack viruses, fungi, organ transplants, or cancer cells is called _____.

2. The immune response that produces antibodies to kill pathogens and recognize them in the future is called _____.

3. The immunity that follows the administration of vaccines is called _____.

4. The short-term immunity provided to a newborn that occurs when antibodies pass to a fetus from the mother is called _____.

5. The immunity that results from contracting an infectious agent and experiencing either an acute or a subclinical infectious disease is called _____.

6. The immunity achieved through administration of ready-made antibodies, such as gamma-globulin, is called _____.

Short Answer

1. The following are the five common stages of many infectious diseases: acute, prodromal, declining, convalescent, incubation. Place the stages in the proper order in the table below, starting with initial infection with a pathogen, and then describe the identifying characteristics and symptoms associated with each.

Order	Stage	Characteristics and Symptoms
1	_____	_____
		_____
		_____
		_____
2	_____	_____
		_____
		_____
		_____
		_____
		_____
3	_____	_____
		_____
		_____
		_____
		_____
		_____
		_____

4   _____   _____
                       _____
                       _____
5   _____   _____
                       _____
                       _____
                       _____
                       _____

2. For each vaccine listed below, identify the disease for which the vaccine provides immunity.

Vaccine	Disease
DTaP	_____
HBV	_____
MMR	_____
Hib	_____
IPV	_____

3. A susceptible host is a person who is not resistant or immune to a pathogenic organism and is, therefore, able to contract the pathogenic organism and experience development of an infection. List the five reasons a person may be susceptible.

_____

_____

_____

4. Susceptibility of a person depends on several factors, such as occupation or lifestyle environment, youth or advanced age, poor psychological health, poor physical condition, presence of underlying disease, the number of pathogens exposed to, and the duration of exposure. For each example given, identify the correct factor of susceptibility.

Example	Susceptibility Factor
A. Dr. Angie Esposito is physically worn down by working double shifts at Inner City Health Care. Although she loves the excitement of working intensely with patients in an urgent care setting, flu season is coming and Dr. Esposito is worried that she will become ill.	_____
B. Significantly overweight and a heavy smoker, Herb Fowler is prone to colds that just will not go away; Dr. Winston Lewis is treating Herb for a case of chronic bronchitis.	_____
C. Mary O'Keefe's 3-year-old son, Chris, and several other members of his play group come down with chickenpox after playing with a child infected with the disease, caused by the varicella zoster virus.	_____
D. Pneumocystis pneumonia is an infection common to patients who have full-blown cases of AIDS.	_____
E. Jim Marshall, stressed out by the pressure to complete an architectural design ahead of schedule and on a tight budget, is depressed and angry when he gets laid up with the flu and misses two days of work.	_____

F. Margaret Thomas's college-age niece is caught in an epidemic of scabies that sweeps through her dorm floor and places the students in temporary isolation until the outbreak is controlled.

_____

_____

G. While vacationing at a remote spot in Mexico, Bill Schwartz eats almost a pound of shrimp at a local restaurant; the next day, he experiences severe diarrhea and vomiting. He is diagnosed with cholera, caused by the *Vibrio cholerae* bacterium harbored in the shellfish he ate.

_____

_____

_____

5. For each infectious disease listed below, identify the agent of transmission (virus, bacteria, fungus, etc.), at least one route of transmission, and common symptoms.

Disease	Agent	Route	Symptoms
AIDS	_____	_____	_____
	_____	_____	_____
	_____	_____	_____
TB	_____	_____	_____
	_____	_____	_____
	_____	_____	_____
	_____	_____	_____
Gastroenteritis	_____	_____	_____
	_____	_____	_____
Hepatitis B	_____	_____	_____
	_____	_____	_____
	_____	_____	_____
Chickenpox	_____	_____	_____
	_____	_____	_____
Influenza	_____	_____	_____
	_____	_____	_____
	_____	_____	_____

6. Describe three methods of medical asepsis used to reduce the presence of pathogens in an ambulatory care setting.

_____

_____

_____

_____

_____

_____

_____

7. Place an X next to each statement below that represents the appropriate use of medical asepsis in the ambulatory care setting.

____ Joe Guerrero, CMA (AAMA), washes his hands before performing the transfer of patient Lenore McDonell from the wheelchair to the examination table.

____ Wanda Slawson, CMA (AAMA), runs a clean sheet of disposable paper over the examination table to prepare the room for the next patient. She picks up the cloth gown that she does not think patient Lydia Renzi used and places it on the examination table for the next patient to use.

____ After performing a venipuncture procedure on patient Leo McKay, Bruce Goldman, CMA (AAMA), tells Leo he can just dispose of the gauze pad he has been holding on the venipuncture site in the trash can.

____ Anna Preciado, CMA (AAMA), moving quickly to assist a patient who may be about to faint, accidentally bumps into a sterile tray of instruments, knocking some of them to the floor. The patient, who is bent over in front of Anna, picks the instruments up off the floor and places them back on the tray in the sterile field. "You dropped these," he says.

____ After assisting in the removal of an infected sebaceous cyst from a patient, clinical medical assistant Audrey Jones cleans, dresses, and bandages the wound as directed by Dr. Winston Lewis. She then disposes of all contaminated items following Standard Precautions and OSHA guidelines, and properly removes personal protective equipment (PPE), removes her gloves, and washes her hands.

8. For each item in Question 7 that does not reflect proper techniques of medical asepsis, explain what went wrong and how the error should be corrected.

_____

_____

_____

_____

_____

_____

_____

_____

_____

_____

_____

CERTIFICATION REVIEW

These questions are designed to mimic the certification examination. Select the best response.

1. Susceptibility to an infectious microorganism depends on all of the following *except:*

    a. number and specific types of pathogens

    b. duration of exposure to the pathogen

    c. indirect contact

    d. general physical condition

2. The body's natural way of responding when invaded by a pathogen is:

    a. inflammation

    b. septicemia

    c. immunosuppression

    d. immunization

3. The greatest natural barrier is:

    a. intact skin

    b. cilia

    c. hydrochloric acid

    d. mucous membranes

4. Specialized antibodies that can render a pathogen unable to reproduce or continue to grow are called:

    a. antigens

    b. immunoglobulins

    c. pathogenic toxins

    d. spores

LEARNING APPLICATIONS

Hands-on Activities

Complete the following forms with the indicated information.

1. You tested the eyewash station on the first of this month. Complete the Eyewash Testing Log below in the next space.

Tested by:	Date	Assessment Action taken
Janie Carter, RN	August 14, 20xx	Flushed until clear, working appropriately.
B. Abbott, RMA	September 16, 20xx	Flushed until clear, working properly.
Joe Guerrero, CMA (AAMA)	October 10, 20xx	Flushed until clear, working appropriately.

2. You checked the emergency cleanup spill kits in all your exam rooms and in the clinical laboratory. You made sure they were complete, had not expired, were intact without tears, and were ready to use when needed. Make notation of your checks on the following form.

Location	Checked by	Date	Assessment - Action Taken
Exam Room #1			
Exam Room #2			
Exam Room #3			
Lab Staion #1			
Lab Kit #2			

3. You were exposed to a patient's blood through an accidental needlestick. Fill out the following form.

OSHA's Form 301
Injury and Illness Incident Report

U.S. Department of Labor

Occupational Safety and Health Administration

Form approved OMB no. 1218-0176

Attention: This form contains information relating to employee health and must be used in a manner that protects the confidentiality of employees to the extent possible while the information is being used for occupational safety and health purposes.

This *Injury and Illness Incident Report* is one of the first forms you must fill out when a recordable work-related injury or illness has occurred. Together with the *Log of Work-Related Injuries and Illnesses* and the accompanying *Summary*, these forms help the employer and OSHA develop a picture of the extent and severity of work-related incidents.

Within 7 calendar days after you receive information that a recordable work-related injury or illness has occurred, you must fill out this form or an equivalent. Some state workers' compensation, insurance, or other reports may be acceptable substitutes. To be considered an equivalent form, any substitute must contain all the information asked for on this form.

According to Public Law 91-596 and 29 CFR 1904, OSHA's recordkeeping rule, you must keep this form on file for 5 years following the year to which it pertains.

If you need additional copies of this form, you may photocopy and use as many as you need.

Completed by _____

Title _____

Phone (_____) _____ – _____   Date ___ / ___ / ___

Information about the employee

1) Full name _____

2) Street _____

City _____ State _____ ZIP _____

3) Date of birth ___ / ___ / ___

4) Date hired ___ / ___ / ___

5) ☐ Male ☐ Female

Information about the physician or other health care professional

6) Name of physician or other health care professional _____

7) If treatment was given away from the worksite, where was it given?

Facility _____

Street _____

City _____ State _____ ZIP _____

8) Was employee treated in an emergency room?
☐ Yes ☐ No

9) Was employee hospitalized overnight as an in-patient?
☐ Yes ☐ No

Information about the case

10) Case number from the Log _____ *(Transfer the case number from the Log after you record the case.)*

11) Date of injury or illness ___ / ___ / ___

12) Time employee began work _____ AM / PM

13) Time of event _____ AM / PM ☐ Check if time cannot be determined

14) **What was the employee doing just before the incident occurred?** Describe the activity, as well as the tools, equipment, or material the employee was using. Be specific. *Examples:* "climbing a ladder while carrying roofing materials"; "spraying chlorine from hand sprayer"; "daily computer key-entry."

15) **What happened?** Tell us how the injury occurred. *Examples:* "When ladder slipped on wet floor, worker fell 20 feet"; "Worker was sprayed with chlorine when gasket broke during replacement"; "Worker developed soreness in wrist over time."

16) **What was the injury or illness?** Tell us the part of the body that was affected and how it was affected; be more specific than "hurt," "pain," or sore." *Examples:* "strained back"; "chemical burn, hand"; "carpal tunnel syndrome."

17) **What object or substance directly harmed the employee?** *Examples:* "concrete floor"; "chlorine"; "radial arm saw." *If this question does not apply to the incident, leave it blank.*

18) **If the employee died, when did death occur?** Date of death ___ / ___ / ___

Public reporting burden for this collection of information is estimated to average 22 minutes per response, including time for reviewing instructions, searching existing data sources, gathering and maintaining the data needed, and completing and reviewing the collection of information. Persons are not required to respond to the collection of information unless it displays a current valid OMB control number. If you have any comments about this estimate or any other aspects of this data collection, including suggestions for reducing this burden, contact: US Department of Labor, OSHA Office of Statistical Analysis, Room N-3644, 200 Constitution Avenue, NW, Washington, DC 20210. Do not send the completed forms to this office.

CASE STUDY 1

Veronica Hernandez, a medical assisting intern at the Northborough Family Medical Group of Drs. Winston Lewis and Elizabeth King, attends to patient procedures and examinations under the supervision of office manager Jacquie Cavanaugh, CMA (AAMA). Although Veronica is careful to follow all infection control methods during patient care, severe dermatitis has developed on her hands. She is concerned that this condition, which has not responded to creams and lotions, is related to the latex gloves she wears during procedures.

CASE STUDY REVIEW QUESTIONS

1. Discuss the possible causes of Veronica's symptoms.

_____

_____

_____

_____

_____

2. Suggest a course of action that both addresses Veronica's condition and maintains the proper degree of asepsis.

_____

_____

_____

_____

_____

CASE STUDY 2

One-year-old Marissa O'Keefe is a patient at the practice of Drs. Lewis and King. During her well-baby check, Joe Guerrero, CMA (AAMA), gives Marissa an MMR vaccination and is about to administer the DTaP when Marissa's mother voices concerns about the safety of the vaccinations.

CASE STUDY REVIEW QUESTIONS

1. Should Joe continue to administer the DTaP even though the mother is concerned?

_____

_____

_____

_____

_____

continues

2. What is Joe's best therapeutic response?

_____

_____

_____

_____

_____

_____

CHAPTER POST-TEST

Perform this test without looking at your book. If an answer is "false," rewrite the sentence to make it true.

1. The single most important action you can take to avoid contracting a communicable disease is to:

    a. mingle with people in crowded areas so you create immunities

    b. wear a mask when in public

    c. wear gloves at all times

    d. wash hands frequently

2. Disinfection is a way to:

    a. clean hands

    b. prepare the patient's skin for surgery

    c. clean inanimate objects, such as countertops

    d. sterilize

3. True or False? The difference between sterilizing and disinfecting is that disinfection gets rid of all microbes and their spores, whereas sterilization gets rid of all surface microbes, but not their spores.

    _____

    _____

4. Epidemiology is:

    a. the study of communicable diseases only

    b. the study of diseases and other conditions and their patterns

    c. the study of *epi-,* or surfaces

    d. the study of bugs

5. The word *pathogen* means:

    a. all "germs" or microorganisms

    b. viruses only

    c. only those microorganisms that cause diseases

    d. all of the above

SELF-ASSESSMENT

As you answer the following questions, think about how you have changed your awareness of disease prevention because of what you have learned in this chapter.

1. Are you always 100% careful to wash your hands after using the restroom?

_____

_____

_____

_____

2. How does it make you feel when you see others leaving a public restroom without washing their hands?

_____

_____

_____

_____

3. Are you always careful to wash your hands just before eating? Even if you are in a car and there is not a sink handy? What can you do in that case?

_____

_____

_____

_____

4. Besides washing your hands and avoiding direct contact with sick people, what do you suppose is the other single most important action you can take to stay healthy?

_____

_____

_____

_____

5. Do you think stress can make you sick? If so, how do you suppose that happens?

_____

_____

_____

_____

_____

_____

CHAPTER **23**

The Patient History and Documentation

CHAPTER PRE-TEST

Perform this test without looking at your book. If an answer is "false," rewrite the sentence to make it true.

1. True or False? To "diagnose" is to give a name to the condition or disease a patient has.

_____

_____

2. True or False? Subjective statements can be described as "opinion."

_____

_____

3. When a patient "complains" of something, he or she is:

   a. just whining

   b. filing a lawsuit

   c. explaining his or her symptoms

   d. gossiping

4. True or False? Once a medical assistant has asked a patient whether he or she has any allergies, and the information has been recorded, the medical assistant does not need to keep asking.

_____

_____

5. True or False? If a disease is familial, that means it is communicable to close family members living in the same house.

_____

_____

VOCABULARY BUILDER

Misspelled Words

Find the words below that are misspelled; circle them, and correctly spell them in the spaces provided. Then, insert one of the correct vocabulary terms into the sentences below. Each word will be used once.

allergy's	clinical diagnosus	SOAP
chart	famileal	SOMR
CHEDDAR	objective	subjective
chief complaint	POMR	

_____   _____   _____

1. The _____ is the main reason the patient has come to the doctor.

2. _____ diseases are those diseases or conditions with genetic links such as breast and colon cancers, coronary artery disease, diabetes mellitus, and hypertension.

3. Mary O'Keefe calls Dr. King's office to schedule an emergency appointment and tells Ellen Armstrong, CMA (AAMA), that her 3-year-old son Chris awakened during the night with extreme pain in his right ear. This is a _____ complaint, as it is known by the patient but cannot be seen or measured by the provider.

4. Dr. King examines 3-year-old Chris O'Keefe's right ear with an otoscope and observes that the ear is inflamed; the ear is also draining. Since these conditions can be visualized, they are called _____ signs.

5. When a 19-year-old young woman comes into Inner City Health Care with extreme abdominal pain localized to the lower right quadrant, vomiting, slight fever, and loss of appetite, Dr. Whitney orders a CBC, a urinalysis, and an abdominal ultrasound to determine a _____ between possible diagnoses of acute appendicitis and an ovarian cyst.

6. Dr. Whitney confirms a _____ of acute appendicitis for the female emergency patient, based on subjective and objective information from the patient's history, the findings of the physical examination, and the results of the laboratory tests ordered.

7. A patient's file containing medical history and treatments kept by the provider is called the patient _____.

8. _____ is a traditional form of charting that consists of a chronological set of notes for each visit, beginning with the patient's first visit.

9. The charting method that lists patient data in the following order: subjective, objective, assessment, plan, is referred to as _____ charting.

10. Acquired abnormal immune responses to substances (allergens) that do not normally cause reactions are called _____.

11. The most efficient way of recording chart notes, especially in multiprovider clinics or practices, is _____.

12. _____ is another more comprehensive approach to charting, which encourages greater detail to SOAP/SOAPER.

LEARNING REVIEW

Reading Chart Notes

> 1/10/XX CC: NVD x 4 days. T: 100°F for 2 days. Loss of appetite.

1. Write what this chart note means.

   _____

   _____

   _____

2. A mistake has been made in the chart note above: three days should be listed instead of four. Using proper procedure for correcting a paper chart, correct the note.

   _____

   _____

3. To practice charting, translate the following statements (A through H) into medical terms as you would document it in a patient's medical record. Use the lines provided.

   A. The patient was examined on January 12, 20XX at Ten fifteen in the morning.

   _____

   _____

   B. The patient says she has had lower abdominal pain on the left side for a week and has been feeling more and more tired.

   _____

   _____

   C. Weight is 135 pounds. Height is 5 feet 4 inches. Temperature is 99.8°F, slightly elevated above normal. Respiration is 19 breaths per minute and is clear. Pulse is 78 beats per minute and is regular. Blood pressure reading is 134 (systolic)/82 (diastolic).

   _____

   _____

   D. The patient describes an increasing urge to urinate with a burning sensation upon urination; pressure in abdomen; lack of energy.

   _____

   _____

   E. The patient has a medical history that is positive for frequent urinary tract infections. The patient was diagnosed with type II diabetes mellitus in 1987 and takes a prescribed dosage of 3 mg of Glynase orally daily in tablet form. The patient quit smoking 20 years ago and has lost 10 pounds in the last 2 years.

   _____

   _____

   _____

F. The patient has no known allergies.

_____

_____

G. There is no change in family history.

_____

_____

H. The patient has less than two glasses of wine per week, does not smoke, and exercises regularly.

_____

_____

Short Answer

1. Every provider/patient interview is a cross-cultural one. List four questions a medical assistant might ask while taking a medical history that would help bridge social and cultural beliefs to obtain accurate information about a patient's condition that the provider will need to give proper care and treatment.

_____

_____

_____

_____

2. List eight possible characteristics of chief complaints.

_____

_____

_____

3. After the history is taken by the medical assistant, the provider will perform a review of systems (ROS). In addition to the patient's general state of health, list 10 body systems the provider will assess during the ROS.

_____

_____

_____

_____

_____

_____

4. True or False? Charts (medical records) belong to the provider, and nobody has a right to see them without a court order.

_____

_____

5. True or False? Abbreviations of medical terms can be confusing from institution to institution, so the Joint Commission has actually created a list of "forbidden" abbreviations.

_____

_____

CERTIFICATION REVIEW

These questions are designed to mimic the certification examination. Select the best response.

1. Which is *not* a component of SOAP charting?

    a. Subjective information

    b. Assessment of symptoms

    c. Symptoms

    d. Plan for treatment

2. POMR stands for:

    a. privacy of medical records

    b. problem-oriented medical record

    c. payment of medical resources

    d. parts of medical records

3. The medical history form includes the social history, medical history, family history, review of systems, and:

    a. insurance information

    b. chief complaint

    c. provider's history

    d. diagnosis and prognosis

4. Primary administrative information includes the patient's full name, telephone numbers, insurance information, and:

    a. addresses

    b. date of birth

    c. vital signs

    d. a. and b.

5. The Continuity of Care Record (CCR):

    a. ensures that a minimum standard of information is to be shared with other providers

    b. will have no effect on the amount of errors made in the patient's chart

    c. is being established by the American Academy of Gerontologists

    d. can be completed only by providers

    e. All of the above

LEARNING APPLICATION

Hands-on Activities

1. Interview students from your school's English-as-a-Second-Language program or someone for whom English is not the primary language. Have them describe diseases or conditions that have bothered them in the past or are bothering them now. Discuss the following questions with classmates:

   a. Was there a problem with communication because of the language differences?

   _____

   _____

   _____

   b. What types of creative communication methods did you use?

   _____

   _____

   _____

   c. Did you find that some people can read another language better than they can "hear" it (or vice-versa)?

   _____

   _____

   _____

2. On a separate piece of paper decode each component of Figure 23-8 in your textbook. Put all the information in lay terms and write out all the abbreviations.

3. Pretend you are a patient and complete the following Health History Questionnaire. You should use "made up" information to protect your privacy, but be sure to put your real name on it for clarification. With another student, take turns role-playing as medical assistant and patient using the forms you have filled out.

CONFIDENTIAL HEALTH HISTORY

Name:_____ Date: _____

Birthdate:_____ Age:_____ Date of last physical examination:_____

Occupation: _____

Reason for visit today: _____

MEDICATIONS List all medications you are currently taking	**ALLERGIES** List all allergies

SYMPTOMS Check (✓) symptoms you currently have or have had in the past year.

GENERAL
- ☐ Chills
- ☐ Depression
- ☐ Dizziness
- ☐ Fainting
- ☐ Fever
- ☐ Forgetfulness
- ☐ Headache
- ☐ Loss of sleep
- ☐ Loss of weight
- ☐ Nervousness
- ☐ Numbness
- ☐ Sweats

MUSCLE/JOINT/BONE
Pain, weakness, numbness in:
- ☐ Arms
- ☐ Back
- ☐ Feet
- ☐ Hands
- ☐ Hips
- ☐ Legs
- ☐ Neck
- ☐ Shoulders

GENITO-URINARY
- ☐ Blood in urine
- ☐ Frequent urination
- ☐ Lack of bladder control
- ☐ Painful urination

GASTROINTESTINAL
- ☐ Appetite poor
- ☐ Bloating
- ☐ Bowel changes
- ☐ Constipation
- ☐ Diarrhea
- ☐ Excessive hunger
- ☐ Excessive thirst
- ☐ Gas
- ☐ Hemorrhoids
- ☐ Indigestion
- ☐ Nausea
- ☐ Rectal bleeding
- ☐ Stomach pain
- ☐ Vomiting
- ☐ Vomiting blood

CARDIOVASCULAR
- ☐ Chest pain
- ☐ High blood pressure
- ☐ Irregular heart beat
- ☐ Low blood pressure
- ☐ Poor circulation
- ☐ Rapid heart beat
- ☐ Swelling of ankles
- ☐ Varicose veins

EYE, EAR, NOSE, THROAT
- ☐ Bleeding gums
- ☐ Blurred vision
- ☐ Crossed eyes
- ☐ Difficulty swallowing
- ☐ Double vision
- ☐ Earache
- ☐ Ear discharge
- ☐ Hay fever
- ☐ Hoarseness
- ☐ Loss of hearing
- ☐ Nosebleeds
- ☐ Persistent cough
- ☐ Ringing in ears
- ☐ Sinus problems
- ☐ Vision - Flashes
- ☐ Vision - Halos

SKIN
- ☐ Bruise easily
- ☐ Hives
- ☐ Itching
- ☐ Change in moles
- ☐ Rash
- ☐ Scars
- ☐ Sores that won't heal

MEN only
- ☐ Breast lump
- ☐ Erection difficulties
- ☐ Lump in testicles
- ☐ Penis discharge
- ☐ Sore on penis
- ☐ Other

WOMEN only
- ☐ Abnormal Pap Smear
- ☐ Bleeding between periods
- ☐ Breast lump
- ☐ Extreme menstrual pain
- ☐ Hot flashes
- ☐ Nipple discharge
- ☐ Painful intercourse
- ☐ Vaginal discharge
- ☐ Other

Date of last menstrual period _____

Date of last Pap Smear _____

Have you had a mammogram? _____

Are you pregnant? _____

Number of children _____

MEDICAL HISTORY Check (✓) the medical conditions you have or have had in the past.

- ☐ AIDS
- ☐ Alcoholism
- ☐ Anemia
- ☐ Anorexia
- ☐ Appendicitis
- ☐ Arthritis
- ☐ Asthma
- ☐ Bleeding Disorders
- ☐ Breast Lump
- ☐ Bronchitis
- ☐ Bulimia
- ☐ Cancer
- ☐ Cataracts

- ☐ Chemical Dependency
- ☐ Chicken Pox
- ☐ Diabetes
- ☐ Emphysema
- ☐ Epilepsy
- ☐ Gall Bladder Disease
- ☐ Glaucoma
- ☐ Goiter
- ☐ Gonorrhea
- ☐ Gout
- ☐ Heart Disease
- ☐ Hepatitis
- ☐ Hernia

- ☐ Herpes
- ☐ High Cholesterol
- ☐ HIV Positive
- ☐ Kidney Disease
- ☐ Liver Disease
- ☐ Measles
- ☐ Migraine Headaches
- ☐ Miscarriage
- ☐ Mononucleosis
- ☐ Multiple Sclerosis
- ☐ Mumps
- ☐ Pacemaker
- ☐ Pneumonia

- ☐ Polio
- ☐ Prostate Problem
- ☐ Psychiatric Care
- ☐ Rheumatic Fever
- ☐ Scarlet Fever
- ☐ Stroke
- ☐ Suicide Attempt
- ☐ Thyroid Problems
- ☐ Tonsillitis
- ☐ Tuberculosis
- ☐ Typhoid Fever
- ☐ Ulcers
- ☐ Vaginal Infections
- ☐ Venereal Disease

CONFIDENTIAL HEALTH HISTORY

HOSPITALIZATIONS

Year	Hospital	Reason for Hospitalization and Outcome

Have you ever had a blood transfusion? ☐ Yes ☐ No
If yes, please give approximate dates: _____

OCCUPATIONAL CONCERNS Check (✓) if your work exposes you to the following:	**HEALTH HABITS** Check (✓) which substances you use and indicate how much you use per day/week.	**PREGNANCY HISTORY**		
		Year of Birth	Sex of Birth	Complications if any
☐ Stress	☐ Caffeine			
☐ Hazardous Substances	☐ Tobacco			
☐ Heavy Lifting	☐ Drugs			
☐ Other	☐ Alcohol			

SERIOUS ILLNESS/INJURIES	DATE	OUTCOME

FAMILY HISTORY Fill in health information about your family.

Relation	Age	State of Health	Age at Death	Cause of Death	Check (✓) if your blood relatives had any of the following Disease	Relationship to you
Father					☐ Arthritis, Gout	
Mother					☐ Asthma, Hay Fever	
Brothers					☐ Cancer	
					☐ Chemical Dependency	
					☐ Diabetes	
					☐ Heart Disease, Strokes	
Sisters					☐ High Blood Pressure	
					☐ Kidney Disease	
					☐ Tuberculosis	
					☐ Other	

I certify that the above information is correct to the best of my knowledge. I will not hold my doctor or any members of his/her staff responsible for any errors or ommisions that I may have made in the completion of this form.

_____   _____
Signature   Date

_____   _____
Reviewed By   Date

CASE STUDY

Yvonne Black is a new patient of Dr. Esposito's at Inner City Health Care. Yvonne is an 88-year-old Italian-born woman who comes to the doctor at the urging of her granddaughter, Kristine, who accompanies her to the clinic. Yvonne's primary care provider has just retired after being her family doctor for over 35 years, and she requested Dr. Esposito because he is of Italian descent. Yvonne has many health problems and wants to describe each of them in great detail, making the intake interview complicated and difficult to perform. To add to the challenge, she is a poor historian when relating dates and events and does not always agree with the records obtained from her former doctor. This upsets Kristine, who wants to correct her, and they end up arguing.

CASE STUDY REVIEW QUESTIONS

1. What communication skills will Liz, the CMA (AAMA), need to get the most accurate information from Yvonne?

_____

_____

_____

_____

_____

_____

_____

_____

_____

2. What can the manner in which the patient relates the information reveal about her?

_____

_____

_____

_____

_____

3. What effect does Kristine have on the process of getting intake information for the patient? Is Kristine helpful or disruptive? What can you do and say to direct the conversation most effectively and efficiently?

_____

_____

_____

_____

_____

_____

CHAPTER POST-TEST

Perform this test without looking at your book. If an answer is "false," rewrite the sentence to make it true.

1. True or False? To "diagnose" means to predict the outcome of a disease or condition.

   _____

   _____

2. True or False? Objective statements can be described as "opinion."

   _____

   _____

3. When a patient "denies" something, he or she is:

   a. just whining

   b. not being truthful

   c. explaining his or her symptoms

   d. trying to blame someone else

4. True or False? Once a medical assistant has asked a patient whether he or she has any allergies, and the information has been recorded, the medical assistant needs to keep asking that patient at every office visit.

   _____

   _____

5. True or False? If a disease is familial, that means it has a pattern of occurring within families and blood relations.

   _____

   _____

SELF-ASSESSMENT

Think about your own personal experiences when answering the following questions. Be as self-reflective as you can.

1. When you are asked to complete a Medical History form, what are some of the emotions that you experience? Do you dread the work (especially if you aren't feeling well)? Are you concerned that you will not know all the answers, have all the dates and numbers, and so on? Are you frustrated because you have filled out so many forms already? Are you ever embarrassed by some of the questions? Do you feel guilty that you will not answer some of the questions honestly? Do you feel stupid if you do not understand all the questions? Do you feel hindered because you did not bring your glasses or you have a sprained wrist or are too sick to fill out the form? Think of other feelings you have that are not listed here.

   _____

   _____

   _____

2. Whenever a patient sees a new doctor or has not been in to the doctor for a while, or even on a periodic basis, a new Medical History form needs to be filled out. There is always paperwork to complete. Can you think of a better/easier/more efficient way to update patient information? Could computers make the job easier? What do you think will happen in the future?

_____

_____

_____

3. Remember your feelings when you ask your patients to fill out the Medical History forms, and be sensitive to their needs. How might you assist them, without dedicating time away from your other duties?

_____

_____

_____

_____

_____

_____

C H A P T E R **24**

Vital Signs and Measurements

CHAPTER PRE-TEST

Perform this test without looking at your book. If an answer is "false," rewrite the sentence to make it true.

1. True or False? Patient weight is measured only to determine how much fat the patient has.

_____

_____

2. True or False? A normal pulse rate is between 60 and 120 beats per minute for adults.

_____

_____

3. True or False? A normal respiration rate for adults is between 12 and 20 breaths per minute.

_____

_____

4. True or False? Blood pressure is the amount of pressure the blood exerts on the inside of veins.

_____

_____

5. True or False? High blood pressure is also called hypertension.

_____

_____

6. True or False? High blood pressure is always caused by inactivity and diet.

_____

_____

VOCABULARY BUILDER

Misspelled Words

Find the words below that are misspelled; underline them, and correctly spell them in the space provided. Then, fill in the blanks below with the appropriate terms from the list.

apnea	emphasema	hypotention
arhythmia	eupnea	orthopnia
baseline	frenulum	rhonchi
bradycardia	hyperpnea	strider
bradypnea	hypertension	systolic
dyspnea	hyperventilation	wheese

_____   _____   _____

_____   _____   _____

1. Tiffany comes to the office of Drs. Lewis and King reporting that she cannot breathe well when she lies down. Joe Guerrero, CMA (AAMA), notes _____ in her chart.

2. Winston Lewis, MD, warns his patient, Herb, that he is in the early stages of _____, a chronic pulmonary condition that causes destruction of the air sacs in the lungs, caused by his smoking.

3. Liz Corbin, CMA (AAMA), writes _____ in Carolyn's chart after she counts her respirations at 45 breaths per minute.

4. Wanda Slawson, CMA (AAMA), is taking Edith's temperature orally and is careful to insert the digital thermometer under her tongue, next to the _____.

5. Marissa is rushed in to see Dr. King after swallowing a coin. Dr. King can clearly hear a crowing _____ whenever the toddler tries to inhale. This indicates to the doctor that the coin is lodged in the upper airway.

6. At a scheduled examination, Lenny's pulse is recorded at 40 beats per minute. This is called _____ in medical terms.

7. Ludmilla has cut her hand and arrives at the Inner City Health Care clinic in an anxious state. She says she is feeling tingly and lightheaded. Bruce Goldman, CMA (AAMA), notes that her respiratory rate is 35 and that Ludmilla is taking deep, rapid breaths. Bruce suspects _____ and calmly has her breathe slowly into her cupped hands until the tingling goes away.

8. Wanda Slawson, CMA (AAMA), can hear a deep snoring sound in the patient's throat when he measures Leo's respirations. This sound is described as _____.

9. Jim's blood pressure is a high 180/98. The number 180 is called the _____ pressure.

10. Dr. Lewis takes careful note of Mr. Marshall's 160/100 blood pressure reading and discusses with him the dangers of _____ and the possible need for lifestyle changes and possible medication to control this condition.

11. Keisha's breathing is noticeably labored at one of her well-child checkups. Joe Guerrero, CMA (AAMA), notes this as _____ in her chart.

12. Three-year-old Chris has had a somewhat persistent chest cold for weeks but has a high-pitched _____ when he exhales, leading Dr. Lewis to consider asthma as a diagnosis.

13. Kareem has normal respirations. This could be described in the chart notes as _____.

14. Liping's breath sounds are normal, but her respiration rate is very slow, only 8 to 9 breaths a minute. This _____ worries Liz Corbin, CMA (AAMA), so she alerts Dr. King immediately.

15. While checking Robert's pulse, Joe Guerrero, CMA (AAMA), notices an obvious irregularity in the pulse. This is known as an _____.

16. When Jamar shares that his wife sometimes stops breathing in her sleep for a couple of minutes, Dr. Lewis becomes concerned that she might be experiencing _____ and recommends that a sleep study be performed.

17. Juanita's resting blood pressure is 60/44. This is _____, and Dr. Rice is concerned about this being a side effect of the prescribed medication Juanita is taking.

18. Dr. Susan Rice orders an ECG on her patient Rebecca, just as a _____ for future reference.

LEARNING REVIEW

Short Answer

1. Temperature, pulse, respiration, and blood pressure are collectively referred to as

_____

_____

2. How is heat produced within the body? What part of the brain maintains the balance between heat production and heat loss? What are ways the body cools itself in hot weather and heats itself in cold weather?

_____

_____

_____

_____

3. List the five ways in which the body loses heat next to each example below.

   a. Ellen climbs into a cold bed.   _____

   b. Anara enjoys her aerobic workout, which causes her to sweat.   _____

   c. On a trip to New York, Richard attends a live studio performance
      where the temperature in the room was kept at about 58 degrees. _____

   d. Christine uses a portable fan when she is working as a seamstress and
      all the sewing machines and irons tend to make the room too warm. _____

   e. Liz performs daily yoga breathing exercises.   _____

4. What is another word for fever?

_____

_____

5. Explain the differences in the patterns of fevers in the list below.

   Remittent:

_____

_____

   Intermittent:

_____

_____

Continuous:

_____

_____

6. Circle the correct words to complete the sentences: A(n) (increase/decrease) in temperature may be caused by several factors, such as eating, medications that increase metabolism, exercise, bacterial infections and exposure to heat, pregnancy, stress, and age. A(n) (increase/decrease) in body temperature may result from fasting, inactivity, medications that decrease metabolism, exposure to cold, and age.

7. An aural temperature is taken where?

_____

_____

8. Write the normal ranges of blood pressures for the following age groups:

   Child, age 10   _____

   Adolescent, age 16   _____

   Adult   _____

9. Define the following terms and explain what each factor has to do with blood pressure and how each affects the pressure.

   Blood volume:

_____

_____

_____

   Elasticity of arterial walls:

_____

_____

_____

_____

   Lumen of the arteries (peripheral resistance):

_____

_____

_____

_____

_____

   Strength of the heart muscle:

_____

_____

_____

_____

   Viscosity of the blood:

_____

_____

_____

10. List four other factors that influence blood pressure that are not listed in Question 9.

_____

_____

11. What is the name of the various sounds sometimes heard during blood pressure measurement?

_____

_____

12. When measuring blood pressure, it is important to not allow the gauge to move faster than

_____

_____

13. List five types of hypertension and explain each type, whether it is curable, and what its treatment(s) and caus(es) are. Then give an example of each.

Type   **Description and Example**

_____   _____

                               _____

                               _____

                               _____

_____   _____

                               _____

                               _____

                               _____

_____   _____

                               _____

                               _____

                               _____

_____   _____

                               _____

_____   _____

14. List and explain three possible causes of hypotension.

_____

_____

_____

_____

_____

_____

15. A very rapid pulse rate is described medically as _____.

16. A very slow pulse rate is described medically as _____.

17. The medical term meaning difficulty and/or painful breathing is _____.

18. Write the normal pulse ranges for the following age groups:

    Birth   _____

    Infants   _____

    Child, age 1 year   _____

    Child, age 7–14 years   _____

    Adult   _____

19. Identify the name of each common pulse site described below and match the site to its proper location on the body in the figure below by placing the correct letter in the space provided.

    a. The site most commonly used for BP reading: _____

    b. The site for blood pressure measurements in the leg: _____

    c. The site commonly used for infant pulse rates: _____

    d. The site used in emergencies and when performing cardiopulmonary resuscitation (CPR): _____

    e. The site used to check for circulation in the lower limbs: _____

    f. The most commonly used site to measure pulse: _____

    g. The site used in an emergency to control bleeding in the leg: _____

20. List and define four characteristics of the pulse.

_____

_____

_____

_____

21. Write the normal range of respiratory rates for each of the following ages.

    Infant   _____

    Child, age 1–7 years   _____

    Adult   _____

22. List and define three characteristics of respiration.

_____

_____

_____

CERTIFICATION REVIEW

These questions are designed to mimic the certification examination. Select the best response.

1. Which of the following is *not* a routine body measurement?

    a. Chest circumference

    b. Head circumference

    c. Ankle circumference

    d. Height

2. In converting inches to feet, which of the following is true?

    a. 62 inches is 5 feet, 2 inches

    b. 62 inches is 6 feet, 2 inches

    c. 62 inches is 6 feet exactly

    d. 62 inches is 5 feet 6 inches

3. When converting Fahrenheit to Celsius, which of the following is the correct formula?

    a. Fahrenheit temperature minus 32 multiplied by 5/9

    b. Fahrenheit temperature multiplied by 5/9 minus 32

    c. Fahrenheit temperature plus 32 multiplied by 5/9

    d. Fahrenheit temperature multiplied by 9/5 plus 32

4. What is considered a normal pulse and respiration rate for an adult?

    a. Pulse of 76, respiration of 20

    b. Pulse of 80, respiration of 18

    c. Pulse of 56, respiration of 16

    d. Pulse of 20, respiration of 60

    e. Both a. and b. are correct.

5. Which of the following is *not* a requirement in order to obtain accurate blood pressure?

   a. The cuff should be the proper size.

   b. The cuff should be placed correctly over the radial artery.

   c. The arm should be above heart level.

   d. The deflation should not be faster than 2 mm/degrees per heartbeat.

   e. The patient should be seated with feet on the floor and back supported.

6. A pulse obtained at the intersection of the fifth intercostal space at the mid-clavicular line on the left chest is called the:

   a. femoral pulse

   b. temporal pulse

   c. brachial pulse

   d. apical pulse

7. Malignant hypertension:

   a. is borderline

   b. is below normal

   c. is life threatening

   d. spreads to other parts of the body

LEARNING APPLICATION

Charting Exercises

Chart the following patient vital signs in the corresponding paper chart record below:

1. On January 4, 20XX you checked Ludmilla in for her office visit at 2:30 PM. Her height was 64 inches, and she weighed 145 pounds. Her temperature taken orally was 99.2 degrees Fahrenheit. You took her pulse rate and respiration rate for 30 seconds and they were 44 and 10, respectively. Her blood pressure measured in her right arm while she was sitting down was 146 over 68. (Be sure to initial your charting.)

_____

_____

2. On March 22nd, you checked Abigail in for her checkup at 10:30 AM. Her height was 66½ inches and she weighed 212 pounds. Her temperature taken orally was 97.8 degrees Fahrenheit, her pulse rate was 90 and irregular twice within 60 seconds. Her respiration rate was 15 in 30 seconds and she was breathing with difficulty. Her blood pressure measured in her right arm while she was sitting down was 190 over 94. You notified Dr. King of her pulse and respirations and stayed with the patient to observe her. (Be sure to initial your charting.)

_____

_____

_____

Hands-on Activities

Perform the following exercises and then measure your pulse and respirations. Chart the measurements in the spaces provided using proper documentation.

1. After three minutes of rest, sitting in a chair with your feet flat on the floor

_____

_____

2. After three minutes of marching in place at a comfortable rate

_____

_____

3. After three minutes of strong aerobic exercise such as jumping jacks or jogging in place

_____

_____

4. Note the variations in the characteristics of your pulse and respirations as you moved from rest to strong activity. Calculate the ratio of respiration to pulse for your resting, active, and aerobic rates listed earlier. Show your results below.

Resting   _____

            _____

Active   _____

            _____

Aerobic   _____

            _____

CASE STUDY 1

Wayne lives near Inner City Health Care in a group home for developmentally delayed adults. Wayne has a history of frequent colds and ear infections. He visits the clinic one morning with pain in both ears. He is also drinking a cup of hot coffee.

CASE STUDY REVIEW QUESTIONS

1. What method would Wanda, the CMA (AAMA), use to take Wayne's temperature?

_____

_____

_____

_____

2. How might Wanda explain to Wayne why she is using the axillary method?

_____

_____

_____

CASE STUDY 2

Henry, who is 4 years old, is rushed to Inner City Health Care. He is bleeding profusely from a cut on his head. "He fell down the stairs," sobs his mother, Juanita. Henry does not seem to be fully conscious and appears confused. Dr. James Whitney attends to Henry's laceration, applying direct pressure on the cut to stop the bleeding. He directs clinical assistant Bruce Goldman to call 911 for emergency services. Then Bruce takes Henry's pulse. "What are you doing?" Juanita asks Bruce. "Why doesn't he wake up?"

CASE STUDY REVIEW QUESTIONS

1. What site would Bruce use to take Henry's pulse?

2. How might Bruce answer Juanita's questions about what he is doing?

CASE STUDY 3

Abigail, who suffers from many problems related to her advanced age, also has type II diabetes. She is very friendly and has a good rapport with everyone in the clinic—all of whom she says are "just like family"—and she is very eager to please the staff. One winter day she comes to the clinic complaining of flu symptoms. When clinical assistant Audrey asks Abigail to step onto the scale to get her weight, Abigail says, "Oh, do we have to? I just don't feel up to it right now."

CASE STUDY REVIEW QUESTION

1. How might Audrey explain to Abigail about why her weight is important at every visit?

CHAPTER POST-TEST

1. True or False? Patient weight is measured sometimes to determine how much fluid the patient is retaining.

_____

_____

2. True or False? A normal pulse rate is between 80 and 100 for adults.

_____

_____

3. True or False? A normal respiration rate is between 16 and 20 for adults.

_____

_____

4. True or False? Blood pressure is the amount of pressure that is exerted on the inside of the arteries.

_____

_____

5. True or False? High blood pressure is also called hypotension.

_____

_____

6. High blood pressure can be lowered by regular exercise, dietary changes, losing weight, and medications.

_____

_____

SELF-ASSESSMENT

As you respond to the following questions, think of how your experiences will affect how you treat your patients.

1. Think of the last time you had your height and weight measured. Did you have enough privacy to make you comfortable?

_____

_____

_____

_____

_____

_____

_____

_____

_____

_____

_____

2. When you had your blood pressure taken, did the medical assistant share your measurements with you? Did you feel comfortable asking questions?

_____

_____

_____

_____

3. Has any health care provider ever discussed any of your vital signs or body measurements with you? Have you been informed of the health factors related to your vital signs or body measurements?

_____

_____

_____

_____

4. Do you still have mercury thermometers in your home? If so, call the health department to find out where you can take them for disposal and then obtain an electronic or digital thermometer for future use at home. How do you think your patients will feel when you encourage them to do the same? Write out exactly what you will say to them to convince them of the importance of replacing all mercury thermometers with a safer alternative. Explain mercury poisoning to them.

_____

_____

_____

_____

_____

_____

_____

_____

_____

CHAPTER **25**

The Physical Examination

CHAPTER PRE-TEST

Perform this test without looking at your book.

1. *(Circle the correct answer)* Palpation/Palpitation is when the patient can feel his or her heartbeat.

2. Which of the following is *not* a method used during a physical examination?

   a. Percussion

   b. Menstruation

   c. Manipulation

   d. Auscultation

3. Which is a component of a routine physical examination?

   a. What the patient looks like

   b. How the patient walks

   c. Whether the patient has bad breath

   d. All of the above

4. Which of the following is *not* a position used in physical examinations of patients?

   a. Lithotomy

   b. Supine

   c. Dorsal recumbent

   d. Reverse Trendelenburg

5. Choose the correct spelling of the instrument used to examine the inside of the eyeball.

   a. Opthalmoscope

   b. Optomescope

   c. Ophthalmoscope

   d. Otoscope

VOCABULARY BUILDER

Misspelled Words

Find the words below that are misspelled; circle them, and correctly spell them in the spaces provided. Then identify the correct vocabulary terms most appropriate for each example below from a patient's physical examination.

ataxia	labirynthitis	symmetry
bruits	pallor	tinnitus
cyanosis	piorrhea	vertigo
jaundice	schleroderma	vertiligo

_____   _____

_____   _____

1. During a physical examination of Louise Kipperley, a 48-year-old woman, Dr. Esposito notices that Louise's facial skin has become tight and atrophied, suggesting possible _____.

2. Leo McKay comes to Inner City Health Care with mouth pain. Dr. Reynolds examines Leo's mouth and discovers _____, which is discharge of pus from the gums around the teeth.

3. Medical assistant Liz Corbin observes the gait of Geraldine Potter, a 36-year-old woman diagnosed with multiple sclerosis. Geraldine's gait is lurching and unsteady, with her feet widely placed. Liz charts this as _____.

4. Annette Samuels is diagnosed with hepatitis B virus (HBV) by Dr. John Pettit. Among Annette's symptoms, noted by Dr. Pettit during the physical examination, was _____, a distinct yellowing of Annette's skin and the whites of her eyes.

5. Lenny Taylor, an older adult man with Alzheimer's disease, is brought to Inner City Health Care by his son George. Apparently, Lenny has had problems breathing. Dr. Whitney observes _____, a bluish color in Lenny's skin.

6. After performing a routine venipuncture procedure on patient Rhoda Au, Bruce Goldman, CMA (AAMA), notices that all color has drained from Rhoda's face. He assumes that her _____ is due to a psychological reaction to the venipuncture, so he has her lie down on the examination table for a few minutes until her color improves.

7. Abigail Johnson's 28-year-old granddaughter Lucy comes in for an examination with Dr. King after observing white patches of depigmentation, or _____, on her hand. "Is this what Michael Jackson had?" she asks Dr. King.

8. While performing a complete physical examination on patient Rowena Lawrence, Dr. King listens for abnormal sounds, or _____, from vital organs while auscultating her abdomen.

9. During a routine physical examination of Lenore McDonnell, a young woman confined to a wheelchair, Dr. Lewis checks for balance or _____ of size, shape, and position of body parts on opposite sides of her body.

10. Mary Tice comes in to see Dr King for ringing in her ears. Dr. King asks her if she is taking large doses of aspirin, which can cause _____.

11. Rowena Lawrence's 6-year-old daughter, Felicia, diagnosed with a case of the mumps, returns with her mother for a reexamination with Dr. Lewis when the child experiences a sensation that the room is spinning, caused by inflammation of the labyrinth, called _____.

12. While her blood was being taken, Susan O'Donnell described the room as spinning and felt lightheaded. This _____ quickly passes in a few minutes.

LEARNING REVIEW

Matching

Match the correct method of examination used by a physician in Column A to the entry in Column B that best describes it.

Column A

_____ 1. Auscultation

_____ 2. Observation or inspection

_____ 3. Manipulation

_____ 4. Mensuration

_____ 5. Percussion

Column B

A. On his physical examination of Charles Williams, Dr. Winston Lewis looks at the patient to assess his general health, posture, body movements, skin, mannerisms, and care in grooming while verbally reviewing Charles's medical history with him.

B. Dr. Mark Woo uses a stethoscope to listen to the bowel sounds that accompany peristalsis.

C. Dr. King performs range of motion exercises on patient Margaret Thomas, who is suspected of having Parkinson's disease.

D. Dr. Rice taps Edith Leonard's chest to feel and hear the hollow quality expected from clear lungs.

E. During Marissa O'Keefe's well-baby visit, chest and head circumference measurements are recorded in the patient's medical record.

Short Answer

1. For each procedure listed below, identify the most likely examination position that will be required during the physician's examination. Use a medical encyclopedia for reference, if necessary.

Examination   **Position**

a. Urinary catheterization   _____

b. Auscultation for audible bowel sounds that are a normal part of the digestive process   _____

c. Colposcopy to observe the cervix under magnified illumination for evidence of precancerous cells, followed by a cone biopsy for laboratory analysis   _____

d. Internal hemorrhoids are examined through the use of a proctoscope   _____

e. Percutaneous renal biopsy to aid in diagnosis of suspected glomerulonephritis   _____

f. An ECG is performed on an older adult woman with angina pectoris   _____

g. A variation of this position is used for patients experiencing shock   _____

h. Proctoscopy to investigate a suspected case of proctitis, inflammation of the rectum   _____

2. Identify each entry below as a piece of medical equipment (ME), a laboratory procedure (LP), a body part (BP), or a patient illness or condition (PI). Then identify the correct component or sequence of the physical examination to which the entry relates. The first two entries have been completed for you as an example.

A. Sphygmomanometer   ME   Vital signs

B. Aphonia   PI   Speech

C. Lymph nodes   _____   _____

D. Edema   _____   _____

E. Anal fissures   _____   _____

F. Emphysema   _____   _____

G. Pharyngeal mirrors   _____   _____

H. Scrotum   _____   _____

I. Areola   _____   _____

J. Electrocardiography   _____   _____

K. Kyphosis   _____   _____

L. Dysphasia   _____   _____

M. Urinalysis   _____   _____

N. Achilles tendon   _____   _____

O. Tympanic membrane   _____   _____

3. Symmetry would be noted by using what method of assessment?

_____

4. What is another term for the supine position or the position assumed when lying face up?

_____

5. *(Circle the correct answer)* Orthostatic hypotension occurs as blood pressure decreases/increases/normalizes.

6. What is the preferred position for administration of an enema or rectal suppositories?

_____

7. Determining the amount of flexion and extension of a patient's extremities would be which form of assessment?

_____

Image Identification

Identify each of the positions shown in the photos below.

A.

_____

B.

_____

C.

_____

D.

_____

E.

_____

F.

_____

G.

_____

CERTIFICATION REVIEW

These questions are designed to mimic the certification examination. Select the best response.

1. A patient having an examination of the abdomen should be placed in which position?

   a. Supine

   b. Prone

   c. Lithotomy

   d. Sims'

2. Listening to the patient's chest as he or she breathes is called:

a. auscultation

b. percussion

c. inspection

d. palpation

3. The process of inspection is also called:

a. percussion

b. measuration

c. observation

d. palpitations

4. Which of the following is *not* a piece of equipment needed in the examination room?

a. Goose-neck lamp

b. Mayo tray

c. Biohazard waste container

d. Adjustable stool

5. Which of the following is *not* a word used to describe skin color?

a. Jaundice

b. Cyanosis

c. Bruits

d. Pallor

LEARNING APPLICATION

Role-Play Exercises

Using the list of patient positions from the book, practice placing your classmates into the various positions for examination. Pay special attention to knee and back problems and any physical limitations patients may have.

CASE STUDY

Kristine Bolt brings her young son Christopher to Inner City Health Care with a suspected case of mumps, which his older sister is just recovering from. As Bruce Goldman, CMA (AAMA), helps the child remove his shirt for the examination, Ian becomes increasingly fearful and begins to cry. Kristine's gentle reprimand to get him to relax is not working. It is obvious the child is feverish and not feeling well.

CASE STUDY REVIEW QUESTIONS

1. What can Bruce do to calm Christopher and make him more comfortable?

   _____

   _____

   _____

   _____

   _____

   _____

2. What should Bruce's therapeutic response be?

   _____

   _____

   _____

   _____

   _____

   _____

CHAPTER POST-TEST

Perform this test without looking at your book.

1. Fill in the blank: _____ is when the physician feels the patient's abdomen.

2. Which of the following is *not* a method used during a physical examination?

   a. Percussion

   b. Manipulation

   c. Auscultation

   d. Symmetry

3. Which is *not* a component of a routine physical examination?

   a. What the patient looks like

   b. How the patient walks

   c. Whether the patient has bad breath

   d. The patient's test results

4. Which of the following is *not* a position used in physical examinations of patients?

   a. Lithotomy

   b. Reverse Trendelenburg

   c. Prone

   d. Dorsal recumbent

5. Choose the correct spelling of the instrument used to examine the inside of the eyeball.

   a. Opthalmoscope

   b. Ophthalmoscope

   c. Optalmascope

   d. Otoscope

SELF-ASSESSMENT

Think about the last time you went to the doctor. As you answer the following questions and remember your personal experience(s), think about how your experience(s) will affect the way you treat your patients in the future. If you have no personal experiences, try to imagine how you would feel and react.

1. Did you have to undress at all? How did that feel? Did you get cold or feel a bit awkward?

   _____

   _____

   _____

   _____

2. When you had your blood pressure taken, did the cuff cause pain or discomfort as it got tighter? Did you say something to the medical assistant? Do you think most people speak up when they are uncomfortable?

   _____

   _____

   _____

   _____

3. Have you ever noticed a sick patient in a public place? What were the clues that told you the patient was sick? Do you think your skills of observation will be enhanced after you complete this chapter?

   _____

   _____

   _____

   _____

Obstetrics and Gynecology

CHAPTER PRE-TEST

Perform this test without looking at your book. If an answer is "false," rewrite the sentence to make it true.

1. True or False? Obstetrics is the branch of medicine that concerns management of pregnancy, childbirth, and the puerperium, whereas gynecology is the study of the diseases of female reproductive organs.

   _____

   _____

2. Which of the following are addressed during the initial prenatal visit and examination?

   a. Genetic diseases/conditions in the family

   b. Kidney and heart diseases/conditions and diabetes

   c. Nutritional deficiencies

   d. All of the above

3. During pregnancy, which of the following is potentially dangerous?

   a. Rapid weight gain

   b. Visual changes

   c. Hypertension

   d. Chill, fever

   e. All of the above

4. True or False? It is recommended that pelvic examinations and Pap smears be performed on all women no later than 21 years of age (or at the onset of sexual activity).

   _____

   _____

5. True or False? Because the provider will perform a breast examination during the annual physical, it is not important for women to perform breast self-examinations on themselves.

   _____

   _____

6. The Pap smear is designed to detect which type of cancer?

a. Cervical

b. Vaginal

c. Ovarian

d. All of the above

e. a. and b. only

VOCABULARY BUILDER

Misspelled Words

Find the words below that are misspelled; circle them, and correctly spell them in the spaces provided. Then fill in the blanks in the following sentences with the correct vocabulary terms from the list.

abortion	gestation	parturation
Braxton-Hicks	gonorrhea	pelvic inflammatory disease
cervical punch biopsy	human papillomavirus	placenta abruption
delation	hysterosalpingogram	placenta previa
dismenorrhea	lochia	preeclampsia
dyspareunia	multigravida	sickle cell anemia
ectopic	neonatal	Tay-Sachs
effacement	nullipara	trichomoniasis

_____   _____   _____

1. Discharge from the uterus of blood, mucus, and tissue during the period after childbirth is called
   _____.

2. The period of development from conception to birth is called _____.

3. Any pregnancy that occurs outside of the uterus is called _____.

4. A _____ is a visual examination of vaginal and cervical tissues using a type of microscope with a magnifying lens and powerful lights.

5. _____ is an infection of the uterus, fallopian tubes, and adjacent pelvic structures.

6. A term that means "painful menses" is _____.

7. _____ occurs when the placenta implants itself low in the uterus and partially or completely covers the cervical os.

8. _____ is the term given to a woman who has not carried a pregnancy to birth.

9. Two types of sexually transmitted diseases are _____, which is caused by bacteria, and _____, which is caused by a virus.

10. _____ is an invasion of a protozoa, often transmitted through sexual contact.

Spelling Review

Choose the correctly spelled words in each row.

1. puerperium   purperium   puerpurium
2. La Maz   Lamaze   Lamase
3. eeclampsia   eclampsia   eclamsia
4. amneocentesis   amniocentisis   amniocentesis
5. coposcopy   colposcapy   colposcopy
6. cryosurgery   criosurgery   crysurgery
7. primogravida   primigravida   Primegravida

LEARNING REVIEW

Matching

Match each female condition or disease in Column A to its description in Column B.

Column A

_____ 1. PID

_____ 2. Menopause

_____ 3. Endometriosis

_____ 4. Ovarian cancer

_____ 5. Ovarian cysts

_____ 6. Dysmenorrhea

Column B

A. Malignant cells found in the ovaries

B. Painful menstruation

C. The end of menstruation

D. Inflammatory disease of the pelvis involving some or all of the reproductive organs

E. Painful condition characterized by endometrial cells adhering to tissues and organs outside of the uterus

F. Cysts located on the ovaries

Labeling

Identify each part of the female reproductive system below. Describe each part and its function in the spaces provided. Use your medical dictionary if needed.

Part	Description and Function
1. _____	_____
	_____
	_____
	_____
	_____
	_____
2. _____	_____
	_____
3. _____	_____
	_____
4. _____	_____
_____	_____
	_____
5. _____	_____
	_____
	_____
	_____
	_____
6. _____	_____
	_____
	_____
7. _____	_____
	_____
8. _____	_____
	_____
9. _____	_____
	_____

Short Answer

1. The obstetric history includes the total number of pregnancies and the number of live births. For each history, give the number of pregnancies and the number of live births.

Obstetric History	Pregnancies	Live Births	Abortions
A. Gravida 2 Para 1 Abortion 1	_____	_____	_____
B. Gravida 6 Para 4 Abortion 2	_____	_____	_____
C. Gravida 3 Para 1 Abortion 2	_____	_____	_____

2. What branch of medicine treats the mother and fetus through all stages of labor, delivery, and postpartum?

_____

_____

3. List at least two signs/symptoms of preeclampsia.

_____

_____

4. A potentially life-threatening disorder during pregnancy that is characterized by hypertension, edema, and proteinuria and may put both mother and fetus in danger is known as what? _____

5. Breast self-examination should be performed at least once every _____.

6. The gynecologic disease in which an infection is caused by a microorganism that may lead to infertility or ectopic pregnancy if not treated is _____.

7. Describe the six types of abortion (interruptions of pregnancy).

_____

_____

_____

_____

_____

_____

_____

8. Fill in the Description, Symptom(s), and Treatment(s) columns below that correspond to the complications of pregnancy listed in the table.

Complication	Description	Symptom(s)	Treatment(s)
Eclampsia			
Preeclampsia			
Gestational diabetes			
Hyperemesis gravidarum			

Placenta
previa
    _____ _____ _____

    _____ _____ _____

    _____ _____ _____

    _____ _____ _____

    _____ _____ _____

    _____ _____ _____

Placenta
abruptio
    _____ _____ _____

    _____ _____ _____

    _____ _____ _____

    _____ _____ _____

    _____ _____ _____

CERTIFICATION REVIEW

These questions are designed to mimic the certification examination. Select the best response.

1. Which of the following are types of abortions?

   a. Spontaneous, complete, incomplete, interrupted, medical

   b. Miscarriage, threatened, induced, voluntary, medical

   c. Induced, spontaneous, postpartum, complete, medical

   d. Complete, threatened, incomplete, induced, missed, spontaneous

   e. Interrupted, complete, induced, medical, voluntary

2. During a prenatal visit, the urine is tested for which two substances?

   a. Drugs, including alcohol, and glucose

   b. Infection and glucose

   c. Glucose and protein

   d. Bilirubin and protein

3. Which of the following is *not* a routine test/procedure performed on pregnant women?

   a. Ultrasound

   b. Amniocentesis

   c. Chorionic villi sampling

   d. Alpha-fetoprotein

   e. Colonoscopy

4. LMP means:

  a. localized medical practices

  b. last menstrual period

  c. localized menstrual pain

  d. limited medical plan

  e. last medical prenatal (examination)

5. A prenatal condition that causes sudden weight gain, an increase in blood pressure, and proteinuria is called:

  a. Rh incompatibility

  b. preeclampsia

  c. hyperemesis gravidarum

  d. gestational diabetes

  e. a. and b.

6. A painful condition characterized by tissue from inside of the uterus adhering to the organs outside the uterus is called:

  a. preeclampsia

  b. endometriosis

  c. metrometriosis

  d. menopause

  e. pelvic inflammatory disease

7. Bartholin glands:

  a. contain mucus for lubrication of the vagina

  b. can become inflamed and infected

  c. are situated on both sides of the vaginal orifice

  d. are similar to the male's Cowper's glands

  e. All of the above

8. Chlamydia, condylomata, HIV, and gonorrhea are all:

  a. complications of pregnancy

  b. diagnosed during the Pap smear and pelvic examination

  c. sexually transmitted

  d. curable

  e. diagnosed through blood tests

LEARNING APPLICATION

CASE STUDY

CASE STUDY REVIEW QUESTION

1. In the office, the provider instructs you that a Pap smear and pelvic examination will be performed on Ms. Smith in Room 1. Describe your role in assisting with these procedures.

_____

_____

_____

_____

_____

_____

_____

CHAPTER POST-TEST

Perform this test without looking at your book. If an answer is "false," rewrite the sentence to make it true.

1. True or False? Obstetrics has to do with female issues, and gynecology has to do with pregnancy.

_____

_____

2. Which of the following are addressed during the initial prenatal visit and examination?

   a. Genetic diseases/conditions in the family

   b. Kidney and heart diseases/conditions and diabetes

   c. Nutritional deficiencies

   d. All of the above

3. During pregnancy, which of the following is potentially dangerous?

   a. Rapid weight gain

   b. Visual changes

   c. Hypertension

   d. Chill, fever

   e. All of the above

4. True or False? It is recommended that pelvic examinations and Pap smears be performed on all women older than 25 years (or at the onset of sexual activity) on an annual basis.

_____

_____

5. True or False? Even though the provider will perform a breast examination during the annual physical, it is still important for women to perform breast self-examinations on themselves.

_____

_____

6. The Pap smear is designed to detect which type of cancer?

   a. Cervical

   b. Ovarian

   c. Vaginal

   d. Breast

   e. All of the above

   f. a. and c. only

SELF-ASSESSMENT

Think about the last time you went to your provider for an examination. As you answer the following questions and remember your personal experiences, think about how your experiences will affect the way you treat your patients in the future. If you have no personal experiences, try to imagine how you would feel and react. All of the following situations may be discussed in small groups with your classmates.

1. Which questions were you asked the last time you went to your provider for a pelvic examination? Try to think of five.

   _____

   _____

   _____

   _____

2. When the provider came into the room, were you dressed and in the examination room? Were you undressed and sitting on the examination table? Were you undressed and lying down? Were you undressed and lying down in the lithotomy position? Which of the previous scenarios would make you the most comfortable? Which would make you the most uncomfortable?

   _____

   _____

   _____

3. How comfortable are you with discussing private information with your provider? How about with your medical assistant? Are you more comfortable with one or the other? Why do you suppose you would be?

   _____

   _____

   _____

CHAPTER **27**

Pediatrics

CHAPTER PRE-TEST

Perform this test without looking at your book. If an answer is "false," rewrite the sentence to make it true.

1. True or False? Pediatrics is the branch of medicine that cares for newborns, infants, children, and adolescents.

_____

_____

2. Toddlers are:

   a. children from birth to 2 years old

   b. children from about 1 to about 3 years old

   c. children from the time they are able to walk until they are in kindergarten

   d. children from about 2 to 5 years old

3. True or False? Measurements of newborn infants consist of length, weight, chest circumference, and head circumference.

_____

_____

4. Normal childhood immunizations include which of the following?

   a. DTaP, MMR, Hib, and HIV

   b. Tetanus, DTaP, MMR, and IPV

   c. IPV, MMR, DTaP, Hib, and HBV

   d. HBV, Hib, pertussis, and HAV

   e. Both c. and d.

5. The preferred site for injections for a child younger than 2 years is:

   a. the vastus lateralis

   b. the gluteus medius

   c. the deltoid

   d. Any of the above is acceptable.

6. Normal pulse and respiration for an 8-year-old child is:

   a. pulse of 80, respiration of 30

   b. pulse of 80, respiration of 12

   c. pulse of 120, respiration of 20

   d. pulse of 86, respiration of 18

   e. none of the above

VOCABULARY BUILDER

Misspelled Words

Find the words below that are misspelled; circle them, and then correctly spell them in the spaces provided.

blood preasure   myringotomy   phynelketonuria
circumfrence   pediatrics   tonsilitis
fontanelle   pediculosis   vacination

_____   _____   _____

_____   _____

Definitions

Define the following vocabulary terms.

1. Exudate _____

   _____

2. Myringotomy _____

   _____

3. Suppurative _____

   _____

4. Tympanostomy _____

   _____

5. Otitis media _____

   _____

6. Tonsillitis _____

   _____

7. Pediculosis _____

   _____

LEARNING REVIEW

Short Answer

1. Mary O'Keefe has called for an emergency appointment with Dr. King for her 3-year-old son, Chris, who awakened during the night with a high fever and severe pain in his right ear, which is draining. Ellen Armstrong, CMA (AAMA), must prepare the examination room for the patient. Based on Chris's symptoms, what equipment will Ellen want to assemble for Dr. King's physical examination of Chris? List the equipment in the order it will most likely be used in the examination.

_____

_____

_____

_____

2. When Mary O'Keefe arrives with her son, Ellen takes them to examination room 2 and prepares the patient for Dr. King's physical examination. Ellen takes and records the child's vital signs: T 102.1°F (Ax); P 115 (AP) bounding, sinus arrhythmia; R 28; 76/42/0, rt. arm, sitting. Ellen tells Mary that Dr. King will be examining Chris's ear and may want to take some laboratory tests.

   A. What method did Ellen use to take Chris's temperature?

   _____

   _____

   _____

   B. What method did Ellen use to measure Chris's pulse? Where on the body is this measured?

   _____

   _____

   _____

   C. Are Chris's vital signs normal?

   _____

   _____

   _____

   _____

   _____

   _____

   _____

   _____

   D. Chris is fussy and disagreeable, but not uncooperative, while Ellen takes his vital signs. What can a medical assistant do to facilitate the measurement of a fussy child's vital signs?

   _____

   _____

   _____

   _____

   _____

3. Ellen assists Dr. King with the physical examination of the patient. After assessing the vital sign measurements taken by the medical assistant, Dr. King examines Chris's ear and lungs. A swab of fluid discharge is taken from the patient's ear. What is the role of the medical assistant during the provider's examination of this patient?

_____

_____

_____

_____

_____

_____

_____

4. Dr. King makes a clinical diagnosis of otitis media for this patient and orders laboratory testing to be performed on the patient's specimen. What criteria are necessary for a provider to make a clinical diagnosis?

_____

_____

_____

_____

_____

5. What is otitis media? Why are children more likely at risk for this condition? How is otitis media commonly treated? What patient education can the health care team offer? (Consult a medical reference or encyclopedia for help in answering this question.)

_____

_____

_____

_____

_____

_____

_____

_____

CERTIFICATION REVIEW

These questions are designed to mimic the certification examination. Select the best response.

1. The head circumference of a newborn should range between:

    a. 12.5 and 14.5 inches

    b. 14.5 and 16.5 inches

    c. 16.5 and 18.5 inches

    d. 18.5 and 20.5 inches

2. The axillary temperature is taken in the:

   a. rectum

   b. mouth

   c. armpit

   d. ear

3. The respiratory rate of a 1-year-old child should range between _____ breaths per minute.

   a. 20 and 30

   b. 20 and 40

   c. 16 and 20

   d. 12 and 20

4. Otitis media is:

   a. an inflammation of the middle ear

   b. an infestation of parasitic lice

   c. a spasm of the bronchi

   d. an infection of the tonsils

LEARNING APPLICATION

CASE STUDY

The following is a true story of a young boy (about 8 years of age) who came in to the office with testicular torsion. This is when the testicle twists on its cord and often becomes ischemic, resulting in tissue death. The surgeon needs to explore the area to determine if the testicle can be saved or if it needs to be removed. The testicle is usually quite swollen and tender. When the child was told that he needed to go to the surgery center and that the doctor would take care of his problem and make him feel better, he began to cry. He was inconsolable. Why do you think he was so upset? Here are some options to discuss with fellow classmates:

1. He was afraid of the pain.

2. He was afraid of the surgery.

3. He was embarrassed.

4. Other?

CASE STUDY REVIEW QUESTION

1. Discuss what you could do as a medical assistant to help the boy and his parents with all of the above possible scenarios. The reason the child was afraid might surprise you and reminds us all to be careful not to assume we know what a patient is thinking.

   _____

   _____

   _____

   _____

CHAPTER POST-TEST

Perform this test without looking at your book. If an answer is "false," rewrite the sentence to make it true.

1. True or False? Pediatrics is the practice of medicine with children from birth through age 14.

   _____

   _____

2. Toddlers are children from:

   a. about 1 to 3 years old

   b. birth to 2 years old

   c. the time they are able to walk until they are in kindergarten

   d. about 2 to 5 years old

3. True or False? Measurements of babies consist of chest circumference, head circumference, length, and weight.

   _____

   _____

4. Normal childhood immunizations include which of the following?

   a. MMR, tetanus, DTaP, and IPV

   b. Hib, DTaP, MMR, and HIV

   c. IPV, MMR, DTaP, Hib, and HBV

   d. HBV, Hib, pertussis, and HAV

   e. Both c. and d.

5. The preferred site for injections for a child younger than 2 years is:

   a. the vastus lateralis

   b. the gluteus medius

   c. the deltoid

   d. Any of the above sites is acceptable.

6. Normal pulse and respiration for a child who is 8 years old is:

   a. respiration of 30, pulse of 80

   b. respiration of 18, pulse of 86

   c. respiration of 12, pulse of 80

   d. respiration of 20, pulse of 120

   e. none of the above

SELF-ASSESSMENT

As you respond to the following questions, think of how your experiences will affect how you treat your patients.

1. Think of your first memory of going to the doctor's office or getting any medical treatment. Think of how you felt from what you can remember. You may have more than one vivid memory, or you may have to think really hard to come up with any memories. Maybe your memories are not from a hospital or doctor's office; that is, maybe you received medical care from your parents, grandparents, or a neighbor. Your memories might not be exactly accurate, but they are a child's perception, and the feelings are real. This awareness can help you interact well with your young patients. Circle all of the words from the following list that come to mind as you take this mental journey back in time (if you have more than one incident to remember, use different colored inks to circle the words). You may even add a couple of your own descriptors if necessary.

helpless	pain	invaded
embarrassed	guilty	angry
alone	afraid of being punished	afraid of what was happening
afraid of pain	happy with the attention	dizzy
relieved	loved	powerless
excited	safe	afraid of the blood
stupid	other: _____	other: _____

Each of our memories will be different, and we will all have different feelings about them. Try to keep this in mind as you treat your young patients. Try to respect what feelings they have and strive to make them comfortable. Reassure them as much as you can.

_____

_____

_____

_____

CHAPTER **2 8**

Male Reproductive System

CHAPTER PRE-TEST

Perform this test without looking at your book. If an answer is "false," rewrite the sentence to make it true.

1. The most common disease afflicting men older than 50 years is:

   a. prostate cancer

   b. benign prostatic hypertrophy (BPH)

   c. epididymitis

   d. testicular cancer

2. ED stands for:

   a. erectile disorder

   b. erectile dysfunction

   c. elemental disease

   d. epididymal disorder

3. Which of the following is *not* a sexually transmitted disease (STD) that afflicts men?

   a. Genital herpes

   b. Chlamydia

   c. Gonorrhea

   d. Epididymis

4. Vasectomy consists of:

   a. dissection of the seminal vesicles

   b. dissection of the vas deferens

   c. dissection of the testicles

   d. removal of the epididymis

5. True or False? Because of the latest discoveries in medications, ED can always be cured.

   _____

   _____

VOCABULARY BUILDER

Misspelled Words and Definitions

Find the words in Column A below that are misspelled; circle them, and correctly spell them in the space provided. Then match the following correct vocabulary terms listed in Column A with their corresponding definitions listed in Column B.

Column A	Correct Spelling	Column B
____ 1. Chriptorchidism	_____	A. Urine held in the bladder; inability to empty the bladder
____ 2. Intervenous pyelogram	_____	
____ 3. Orchectomy	_____	B. Amount of urine remaining in bladder immediately after voiding; seen with hyperplasia of prostate
____ 4. Residual	_____	
____ 5. Retention	_____	C. Undescended testicle
____ 6. Transluminator	_____	D. X-ray of the kidneys, ureter, and bladder using a contrast medium
____ 7. Transureteral resection	_____	
		E. Instrument used to inspect a cavity or organ by passing a light through the walls
		F. Removal of prostate tissue using a device inserted through the urethra
		G. Surgical excision of a testicle

LEARNING REVIEW

Short Answer

1. Identify each part of the male reproductive system below. Describe each part and its function in the space provided. Then, using the textbook, a medical dictionary, or the Internet, list at least one common disorder that would adversely affect the part described.

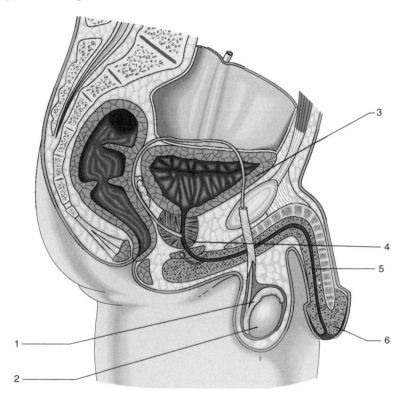

	Part	**Common Disorder(s)**
1.	_____	_____
2.	_____	_____
3.	_____	_____
4.	_____	_____
5.	_____	_____
6.	_____	_____

2. List at least two symptoms of a benign hypertrophic prostate gland.

_____

_____

_____

3. The third leading cause of cancer deaths among men is _____.

4. Name at least two sexually transmitted diseases.

_____

_____

5. PSA tests should be performed _____ beginning at age 40.

CERTIFICATION REVIEW

These questions are designed to mimic the certification examination. Select the best response.

1. Testicular cancer is one of the leading causes of death in men younger than:

   a. 25

   b. 60

   c. 40

   d. 50

2. Male individuals from the onset of puberty should examine their testicles every:

   a. 6 months

   b. year

   c. month

   d. 3 months

3. BPH is a condition of the prostate. It stands for:

   a. benign prostatic hypertrophy

   b. benign prostatic hyperplasia

   c. beginning prostate hyperactivity

   d. benign prostate hyperactivity

4. The best way to determine that a patient has prostate cancer is by a(n):

   a. biopsy of the prostate

   b. PSA blood test

   c. rectal examination

   d. X-ray

5. Which of the following STDs is *not* treated with antibiotics?

   a. Chlamydia

   b. Gonorrhea

   c. Syphilis

   d. Genital herpes

   e. None of the above

LEARNING APPLICATION

○ CASE STUDY

CASE STUDY REVIEW QUESTION

1. Mr. Jones, a 75-year-old patient, has just been diagnosed with prostatic cancer. The provider has explained what is to be expected, but Mr. Jones is upset and asks you for your help in understanding the disease and treatment. How will you help him?

_____

_____

_____

_____

_____

_____

_____

CHAPTER POST-TEST

Perform this test without looking at your book.

1. In men older than 50 years, a common disease condition is:

   a. prostate cancer

   b. BPH

   c. epididymitis

   d. testicular cancer

2. ED stands for:

   a. erectile dysfunction

   b. erectile disorder

   c. erectile disease

   d. epididymal disorder

3. Which of the following is an STD that can afflict men?

   a. Chlamydia

   b. Balanitis

   c. Peyronie's

   d. Epididymis

4. The dissection of the vas deferens is called a:

   a. vas-deferenectomy

   b. vasotomy

   c. vasectomy

   d. deferenectomy

SELF-ASSESSMENT

How do you think you will feel when assisting with a genitourinary examination or procedure on a male patient? Do you think it will be easier if the patient is much younger or much older than you are? Do you think older medical assistants feel more comfortable assisting with these types of examinations, regardless of their professional experience? Do you think you will become more comfortable with time? Do you think your male patient is also uncomfortable? After giving these questions some thought, answer the following questions. Discuss your ideas with other students. Discuss your ideas with male friends, family members, or classmates to gain more perspectives.

1. Do you think your behavior or attitude will have anything to do with your patients' comfort level?

   _____

   _____

   _____

   _____

2. What might you do to make yourself more comfortable during a male genitourinary examination/procedure?

   _____

   _____

   _____

   _____

3. What might you do to make your patient more comfortable?

   _____

   _____

   _____

   _____

Name _____ Date _____ Score _____

Gerontology

CHAPTER PRE-TEST

Perform this test without looking at your book. If an answer is "false," rewrite the sentence to make it true.

1. True or False? Older adults are healthier today than they were a generation ago.

_____

_____

2. True or False? Chronic diseases are just a part of what will happen as we age.

_____

_____

3. True or False? To be old is to be sick, weak, and confused.

_____

_____

4. True or False? Every system in the body undergoes changes as people age.

_____

_____

5. True or False? The senses of sight, hearing, taste, and smell diminish with age.

_____

_____

VOCABULARY BUILDER

Misspelled Words and Definitions

Find the words in Column A below that are misspelled; circle them, and correctly spell them in the space provided. Then match the following correct vocabulary terms listed in Column A with their corresponding definitions listed in Column B.

Column A	Correct Spelling	Column B
____ 1. Arterialsclerosis	_____	A. The branch of medicine that is concerned with the problems of older adults
____ 2. Dementia	_____	B. Disease marked by degeneration of the macular area of the retina of the eye
____ 3. Geriatrics	_____	C. Progressive loss of hearing ability caused by the normal aging process
____ 4. Incontinance	_____	D. Temporary loss of blood to the brain, causing stroke-like symptoms
____ 5. Macular degeneration	_____	E. Urine remaining in the bladder after urination
____ 6. Pernicous anemia	_____	F. Loss of the ability to retain urine in the bladder
____ 7. Presbycusis	_____	G. Disorder involving the stomach that causes a deficiency of red blood cells
____ 8. Residule urine	_____	H. Decrease in cognitive abilities, especially memory impairment, often associated with Alzheimer's and Parkinson's diseases
____ 9. Transient ischemic attack	_____	I. Disease that leads to thickening, hardening, and loss of elasticity of the arteries

LEARNING REVIEW

True or False?

Tell whether each statement below is true or false. If an answer is "false," rewrite the sentence to make it true.

____ 1. When going over medications with geriatric patients, it is helpful for them to bring all their medications with them in their original containers.

_____

_____

____ 2. If you suggest memory joggers (such as use of a calendar for appointments and making lists) to your geriatric patients, you will insult their intelligence.

_____

_____

___ 3. Every system in the body is going to be affected by aging.

_____

_____

___ 4. Older adult patients have a heightened sense of pain compared with younger patients.

_____

_____

___ 5. True or False? There is not much a person can do to counteract the effects of aging.

_____

_____

Short Answer

1. List at least five ways to improve communication with the geriatric patient.

_____

_____

_____

_____

_____

_____

_____

_____

_____

2. Why is gerontology becoming more recognized?

_____

_____

3. Why does food become less appealing as one ages, often decreasing the desire to eat and causing weight loss?

_____

_____

_____

4. Fill in the chart below, listing two problems that might occur with each system as people age. **The first row has been filled out as an example for you.**

A. Vision and hearing	Dry, red, irritated eyes; sensitivity to light; inability to see clearly; inability to tell colors apart; inability to see small print; loss of hearing
B. Taste and smell	_____ _____
C. Integumentary system	_____ _____

D. Nervous system

_____

_____

_____

_____

E. Musculoskeletal system

_____

_____

_____

F. Respiratory system

_____

_____

G. Cardiovascular system

_____

_____

_____

_____

H. Gastrointestinal system

_____

_____

_____

I. Urinary system

_____

_____

_____

J. Reproductive system

_____

_____

_____

CERTIFICATION REVIEW

These questions are designed to mimic the certification examination. Select the best response.

1. When giving instructions to older adults, it is always a good idea to *(circle all that apply)*:

   a. speak really loud

   b. write them in large print

   c. have patients repeat the instructions back to you if you think they did not understand completely

   d. a. and b.

   e. a., b., and c.

2. Dementia can include:

   a. memory loss

   b. confusion

   c. depression and agitation

   d. all of the above

3. The nervous system is affected by aging, resulting in all of the following *except*:

  a. insomnia

  b. problems with balance

  c. increased pain sensation

  d. problems with temperature regulation

4. The buildup of plaque in blood vessels is called:

  a. incontinence

  b. heart attack

  c. arteriosclerosis

  d. cardiopulmonary dysfunction

5. The progressive loss of hearing ability caused by the normal aging process is called:

  a. senility

  b. presbycusis

  c. deafness

  d. audio deficiency

LEARNING APPLICATION

CASE STUDY 1

CASE STUDY REVIEW QUESTION

1. Sam Jones, 84 years old, has been examined by the provider and is ready to leave the office. Mr. Jones tells you that he is having trouble remembering to take the many medications the doctor has given him. As a medical assistant, what can you do to help him remember to take his medication?

_____

_____

_____

_____

_____

CASE STUDY 2

CASE STUDY REVIEW QUESTION

1. Sandy Jones, granddaughter of Sam Jones, has come to the office with her grandfather. She tells you that she is concerned because of her grandfather's recent weight loss. She shares with you that he is not eating well. Mr. Jones is 84 and lives alone. How will you respond to Sandy? Can you think of some suggestions for them?

_____

_____

_____

_____

_____

_____

_____

_____

_____

_____

_____

_____

CHAPTER POST-TEST

Perform this test without looking at your book. If an answer is "false," rewrite the sentence to make it true.

1. True or False? Older adults are less healthy today than they were a generation ago.

_____

_____

2. True or False? Chronic diseases do not have to be a normal part of aging.

_____

_____

3. True or False? Memory loss is Alzheimer's.

_____

_____

4. True or False? Few changes occur as people age.

_____

_____

5. True or False? As people age, their senses of sight, hearing, taste, and smell diminish.

_____

_____

6. True or False? There is much a person can do to counteract the effects of aging.

_____

_____

SELF-ASSESSMENT

Without looking in the textbook, list 15 adjectives that describe older adults. Then list 15 adjectives that describe young adults. As you make your list, consider your personal biases toward older adults. Consider the differences in the two lists and think of why you chose those descriptors. When you are finished, discuss your lists with classmates. Share stories about people in your lives who are extraordinarily healthy and happy as they age. Think about the prejudices and assumptions you carry toward aging patients. Try to remember these as you work with those patients. It might be a good idea to create a list of tips to remember about geriatrics and keep it posted by your workstation.

_____

_____

_____

_____

C H A P T E R **30**

Examinations and Procedures of Body Systems

CHAPTER PRE-TEST

Perform this test without looking at your book. If an answer is "false," rewrite the sentence to make it true.

1. True or False? Urinary catheterization is performed only in hospitals during surgeries.

   _____

   _____

2. True or False? Instillation and irrigation mean the same thing.

   _____

   _____

3. An upper GI series (barium swallow) is used to examine the:

   a. entire large intestine

   b. stomach and entire small intestine

   c. esophagus, stomach and part of the small intestine

   d. esophagus, stomach, and small and large intestines

4. True or False? To test visual acuity, the patient must be able to recognize the letters of the English alphabet.

   _____

   _____

5. Medical assistants cannot remove casts.

   _____

   _____

6. True or False? Pulse oximetry is a way of counting the pulse at the wrist to determine the heart rate.

   _____

   _____

VOCABULARY BUILDER

Misspelled Words I

Find the words below that are misspelled; circle them, and correctly spell them in the spaces provided. Then fill in the blanks in the sentences below with the correct vocabulary terms listed below with their proper definitions.

alveoli	biopsy	comedome
aphasia	bronchi	demyelination
aurical	carbuncle	erythemia

_____   _____   _____

1. A _____ is an inflammation of the skin and deeper tissues that terminates in slough and suppuration.

2. _____ is a form of macula showing diffused redness of the skin.

3. Destruction or removal of the myelin sheath is _____.

4. The _____ are the two main branches leading from the trachea to the lungs.

5. The provider obtains a representative tissue sample for microscopic examination during a _____.

6. _____ is the absence or impairment of the ability to communicate through speech.

7. _____ are air sacs in the lungs.

8. The typical small lesion of acne vulgaris is _____.

9. The _____ is the portion of the external ear that is not connected to the head.

Misspelled Words II

Find the words in Column A that are misspelled; circle them, and then correctly spell them in the spaces provided. Then match each of the correct vocabulary terms listed below with its proper definition.

	Column A	Correct Spelling	Column B
___	1. Akinesia	_____	A. A device for producing a fine spray
___	2. Vescicle	_____	B. A device used to close or obstruct an eye
___	3. Spirometer	_____	C. A wound, an injury, or any pathologic change in body tissue
___	4. Ossicle	_____	D. A device for examining the interior of the eye
___	5. Opthalmoscope	_____	E. A collection of urine in the renal pelvis caused by obstructed outflow forming a cyst by distention or atrophy
___	6. Ocluder	_____	F. Small raised skin lesion containing fluid
___	7. Obturator	_____	G. A small bone such as the malleus, incus, and stapes
___	8. Nebulizer	_____	H. A manner of walking
___	9. Lesion	_____	I. A device used to close or block a canal, vessel, or passage of the body
___	10. Hydronephrosis	_____	J. Complete or partial loss of muscle movement
___	11. Gate	_____	K. An instrument used to measure and record the volume of inhaled and exhaled air

LEARNING REVIEW

Multiple Choice

1. Common symptoms of urinary tract diseases and disorders are:

   a. dysuria, proteinuria, hematuria, and frequency

   b. dysuria, frequency, oliguria, and headache

   c. hematuria, pain, frequency, and headache

   d. frequency, hematuria, vaginal discharge, and dysuria

2. Cystitis is another name for what disorder?

   a. Kidney cysts

   b. Gallbladder disease

   c. Multiple cysts of the breasts or other area

   d. Bladder inflammation

3. UTI means:

   a. urinary tract infection

   b. urinary tract inflammation

   c. urinary tract involvement

   d. urinary treatment initiated

4. The medical term meaning "hidden" is:

   a. cult

   b. occult

   c. crypt

   d. retro

5. Which of the following is(are) an eating disorder(s)?

   a. Bulimia

   b. Anorexia nervosa

   c. Diverticulosis

   d. Crohn's disease

   e. a. and b.

6. The medical condition of having an increase in intraocular pressure is called:

   a. glaucoma

   b. retinal detachment

   c. cataract

   d. macular degeneration

7. Ear lavage or irrigation is performed for:

   a. impacted sebum

   b. impacted cerumen

   c. impacted lacrimal glands

   d. otitis media

8. The leading cause of blindness in the United States is:

   a. retinal detachment

   b. cataract

   c. glaucoma

   d. diabetes

9. A cholecystectogram is a test for:

   a. kidney stones

   b. diseases of the gallbladder

   c. diseases of the blood vessels

   d. gastrointestinal disorders

10. Which of the following is not determined by a chest radiograph?

    a. Bronchitis

    b. Pneumonia

    c. Pharyngitis

    d. Tuberculosis

11. Coronary artery bypass surgery might be used to help prevent which of the following cardiovascular conditions?

    a. Myocardial infarction

    b. Pericarditis

    c. Thrombophlebitis

    d. Coronary artery disease

12. Which of the following cardiovascular diseases may be treated with antibiotics?

    a. Thrombophlebitis

    b. Pericarditis

    c. Angina pectoris

    d. Valve stenosis

13. Which of the following diseases is caused by a lack of dopamine?

    a. Epilepsy

    b. Depression

    c. Reye's syndrome

    d. Parkinson's disease

14. Shingles is a type of:

    a. herpes

    b. psoriasis

    c. dermatitis

    d. acne

15. The type of disease in which the white blood cells become prolific is:

    a. anemia

    b. infectious mononucleosis

    c. leukemia

    d. lymphedema

Labeling

1. Identify the parts of the digestive system.

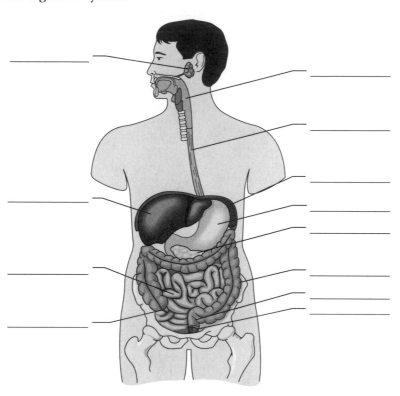

2. Identify the parts of the eye.

3. Identify the parts of the ear.

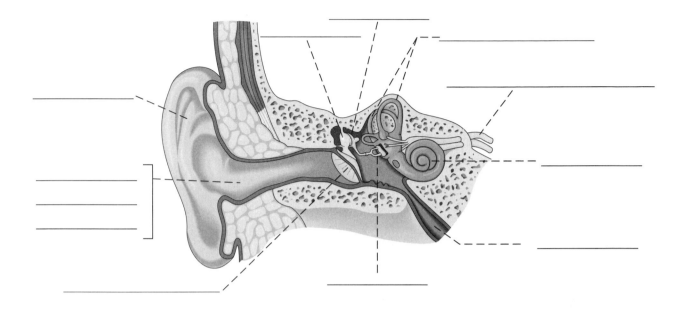

CERTIFICATION REVIEW

These questions are designed to mimic the certification examination. Select the best response.

1. Bacteria that reach the urinary tract through the blood cause _____ infection.

   a. homogenous

   b. hematogenous

   c. ascending

   d. descending

2. High levels of nitrogenous waste in the blood may result in:

   a. polyuria

   b. oliguria

   c. uremia

   d. pyuria

3. A sigmoidoscopy is a diagnostic examination of:

   a. the inner ear

   b. the bladder

   c. a part of the colon

   d. the eye

4. Guaiac slides are used to detect:

   a. occult blood in the stool

   b. the type of bacteria found in otitis media

   c. thrush of the mucous membranes of the mouth

   d. cholelithiasis

5. A diagnostic test done to determine the presence of stones, duct obstruction, or inflammation of the gall-bladder is called a:

   a. barium enema

   b. barium swallow

   c. cholecystogram

   d. gastroscopy

LEARNING APPLICATION

C A S E   S T U D Y

CASE STUDY REVIEW QUESTIONS

1. While visiting with family members, your elderly aunt shares with you that she has noticed that her stools are black. This has been happening off and on for several months and now she says her "belly feels swollen" and she is constipated a lot, which is not normal for her. How will you respond?

   _____

   _____

   _____

2. Your aunt becomes alarmed and says she is afraid of what they will do to her; maybe she will need surgery, and she cannot leave her husband alone, and what if it is cancer. She obviously has many concerns and is quite worried. How can you assist her?

   _____

   _____

   _____

   _____

   _____

   _____

   _____

   _____

CHAPTER POST-TEST

Perform this test without looking at your book. If an answer is "false," rewrite the sentence to make it true.

1. True or False? Urinary catheterization often is performed in clinics, hospitals, and surgery centers.

_____

_____

2. True or False? Instillation and irrigation are different procedures.

_____

_____

3. An upper GI series (barium swallow) is used to examine:

   a. the esophagus, the stomach, and the small and large intestines

   b. both the small and the large intestine

   c. the stomach and the entire small intestine

   d. the esophagus, stomach and part of the small intestine

4. True or False? To test visual acuity, the patient does not need to recognize the letters of the English alphabet.

_____

_____

5. True or False? Medical assistants often remove casts.

_____

_____

6. True or False? Pulse oximetry is used to determine the oxygen concentration of the blood in a noninvasive way.

_____

_____

SELF-ASSESSMENT

Think of a time when you or a close family member had to go to the provider's office and then go through a diagnostic procedure or test for a medical disorder or a disease. Fill in the following outline with as much information as you can remember.

1. What were the patient's symptoms? Try to list two or three.

_____

_____

_____

_____

_____

2. Describe how the disease started. (Suddenly? Gradually? Over time? Related to an injury?)

_____

_____

_____

_____

3. Did the patient go to the emergency department or to the provider's office first?

_____

_____

_____

_____

4. Did the provider, or his or her staff, clearly explain the test or procedure to the patient or the patient's family?

_____

_____

_____

_____

5. What were some of the feelings that you had during the process? List two or three.

_____

_____

_____

_____

6. Could the medical assistant and doctor have reassured you better or kept you better informed, or did they do a good job of answering your questions and meeting your needs and the needs of the patient?

_____

_____

_____

_____

7. How will your experience influence your interaction with your patients when you are assisting with a diagnostic test or procedure? What will you pay special attention to that you might not have if you had not had the experience described above?

_____

_____

_____

_____

C H A P T E R **3 1**

Assisting with Office/ Ambulatory Surgery

CHAPTER PRE-TEST

Perform this test without looking at your book. If an answer is "false," rewrite the sentence to make it true.

1. True or False? The anesthesia used in ambulatory care surgery is different from anesthesia used in major surgeries.

   _____

   _____

2. True or False? "Dressing" and "bandage" are different words that mean the same thing.

   _____

   _____

3. True or False? "Inflammation" means infection.

   _____

   _____

4. The signs of inflammation are:

   a. redness, drainage, pain, and swelling

   b. redness, pain, and swelling

   c. redness, pain, swelling, and tenderness

   d. redness, pain, swelling, and warmth

5. True or False? A sterile item is free from all microorganisms and their spores.

   _____

   _____

6. True or False? Only major surgeries require the patient to sign an informed consent form.

   _____

   _____

VOCABULARY BUILDER

Misspelled Words

Find the words in Column A that are misspelled; circle them, and correctly spell them in the spaces provided. Then match each of the vocabulary terms below with the correct definition in Column B.

	Column A	Correct Spelling	Column B
____	1. Inflamation	_____	A. The trade name for povidone-iodine, a topical anti-infective
____	2. Ephinephrine	_____	
____	3. Ligature	_____	B. A toxic preparation important as a germicide and local astringent
____	4. Sodium hydroxide	_____	
____	5. Hibeclens®	_____	C. Partial or complete loss of sensation, with or without loss of consciousness
____	6. Anestesia	_____	D. A hormone secreted by the adrenal medulla in response to stimulation of the sympathetic nervous system; used in conjunction with a local anesthetic. It constricts blood vessels to help lessen bleeding during ambulatory surgery.
____	7. Betadine	_____	
____	8. Silver nitrate	_____	
____	9. Isopryl alcohol	_____	
____	10. Hydrogen proxide	_____	
____	11. Strictures	_____	E. A condition free from germs, infection, and any form of life
____	12. Tetnus	_____	
____	13. Surgical asepsis	_____	F. A narrowing or constriction of the lumen of a tube, duct, or hollow organ

G. Trade name for chlorhexidine gluconate, a topical antiseptic

H. A thread or wire for tying a blood vessel or other structure to constrict or fasten it

I. The nonspecific immune response that occurs in reaction to any type of bodily injury

J. NaOH, a caustic antacid used in detergents and other chemical compounds

K. An acute infectious disease of the central nervous system (CNS) caused by an exotoxin

L. A clean, flammable liquid used in medical preparations for external use

M. Used in aqueous solution as a mild antiseptic, germicide, and cleansing agent

Definitions

Match the vocabulary words below with their correct definitions.

＿＿＿	1. Allergies	＿＿＿	9. Informed consent
＿＿＿	2. Antibacterial	＿＿＿	10. Liquid nitrogen
＿＿＿	3. Approximate	＿＿＿	11. Mayo stand/instrument tray
＿＿＿	4. Bandage	＿＿＿	12. Ratchets
＿＿＿	5. Cautery	＿＿＿	13. Surgery cards/computer
＿＿＿	6. Contamination	＿＿＿	14. Suture
＿＿＿	7. Dressings	＿＿＿	15. Swaged/atraumatic
＿＿＿	8. Infection		

A. To bring together the edges of a wound

B. A written reference for surgeries and procedures

C. Gauze or other material applied directly to a wound to absorb secretions and for protection

D. A surgical needle is attached to a length of suture material

E. Surgical material or thread; may describe the act of sewing with the surgical material and needle

F. Being sensitive to a normally harmless substance that causes an autoimmune reaction

G. An invasion of pathogens into living tissue

H. A voluntary agreement to have a procedure or surgery after a patient has been informed about the risks and benefits

I. A portable metal tray table used for setting up a sterile field for minor surgery and procedures

J. Capable of destroying bacteria

K. Commonly and incorrectly referred to as "dry ice"; a volatile freezing agent used to destroy unwanted tissue such as warts

L. The locking mechanisms on the handles of many surgical instruments

M. The destruction of tissue by burning

N. Gauze or other material applied over a dressing to protect and immobilize

O. To make something unclean, often used to describe a sterile area being made "unsterile" or exposing a clean area to a pathogenic substance

LEARNING REVIEW

True or False?

Identify each statement as true or false. If an answer is "false," rewrite the sentence to make it true.

＿＿＿ 1. Suture material may also be called ligature.

＿＿＿

＿＿＿

____ 2. The word *ligature* means "to tie."

_____

_____

____ 3. Tissue forceps have teeth; dressing forceps do not.

_____

_____

____ 4. Epinephrine causes blood vessels to dilate.

_____

_____

____ 5. Sterile technique is a term used interchangeably for surgical asepsis.

_____

_____

Short Answer

1. Identify each entry below as an example that follows strict sterile principles or in which the sterile area, field, or tray is contaminated. Write "sterile" or "contaminated" in the spaces provided. If the entry is "contaminated," write what was done to render it contaminated.

   A. Bruce Goldman, CMA (AAMA), collects used instruments handed to him by Dr. Mark Woo during a minor surgical procedure to excise an infected sebaceous cyst by placing the instruments in a separate container or area out of view of the patient.

   _____

   _____

   B. Ellen Armstrong, CMA (AAMA), sets up a sterile field for a minor surgical procedure. After setting up the field, she remembers that a sterile solution is required and leaves the room to obtain the solution to be poured into a sterile cup.

   _____

   _____

   _____

   C. Wanda Slawson, CMA (AAMA), removes a dressing from a wound on a patient's arm and reaches over the sterile field to discard the used dressing in a biohazard waste container she has placed on the other side of the sterile field that she set up for the procedure.

   _____

   _____

   _____

   D. Patient Edith Leonard will not stop talking and asking questions as Liz Corbin, CMA (AAMA), removes sutures from a small wound on Edith's arm sustained during a recent fall. The medical assistant is careful to time her responses to Edith so that she is not talking when she is working directly over the sterile field.

   _____

   _____

E. Anna Preciado, CMA (AAMA), applies sterile gloves in preparation to assist Dr. Lewis with a minor surgical procedure. During the procedure, she comforts the patient and assists the physician as required. When Anna's hands are not in use, she keeps them down at her sides, careful not to touch her gloved hands to her clothing or any other nonsterile item.

_____

_____

_____

_____

2. Living tissue surfaces, such as skin, cannot be sterilized. Name two examples of ways that skin can be rid of as many pathogens as possible before the use of a sterile covering.

_____

_____

_____

3. Identify and describe the most widely used method of sterilization in the ambulatory care setting.

_____

_____

_____

_____

_____

4. List six general rules that ensure proper sterilization when using an autoclave.

_____

_____

_____

_____

_____

_____

5. Identify the recommended requirements for effective sterilization in an autoclave.

Temperature   _____

Time for sterilization of unwrapped items   _____

Time for sterilization of loosely wrapped items   _____

Time for sterilization of tightly wrapped items   _____

Frequency of draining of water and cleaning of autoclave   _____

Matching I

Match the following equipment with the correct aseptic method. For each instrument or item below, identify the method used for proper asepsis: chemical disinfection (CD), chemical sterilization (CS), or steam sterilization (SS) in an autoclave.

_____ 1. Percussion hammer

_____ 2. Wrapped surgical instruments

_____ 3. Stethoscopes

_____ 4. Fiber-optic endoscopes

_____ 5. Countertops

_____ 6. Wheelchairs

_____ 7. Gynecologic instruments

_____ 8. Examination tables

Matching II

Identify each action that follows as an action appropriate to medical aseptic hand washing technique (MAH) or surgical aseptic hand washing technique (SAH).

_____ 1. Do not apply lotion.

_____ 2. Glove for sterility.

_____ 3. 1 minute duration

_____ 4. Hold hands up during washing and rinsing.

_____ 5. Apply lotion.

_____ 6. Wash hands, wrists, and forearms to the elbows.

_____ 7. Hold hands down during rinsing.

_____ 8. 3- to 6-minute duration

CERTIFICATION REVIEW

These questions are designed to mimic the certification examination. Select the best response.

1. Surgical instruments that have opposing cutting edges are classified as:

   a. hemostats

   b. probes

   c. scissors

   d. scalpels

2. Surgical instruments that have ratchets are used for:

   a. cutting

   b. clamping

   c. probing

   d. exploring

   e. opening

3. Thumb forceps may also be called:

   a. pickups

   b. towel clamps

   c. hemostats

   d. Allis forceps

4. The recommended temperature for effective sterilization in an autoclave is:

   a. 212°F

   b. 270°F

   c. 150°F

   d. 220°F

5. An acceptable border between a sterile and a nonsterile area is:

   a. 1 inch

   b. 2 inches

   c. 4 inches

   d. 5 inches

6. The preferred length for suture material because it is manageable yet long enough to complete most suture procedures is:

   a. 10 inches

   b. 8 inches

   c. 12 inches

   d. 18 inches

7. Suture material that is used when more time is needed for healing is coated with:

   a. magnesium

   b. chromium

   c. calcium

   d. iodine

8. Application of a caustic chemical or destructive heat that burns tissue is called:

   a. cryotherapy

   b. evisceration

   c. approximation

   d. cauterization

9. Mechanism located between the rings of the handles of surgical instruments that is used for locking the instrument is called the:

   a. serration

   b. box-lock

   c. ratchet

   d. probe

LEARNING APPLICATION

Preparing Surgical Packs

Pretend the areas outlined below are labels on surgical packs that you have just wrapped. Label them with the proper information.

a. Iris scissors and 4 × 4 gauze.

b. Needle driver and a #3 scalpel handle.

c. Thumb tissue forceps and a #3 scalpel handle.

CASE STUDY 1

Joyanna Evans, CMA (AAMA), is responsible for maintaining and cleaning the autoclave at Inner City Health Care. Because this equipment is used every day to sterilize instruments, Joyanna cleans the inner chamber of the autoclave daily. Once a week she gives the autoclave a thorough cleaning.

CASE STUDY REVIEW QUESTIONS

1. Describe Joyanna's daily cleaning procedure.

   _____

   _____

   _____

   _____

2. Describe Joyanna's weekly cleaning procedure.

   _____

   _____

   _____

   _____

   _____

   _____

3. Why is proper maintenance and cleaning of the autoclave important?

   _____

   _____

   _____

   _____

CASE STUDY 2

Joyanna works with a variety of instruments and supplies as she assists in ambulatory care surgery. Answer the following questions related to surgical instruments and supplies.

CASE STUDY REVIEW QUESTIONS

1. From the selection that follows, identify each instrument by name. In the spaces provided, give a brief description of each instrument's use.

Instrument	Instrument Name	Uses

continues

_____   _____
_____   _____
                           _____
                           _____
                           _____

_____   _____
_____   _____
                           _____
                           _____
                           _____
                           _____
                           _____
                           _____

_____   _____
_____   _____
                           _____
                           _____
                           _____
                           _____

_____   _____
_____   _____
                           _____
                           _____
                           _____

2. Joyanna will be removing stitches today. Which two instruments from above will she need for removing sutures?

_____

_____

_____

CHAPTER POST-TEST

Perform this test without looking at your book. If an answer is "false," rewrite the sentence to make it true.

1. True or False? Anesthetics used in ambulatory care surgery are different from anesthetics used in major surgeries.

_____

_____

2. True or False? Dressings and bandages differ in that bandages are sterile and dressings are not.

_____

_____

3. True or False? Inflamed wounds are always infected.

_____

_____

4. The cardinal signs of inflammation are:

    a. redness, pain, swelling, and tenderness

    b. redness, drainage, pain, and swelling

    c. redness, pain, and swelling

    d. redness, pain, swelling, and warmth

5. True or False? A sterile item is free from all viruses and their spores.

_____

_____

6. True or False? Patients are required to sign an informed consent form only if they are having major surgery.

_____

_____

7. True or False? Patients must be told, in writing, all the things that can go wrong in a surgery and what other options they have besides surgery.

_____

_____

SELF-ASSESSMENT

Think of a time when you or a family member experienced a surgical event. If you have not had a personal surgical experience, interview a friend or family member and gather answers to the following questions.

1. Did the doctor or his or her staff explain the procedure clearly?

_____

_____

_____

_____

2. Were your questions answered to your satisfaction?

_____

_____

_____

_____

3. What was of greatest concern to you (financial concerns, pain, recovery, results, etc.)?

_____

_____

_____

_____

4. Did the recovery go as expected?

_____

_____

_____

_____

5. Were the results what you expected?

_____

_____

_____

_____

6. What could have made the experience better?

_____

_____

_____

_____

Diagnostic Imaging

CHAPTER PRE-TEST

Perform this test without looking at your book. If an answer is "false," rewrite the sentence to make it true.

1. True or False? Medical assistants may perform limited radiograph procedures in all states.

   _____

   _____

2. True or False? X-rays for fractures require no special patient preparation.

   _____

   _____

3. True or False? Radiopaque means that X-rays cannot penetrate it.

   _____

   _____

4. True or False? Ultrasound uses no X-rays and can view organs while they are in motion.

   _____

   _____

5. MRI stands for:

   a. magnetic realistic imaging

   b. magnetic resonance imaging

   c. magnetic ray imaging

   d. magnetic radiologic imagining

6. True or False? Radiation as a treatment for tumors uses X-rays to kill cancer cells.

   _____

   _____

VOCABULARY BUILDER

Misspelled Words

Find the words below that are misspelled; circle them, and correctly spell them in the spaces provided. Then write the following correct vocabulary terms next to their corresponding definitions.

computerized tomography	magnetic resonance imaging	radialpaque
dosimeter	MRA	radiolucent
flat plate	noninvasive	transducer
flouroscopy	position emission tomography	

_____ _____ _____

_____

_____   1. Use of fluorescent screen that shows the images of objects inserted between the tube and the screen

_____   2. Sound waves emitted from its head during ultrasound

_____   3. A noninvasive procedure where the patient lies inside a cylinder-shaped machine, or an open-bore machine, in which there is an electromagnet

_____   4. A noninvasive procedure that uses a small amount of radiation and beams that produce a series of cross-sectional images

_____   5. A radiographic procedure using a computer and radioactive substance

_____   6. Term a structure is called if X-rays do not penetrate it.

_____   7. "Plain" films

_____   8. Small, badgelike device worn above the waist which measures the amount of X-ray a person is exposed to

_____   9. Not entering the body

_____ 10. Term a structure is called if X-rays penetrate it easily

_____ 11. MRI for arteries and veins

LEARNING REVIEW

Short Answer

1. Describe the positions used during X-rays and include the direction of the X-rays, if applicable.

Position	Description	Direction of X-rays
Anteroposterior view (AP)	_____	_____
	_____	_____
	_____	_____
Posteroanterior view (PA)	_____	_____
	_____	_____
	_____	_____

Lateral view   _____   _____

                                      _____   _____

                                      _____   _____

Right lateral view (RL)   _____   _____

                                      _____   _____

                                      _____   _____

Left lateral view (LL)   _____   _____

                                      _____   _____

                                      _____   _____

Oblique view   _____   _____

                                      _____   _____

                                      _____   _____

Supine view   _____   _____

                                      _____   _____

                                      _____   _____

Prone view   _____   _____

                                      _____   _____

                                      _____   _____

2. For each radiologic test listed below, explain the purpose of the test.

Test   **Purpose**

Angiography   _____

                            _____

Barium swallow   _____
(upper GI series)
                            _____

Barium enema   _____
(lower GI series)
                            _____

Cholangiography   _____

                            _____

Cholecystography   _____

                            _____

Cystography   _____

                            _____

Hysterosalpingography   _____

                            _____

Intravenous pyelography (IVP)

_____

_____

Mammography

_____

_____

Retrograde pyelography

_____

_____

3. Describe the patient preparation needed for each test: before, during, and after. *NOTE*: instructions to the following exams may differ depending on the facility and technology involved.

Test   **Patient Preparation**

Angiography

_____

_____

Barium swallow (upper GI series)

_____

_____

_____

_____

Barium enema (lower GI series)

_____

_____

_____

_____

_____

_____

_____

_____

_____

Cholangiography

_____

_____

_____

Cholecystography

_____

_____

_____

_____

Cystography

_____

_____

_____

Hysterosalpingography

_____

_____

_____

Intravenous pyelography (IVP)

_____

_____

_____

Mammography

_____

_____

_____

Retrograde pyelography

_____

_____

4. Why is exposure to radiation dangerous?

_____

_____

_____

5. What test is performed to study the colon for disease?

_____

_____

CERTIFICATION REVIEW

These questions are designed to mimic the certification examination. Select the best response.

1. If a patient needs to be NPO before a radiologic procedure and the patient drinks a glass of water 3 hours before the appointment, what must you do?

   a. Water is allowed but nothing else.

   b. The procedure will need to be rescheduled.

   c. The patient needs a clearer explanation of what NPO means.

   d. Three hours is long enough for the water to be through the patient's system.

   e. b. and c.

2. Possible side effects of radiation include:

   a. hair loss, weight loss, nausea, and diarrhea

   b. hair loss, nausea, dizziness, and diarrhea

   c. nausea and vomiting, inflammation of the mouth, and hair loss

   d. all of the above

3. Palliative means:

   a. relieving symptoms, as well as curing

   b. curing but not offering much relief of symptoms

   c. placebo, or an agent that does nothing but the patient thinks it helps

   d. agents, such as pain relievers, used to relieve or alleviate painful or uncomfortable symptoms but do not cure the condition

4. When storing and safeguarding radiographs:

   a. they must be protected from light, heat, and moisture

   b. the environment is of little concern; they are basically plastic and can be wiped clean

   c. they must be kept in a cool, dry place

   d. a. and c.

5. What part of the X-ray machine produces X-rays?

   a. The control panel

   b. The tube

   c. The table

   d. The particle beam

6. Diagnostic imaging:

   a. is accessible to all offices and hospitals

   b. is an inexpensive form of testing

   c. results are easy to read

   d. results can be stored on computer systems

CASE STUDY

You begin working in an office where X-ray procedures are done. The provider has informed you that he will teach you the procedure for taking X-rays. In your state, special education and licensure are needed for a medical assistant to perform X-ray procedures. You also notice that no one in the office wears a dosimeter, although all are near the X-ray room during the day. Lead aprons are also not used on patients during X-ray procedures.

CASE STUDY REVIEW QUESTION

1. How will you handle this situation?

   _____

   _____

   _____

   _____

   _____

   _____

   _____

CHAPTER POST-TEST

Perform this test without looking at your book. If an answer is "false," rewrite the sentence to make it true.

1. True or False? Medical assistants and other health care professionals may perform limited X-ray procedures in most states.

_____

_____

2. True or False? X-rays for fractures require special patient preparation.

_____

_____

3. True or False? Radiopaque means that X-rays can penetrate a body part.

_____

_____

4. True or False? Ultrasound uses X-rays and can view organs while they are in motion.

_____

_____

5. MRI stands for:

   a. magnetic realistic imaging

   b. machine for radiologic imagining

   c. magnetic resonance imaging

   d. magnetic ray imaging

6. True or False? Radiation as a treatment for malignant tumors uses X-rays and radiopharmaceuticals to kill cancer cells.

_____

_____

SELF-ASSESSMENT

As a clinical medical assistant, if you are taking X-rays or assisting with X-ray procedures, what protective measures would you take? Would the patient take the same precautions? Why would you need more precautions than the patient?

_____

_____

_____

_____

_____

C H A P T E R **3 3**

Rehabilitation and Therapeutic Modalities

CHAPTER PRE-TEST

Perform this test without looking at your book. If an answer is "false," rewrite the sentence to make it true.

1. True or False? To adduct is to move away from the midline.

_____

_____

2. True or False? Range of motion is measured in inches.

_____

_____

3. True or False? When lifting a heavy object, always bend from the waist and keep the object close to your body.

_____

_____

4. True or False? It helps to have patients put their arms around your neck when you lift them.

_____

_____

5. True or False? If a patient falls, you should protect his or her head, but otherwise, let the patient fall.

_____

_____

6. True or False? Medical assistants often perform range-of-motion exercises on patients in the office.

_____

_____

VOCABULARY BUILDER

Misspelled Words

Find the words below that are misspelled; circle them, and correctly spell them in the spaces provided. Then write the correct vocabulary terms next to the example below that best describes it.

activities of daily living	gait	range of motion
ambulation	gait belt	thermaltherapy
assistive devices	goniometer	ultrasound
atrophy	goniometry	vasoconstriction
body mechanics	hemaplegia	vasodialation
contractures	modality	
criotherapy	muscle testing	

_____   _____   _____

_____

_____   1. Patient Lenore McDonell, confined to a wheelchair since early childhood, receives continuing physical therapy to minimize the effects of any decrease of mobility and/or shrinkage of muscle tissue in her legs caused by inactivity.

_____   2. When examining a new patient, a physical therapist must determine which of the physical agents, such as heat, cold, light, water, and electricity, will be most beneficial in treating the patient's condition.

_____   3. As Margaret Thomas, diagnosed with Parkinson's disease, began to experience balance problems and difficulties in walking, her physical therapist prescribed the use of high-frequency sound waves to generate heat in the deep tissue of her right leg, producing a therapeutic effect.

_____   4. Cold applications may be used to constrict blood vessels to slow or stop the flow of blood to an area.

_____   5. Lenny Taylor, suffering the early stages of dementia from Alzheimer's disease, works with an occupational therapist to practice methods of making these everyday tasks easier to perform.

_____   6. Heat is a modality that creates a therapeutic effect by causing blood vessels to dilate, thereby increasing circulation to an area and accelerating the healing process.

_____   7. When construction worker Jaime VanBeek suffers a shoulder injury on the job, Dr. James Whitney performs this test for assessing the motion, strength, and task potential of the muscle group, tendons, and associated tissues.

_____   8. Dr. Winston Lewis recommends this heat modality to help relieve Herb Fowler's chronic lower back pain, which is caused by strain on the back muscles created by the patient's overweight condition.

_____   9. When patient Linda Maier comes to Inner City Health Care describing a sore back and several recent falls, Dr. Whitney asks clinical medical assistant Bruce Goldman to secure a gait belt around Linda's waist and have her walk across the room. With Bruce staying a step behind her and slightly to the side, Dr. Whitney carefully observes Linda's progress when performing this task.

_____   10. As a muscle atrophies, shrinking and losing its strength, joints become stiff and experience development of these deformities. Without constant exercise, the musculoskeletal system deteriorates.

_____ 11. Dr. Susan Rice recommends that patient Linda Maier begin to use a walker at home to prevent further falls. Bruce Goldman, CMA (AAMA), secures this safety device around Linda's waist and positions her inside the walker as he gives her verbal instructions to begin the procedure of learning to ambulate with a walker.

_____ 12. Older adult patient Abigail Johnson is afraid that because she has diabetes mellitus she is at increased risk for stroke. "I don't want to end up a vegetable and a burden to my family," she tells Dr. Elizabeth King, "all paralyzed on one side like that."

_____ 13. Clinical medical assistant Joe Guerrero applies this practice of using certain key muscle groups together with correct body alignment to avoid injury when assisting patient Lenore McDonell in performing a transfer from her wheelchair to the examination table.

_____ 14. Margaret Thomas's neurologist uses this instrument to measure the angle of her shoulder joint's ROM during a follow-up examination for Parkinson's disease.

_____ 15. Dr. Mark Woo chooses this cold modality to treat the sprained wrist of an emergency patient, reducing inflammation.

_____ 16. Canes, walkers, and crutches are examples of walking aids.

_____ 17. When lying flat with arms at the sides, the average person should be able to move from a 20-degree hyperextension of the elbow joint to a 150-degree flexion.

_____ 18. A physical therapist uses the measurement of joint motion to help evaluate a patient's ROM.

Matching

Match each of the joint movement terminology listed below to its proper definition.

1. Extension _____   A. Moving the arm so the palm is up

2. Circumduction _____   B. Moving a body part outward

3. Plantar flexion _____   C. Straightening of a body part

4. Dorsiflexion _____   D. Motion toward the midline of the body

5. Eversion _____   E. Moving a body part inward

6. Adduction _____   F. Turning a body part around its axis

7. Hyperextension _____   G. A position of maximum extension, or extending a body part beyond its normal limits

8. Flexion _____

9. Inversion _____   H. Motion away from the midline of the body

   I. Circular motion of a body part

10. Pronation _____

   J. Moving the arm so the palm is down

11. Supination _____

   K. Moving the foot downward at the ankle

12. Rotation _____

   L. Moving the foot upward at the ankle joint

13. Abduction _____

   M. Bending of a body part

LEARNING REVIEW

1. Some patients require assistive devices to ambulate. Name each assistive device shown below, then name the physical conditions each style is best suited to be used with as part of a physician's treatment plan. The first row has been completed for you as an example.

Name

Standard cane

Uses

The standard cane is good for patients

with only one good arm, lateral instability,

or balance conditions.

Name   **Uses**

_____   _____

_____   _____

                            _____

                            _____

                            _____

                            _____

_____   _____

_____   _____

                            _____

_____   _____

_____   _____

                            _____

                            _____

2. Name four types of exercise programs that are used for therapeutic or preventative purposes.

_____

_____

3. Using the four types of exercise programs identified above, match each one to the example below that best describes it.

_____ Pat Tidmarsh, who is suffering a sports injury to the muscles surrounding the knee, performs exercises with the help of a rubber exercise band.

_____ Lourdes Austen performs self-directed exercises at home to improve the ROM and increase strength in her left arm, after lumpectomy and axillary lymph node dissection.

_____ Lenore McDonell, who is confined to a wheelchair and unable to move her legs voluntarily, works regularly with a physical therapist to avoid atrophy and contractures in the legs and to improve overall circulation.

_____ Luanne Moore, who is recovering from a shoulder injury, rebuilds upper body strength with a daily regimen of push-ups, first against the wall and then on the floor.

4. Therapeutic exercise is not the only way to treat painful joints or tissues. Many patients respond well to the therapeutic modalities of heat and cold, thermotherapy and cryotherapy. List six precautions that medical assistants must take when applying heat or cold modalities.

_____

_____

_____

_____

_____

_____

_____

_____

_____

_____

_____

_____

5. Identify each modality listed below as either a dry heat therapy (DHT), a moist heat therapy (MHT), a moist cold therapy (MCT), or a dry cold therapy (DCT) by placing the proper letters in the space provided. Then identify whether the modality can be performed at home by the patient, with or without caregiver assistance, or whether the modality must be performed in a clinical setting under the supervision of a health care professional.

_____   A. Ice pack   _____

_____

_____   B. Paraffin wax bath   _____

_____

_____   C. Cold compress

_____

_____

_____

_____   D. Hot water bottle

_____

_____

_____

_____

_____   E. Warm compress

_____

_____

_____

_____   F. Whirlpool bath

_____

_____

_____

_____

_____   G. Heating pad

_____

_____

_____

_____

_____

_____   H. Warm soak of one
          extremity

_____

_____

_____   I. Warm pack

_____

_____

_____

_____   J. Total body immersion
          in a Hubbard tank

_____

_____

_____

_____

6. For each of the following, identify the proper temperature and correct amount of time the modality should be administered to the patient. The first row has been completed for you as an example.

Modality	Temperature	Time
Aquamatic K-Pad for an older adult patient	Water temperature between 104°F and 113°F (41°C and 46°C)	Administered for no more than 30 minutes
Paraffin wax bath for a patient with rheumatoid arthritis		
An ice pack for a patient with an ankle sprain		
Hot water bottle for an adult patient		
A warm compress to drain pus from a patient's skin infection		
Warm soak of the arm and hand for a patient with osteoarthritis		

7. How do ultrasound waves best travel? What are the special concerns of ultrasound treatment, how long can ultrasound be administered, and who is authorized to perform ultrasound procedures on patients?

_____

_____

_____

_____

_____

CERTIFICATION REVIEW

These questions are designed to mimic the certification examination. Select the best response.

1. When lifting or carrying heavy objects, you should rely on the following muscle groups:

   a. abdominal

   b. thoracic

   c. legs and arms

   d. back

2. The type of assistive device that does not require much upper body strength but is not recommended for older adults is the:

   a. walker

   b. cane

   c. crutches

   d. wheelchair

3. When a patient is standing with hands on the grip of a walker, the elbow should be bent at a _____-degree angle.

   a. 90

   b. 45

   c. 15

   d. 30

4. The type of crutch that may be used temporarily while a lower extremity heals is:

   a. axillary

   b. forearm

   c. platform

   d. Lofstrand

5. A quad cane is:

   a. two-legged

   b. four-legged

   c. one-legged

   d. three-legged

LEARNING APPLICATION

CASE STUDY 1

Ellen Armstrong, CMA (AAMA), performs the annual task of assembling and moving inactive patient files into a storage filing area for safekeeping. It is the end of the day and Ellen is tired and eager to finish the job; this task has never been one of Ellen's favorites. When she gets to filling the last of three cartons of files, Ellen moves the carton to a shelf, about shoulder high, in the storage room. She returns and decides to take both of the remaining cartons in one trip. Fatigued, she bends at the waist to pick them up.

CASE STUDY REVIEW QUESTION

1.   Describe the proper lifting technique that Ellen should use.

_____

_____

_____

_____

_____

CASE STUDY 2

After explaining the procedure to the patient and her son, Wanda Slawson, CMA (AAMA), applies a gait belt and performs the transfer of Mary Craig, an older adult blind patient with diabetes mellitus who is suffering from atrophy of the legs, from a car to a wheelchair in the parking lot of Inner City Health Care. Unfortunately, because of Mary's position in the car, the patient must be transferred with her weaker side closest to the wheelchair. The patient panics during the transfer and throws her arms around Wanda's neck as she is lifting and pivoting Mary to the right to position her in the wheelchair. The patient's son, John, rushes forward to grab on to his mother.

CASE STUDY REVIEW QUESTIONS

1.   What is the best action of the medical assistant?

_____

_____

_____

_____

_____

_____

_____

continues

2. What is the best therapeutic response of the medical assistant?

_____

_____

_____

_____

_____

3. Could the situation have been avoided? If so, how? If not, why not?

_____

_____

_____

_____

_____

CASE STUDY 3

Dr. Susan Rice asks Bruce Goldman, CMA (AAMA), to instruct patient Dottie Tate in the use of a walker to prevent further falls at home. Dottie is silent as Dr. Rice leaves the examination room and Bruce proceeds to set the walker correctly. However, when Dottie sees that Bruce must once again put Dottie in a gait belt for her protection—the belt was used earlier in the examination to assess Dottie's ability to ambulate—the patient gets feisty. She is visibly tired and ready to go home. "I'll learn to use the walker if I have to, but I won't wear that infernal contraption. It makes me feel like a baby. And it's such a bother. Who wants to go through all that? We just don't need it."

CASE STUDY REVIEW QUESTIONS

1. What is the best action of the medical assistant?

_____

_____

_____

_____

2. What is the best therapeutic response of the medical assistant?

_____

_____

_____

_____

3. Could the situation have been avoided? If so, how? If not, why not?

_____

_____

_____

_____

CHAPTER POST-TEST

Perform this test without looking at your book. If an answer is "false," rewrite the sentence to make it true.

1. True or False? To abduct is to move away from the midline.

   _____

   _____

2. True or False? ROM is measured in degrees.

   _____

   _____

3. True or False? When lifting heavy objects, always bend from the waist and keep the object close to your body.

   _____

   _____

4. True or False? It helps to have patients put their arms on your shoulders when you help them to ambulate.

   _____

   _____

5. True or False? If a patient falls, you should gently ease him or her to the floor.

   _____

   _____

6. True or False? Medical assistants must be familiar with ROM exercises that will be performed on patients by other members of the health care team.

   _____

   _____

SELF-ASSESSMENT

1. Have you ever considered the field of physical or occupational therapy as a career?

   _____

   _____

   _____

   _____

2. What makes you think you would do well or not do well in those fields?

   _____

   _____

   _____

   _____

3. What do you think you would not care for in working with rehabilitative medicine? What would you like the most?

_____

_____

_____

_____

4. What are some of the skills, talents, interests, and abilities a person would need to have to do well in rehabilitative medicine? List a dozen or more, and then consider and circle all of those that you possess. Which on the list could you learn in a rehabilitative medicine program (insert an S for school), and which would be a natural part of your makeup (insert an N for natural)? Is there a direct relation between the skills, talents, interests, and abilities you possess and those that you marked with an N? Discuss your results with a small group of fellow students. What conclusion(s) did you reach?

_____

_____

_____

_____

CHAPTER **34**

Nutrition in Health and Disease

CHAPTER PRE-TEST

Perform this test without looking at your book. If an answer is "false," rewrite the sentence to make it true.

1. True or False? Homeostasis depends on proper nutrients being made available for the body to use.

_____

_____

2. True or False? Some nutrients provide energy, whereas others help with bodily processes.

_____

_____

3. True or False? Fats, carbohydrates, and proteins provide energy.

_____

_____

4. True or False? Fat-soluble vitamins are those vitamins that need oil to be used and stored.

_____

_____

5. True or False? Water-soluble vitamins are readily depleted, and therefore must be taken in daily.

_____

_____

6. True or False? Antioxidants are those substances that help the body cells recover from the damaging effects of day-to-day living.

_____

_____

7. True or False? Fiber is primarily a carbohydrate and comes only from plant sources.

_____

_____

VOCABULARY BUILDER

Misspelled Words

Find the words below that are misspelled; circle them, and then correctly spell them in the spaces provided. Then fill in the blanks below with the correct vocabulary term from the following list.

absorbtion	digestion	metabolism
amino acids	electrolytes	nutrients
antioxident	elimination	nutrition
basal metabolic rate	extracellular	oxidation
calories	fat-soluble	preservatives
catalist	glycogen	processed foods
cellulose	homostasis	saturated fats
coenzyme	ingestion	trace minerals
diaretics	major minerals	water soluable

_____   _____   _____

_____   _____   _____

1. Artificial flavors, colors, and _____, chemicals that keep food fresh longer, are non-nutritive substances commonly added to processed foods.

2. _____ is the study of the intake of nutrients into the body and how the body processes and uses these nutrients.

3. Toxicity is most likely to occur with _____ vitamins because they are stored in tissues composed of lipids and in the liver and are not carried easily into the bloodstream.

4. The best source of complete proteins are meats and animal products such as milk and eggs; complete proteins contain all eight of the essential _____.

5. Beverages that contain caffeine and alcohol, which are _____, will cause the body to increase urinary output and lose water. These substances should be avoided when performing activities, such as a good physical workout, and entering environments, such as an airplane passenger cabin, that promote dehydration.

6. A _____ is a nonprotein substance that acts with a catalyst to facilitate chemical reactions in the body.

7. _____ is the process of the digestive system involving the transfer of nutrients from the gastrointestinal tract into the bloodstream.

8. Chlorine (Cl) is a mineral with an important _____ function, one that takes place outside the cells of body tissues in the spaces between layers or groups of cells.

9. The total of all changes, or energy, chemical and physical, that takes place in the body is called

_____.

10. Some minerals are considered _____ in that they become ionized and carry a positive or negative charge; these minerals must be carefully balanced in the body.

11. _____ begins at the mouth with chewing and progresses through the gastrointestinal tract to the small intestine.

12. _____ are ingested substances that help the body maintain a state of homeostasis.

13. The process of _____ maintains a constant internal environment of the human body, including such functions as heartbeat, blood pressure, respiration, and body temperature.

14. A _____ facilitates chemical reactions by speeding up the reaction time without the need for a high-energy output.

15. It is always important to analyze the nutritional labels on _____ purchased in the supermarket.

16. Lard is one example of _____, which have been found to increase the level of fats and cholesterol in the blood and are hydrogenated, or contain hydrogen.

17. The ability to reduce _____ is a characteristic of vitamin E that has led some researchers to suggest that vitamin E may slow the aging process, although its true effectiveness has not yet been demonstrated.

18. The excretion of waste through the anus is called _____, the final step of the digestive process.

19. The amount of energy a substance is able to supply is measured in large _____.

20. Potassium is one of the seven _____ found in the body.

21. Vitamins that are _____ must be constantly ingested to maintain proper blood levels, because these vitamins are not easily stored in the body.

22. Vitamin E is a fat-soluble vitamin that belongs to a group of compounds called _____, which counteract the damaging effects of oxidation. Beta-carotene is another substance in this group.

23. Despite their name, _____ are vital to body functioning and include molybdenum and fluorine.

24. _____ begins the digestive process when we put food in our mouths to eat.

25. Children, pregnant women, and people with a lean body mass will have a higher _____ because it takes more energy to fuel the muscles than it does to store fat.

26. A type of carbohydrate, _____, is derived from a plant source and supplies fiber in the human diet.

27. Ingested only in small quantities, _____ is an important carbohydrate form for storage of glucose in the body.

LEARNING REVIEW

1. Vitamins are a class of nutrients in which each specific vitamin has a function entirely of its own. These complex molecules are required by the body in minute quantities. What are the two functions of vitamins in the body?

_____

_____

_____

2. Identify the correct chemical name for each vitamin listed. Then describe what each vitamin does in the body to promote good health.

A. One of the B-complex vitamins, also called nicotinic acid:

_____

_____

B. Vitamin B_1:

_____

_____

C. Vitamin E:

_____

_____

D. Vitamin D:

_____

_____

_____

E. One of the B-complex vitamins, also called folacin:

_____

_____

F. Vitamin A:

_____

_____

_____

_____

G. Vitamin B_{12}:

_____

_____

_____

H. Vitamin C:

_____

_____

I. Vitamin B_2:

_____

_____

_____

J. Vitamin B_6:

_____

_____

_____

3. Nutrients are divided into two groups: those that provide energy and those that do not. Identify the nutrients listed below as providing energy or not providing energy by placing an X in the appropriate column.

	Energy	No Energy
Vitamins		
Carbohydrates		
Fiber		
Minerals		
Lipids (fats)		
Proteins		
Water		

4. What three chemical elements do carbohydrates, fats, and proteins all contain?

_____

_____

5. Name the most important dietary complex carbohydrate. _____

6. Name the only true essential fatty acid in the human diet. _____

7. What additional chemical element does protein alone contain? _____

8. What happens when the body does not have enough carbohydrates or fats in supply as an energy source? What effect does this have on the body?

_____

_____

_____

9. Name two conditions associated with deficiencies in protein.

_____

_____

_____

10. List two distinct ways in which minerals differ from vitamins.

_____

_____

_____

_____

11. For each food source, list the mineral or minerals that each provides.

(1) Eggs: _____

(2) Milk: _____

(3) Cheese: _____

(4) Salmon: _____

(5) Bananas: _____

(6) Green vegetables: _____

12. List six types of fiber that are carbohydrates.

_____

_____

_____

13. What important fiber is *not* a carbohydrate?

_____

_____

14. Americans generally do not consume enough fiber. How much fiber should be consumed each day?

_____

_____

15. Why does brown rice contain more fiber than white rice?

_____

_____

16. What happens when the body takes in more calories than will be expended by the body as energy?

_____

_____

17. What happens when the body uses more energy than the calories it takes in will produce?

_____

_____

_____

18. What is the ideal percentage of total calories for adults that should be consumed as carbohydrates, fats, and proteins?

_____

_____

_____

_____

19. Compare the advantages and disadvantages of the following diets: U.S. southern, Jewish, and Japanese.

_____

_____

_____

_____

_____

_____

_____

_____

_____

20. Obesity is a major health concern in the United States and often begins in childhood. What can you do as a medical assistant to assist parents to help their children avoid obesity?

_____

_____

_____

_____

Matching

For each of the following in Column A, identify the substance as a water-soluble vitamin (WSV), fat-soluble vitamin (FSV), a major mineral (MM), or a trace mineral (TM) in Column B. Then match the substance to the response in Column C that best fits its character or properties. The first one has been completed for you as an example.

Column A	Column B	Column C
H — 1. Sulfur	MM	A. This substance works with potassium to maintain proper water balance and proper pH balance; the two also are involved in nervous muscular conduction and excitability.
___ 2. Vitamin B₁₂	___	
___ 3. Iron	___	B. This substance is part of the pigment rhodopsin found in the eye and is responsible in part for vision, especially night vision.
___ 4. Vitamin K	___	
___ 5. Sodium	___	C. This substance is vital to life because of its role in the heme molecule, which carries oxygen to every cell in the body.
___ 6. Pyridoxine	___	
___ 7. Iodine	___	D. Rickets and osteomalacia are diseases caused by deficiencies in this substance; when deficiencies occur, usually in childhood, malformation of the skeleton is seen.
___ 8. Biotin	___	
___ 9. Retinol	___	E. This member of the B-complex, together with pantothenic acid, is generally responsible for energy metabolism.
___ 10. Vitamin D	___	

F. Because this substance is found only in foods from animal sources, such as liver, kidney, and dairy products, pernicious anemia, the result of deficiencies, may be a problem for some vegetarians.

G. This substance, found in rice, beans, and yeast, is important to protein metabolism.

H. This substance is a component of one of the amino acids and is found in protein; it is also involved in energy metabolism.

I. About half of the body's requirement for this substance is fulfilled through synthesis by intestinal bacteria; bile is required for its absorption into the bloodstream.

J. This substance is found only in the thyroid hormones; without it, the thyroid gland would be unable to regulate the overall metabolism of the body.

CERTIFICATION REVIEW

These questions are designed to mimic the certification examination. Select the best response.

1. Carbohydrates, fats, and proteins have one thing in common. What is it?

   a. High calcium content

   b. Their ability to convert into energy

   c. Low sodium content

   d. All of the above

2. Examples of monosaccharides are:

   a. fructose

   b. sucrose

   c. a. and d.

   d. glucose

3. The compounds composed of carbon, hydrogen, and oxygen that exist as triglycerides in the body are:

   a. fats

   b. fiber

   c. vitamins

   d. minerals

4. The basic structural unit of a protein is:

   a. simple sugar

   b. complex sugar

   c. lipids

   d. amino acids

5. Herbal supplements are also known as:

   a. phytomedicines

   b. antioxidants

   c. amino acids

   d. trans acids

LEARNING APPLICATION

Research Activities

1. Identify each organ of the digestive system below. Describe the healthy functioning of each organ in the space provided. Then, using a medical dictionary or encyclopedia, look up each organ and list one common disorder that would adversely affect the digestive process.

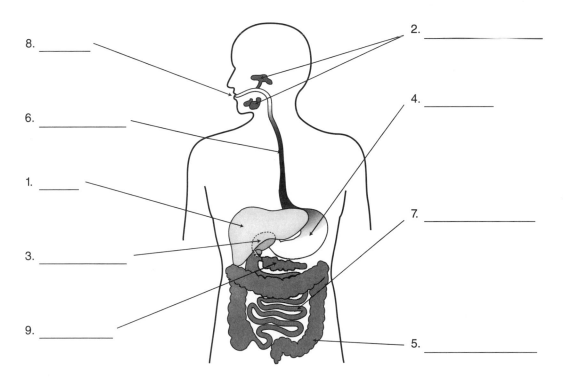

8. _____

2. _____

6. _____

4. _____

1. _____

7. _____

3. _____

9. _____

5. _____

Healthy Function	**Common Disorders**
1. _____	_____
_____	_____
_____	_____
_____	_____
_____	_____
2. _____	_____
_____	_____
_____	_____
_____	_____
3. _____	_____
_____	_____
_____	_____

4. _____   _____
   _____   _____
   _____   _____
   _____   _____
   _____   _____

5. _____   _____
   _____   _____
   _____   _____
   _____   _____

6. _____   _____
   _____   _____
   _____   _____

7. _____   _____
   _____   _____
   _____   _____
   _____   _____
   _____   _____
   _____   _____

8. _____   _____
   _____   _____

9. _____   _____
   _____   _____
   _____   _____
   _____   _____

2. When helping patients modify their diets, medical assistants need to be knowledgeable about the nutrients in the food we eat. The nutritional analysis label on the back or side of a food package is helpful when figuring out the levels of fat, cholesterol, sodium, carbohydrates, protein, and vitamins contained in a particular food. Obtain a food label and answer the following questions.

   A. The percentage of daily values listed on a food label report the amount of a nutrient obtained by eating how many servings of a product? _____

   B. The percentages are based on a _____-calorie diet.

   C. The listing for total carbohydrates is broken down into what two additional listings? Which type of carbohydrate is more beneficial and why?

   _____
   _____
   _____

D. A patient should look for a food product in which the sodium content is relatively low. What is the greatest number of milligrams of sodium a person should eat each day?

_____

_____

E. Why is a high-fiber diet important?

_____

_____

_____

_____

3. Compare the nutrition label from a box of muesli with fruit, nuts, and seeds with the label from a package of pretzel snacks. Which is more nutritious and why? Note that one serving of the muesli, a half cup or 55 grams, is roughly equivalent to 2 servings of pretzels, 14 pretzels or 60 grams.

Muesli

Nutrition Facts
Serving Size: 1/2 cup (55g)
Servings Per Container: about 8

	Cereal	Cereal + 125 mL Vitamin A & D fortified skim milk
Amount Per Serving		
Calories	210	250
Calories from Fat	30	35
	% Daily Value**	
Total Fat 3g*	**5%**	**5%**
Saturated Fat 0.5g	**3%**	**3%**
Cholesterol 0mg	**0%**	**0%**
Sodium 30mg	**1%**	**4%**
Total Carbohydrate 40g	**13%**	**15%**
Dietary Fiber 5g	**21%**	**21%**
Sugars 13g		
Protein 6g		
Vitamin A	0%	8%
Vitamin C	8%	8%
Calcium	4%	20%
Iron	35%	35%
Vitamin D	0%	10%
Thiamine	35%	40%
Riboflavin	25%	35%
Niacin	2%	2%
Vitamin B₆	15%	20%
Folate	10%	10%
Pantothenic Acid	4%	10%

*Amount in Cereal. One half cup skim milk contributes an additional 40 calories. 65 mg sodium, 6g total carbohydrate (6g sugars), and 4g protein.

**Percent Daily Values are based on a 2,000 calorie diet. Your daily values may be higher or lower depending on your calorie needs.

	Calories	2,000	2,500
Total Fat	Less than	65g	80g
Sat Fat	Less than	20g	25g
Cholesterol	Less than	300mg	300mg
Sodium	Less than	2,400mg	2,400mg
Total Carbohydrate		300g	375g
Dietary Fiber		25g	30g

Calories per gram:
Fat 9 • Carbohydrate 4 • Protein 4

Pretzels
Nutrition Facts
Serving Size: 7 Pretzels (30g)
Servings Per Container: 9.4

Amount Per Serving

Calories 120	
Calories from Fat 10	
% Daily Value*	
Total Fat 1g	2%
Saturated Fat 0g	0%
Cholesterol 0g	0%
Sodium 360mg	15%
Total Carbohydrate 24g	8%
Dietary Fiber 1g	4%
Sugars 1g	
Protein 3g	

Vitamin A 0%	Σ Vitamin C 0%
Calcium 0%	Σ Iron 2%

*Percent Daily Values are based on a 2,000 calorie diet. Your daily values may be higher or lower depending on your calorie needs:

	Calories	2,000	2,500
Total Fat	Less than	65g	80g
Sat Fat	Less than	20g	25g
Cholesterol	Less than	300mg	300mg
Sodium	Less than	2,400mg	2,400mg
Total Carbohydrate		300g	375g
Dietary Fiber		25g	30g

Calories per gram:
Fat 9 Σ Carbohydrate 4 Σ Protein 4

Ingredients: Unbleached Wheat Flour, Water, Corn Syrup, Partially Hydrogenated Vegetable Oil (Soybean), Yeast Salt, Bicarbonates and Carbonates of Sodium.

_____

_____

_____

_____

_____

_____

Calorie Calculating Activity

1. An 8-fluid-ounce serving of 1% fat soy milk contains 110 calories with 2 grams of total fat, 20 grams of total carbohydrates, and 4 grams of total protein. Calculate the total number of calories from each energy nutrient; show your calculations in the space provided below.

   Number of calories from fat: _____

   Number of calories from carbohydrates: _____

   Number of calories from protein: _____

   _____

   _____

   _____

2. Now calculate the percentage of total calories due to each energy nutrient.

   Percentage of calories from fat: _____

   Percentage of calories from carbohydrates: _____

   Percentage of calories from protein: _____

   _____

   _____

   _____

3. Compare the percentages of total calories due to fat, carbohydrates, and protein found in soy milk with the percentages you calculated for one serving of peanut butter in the textbook's Critical Thinking box on page 961. How do the percentages relate to the ideal percentages for optimum energy balance in the body?

   _____

   _____

   _____

   _____

   _____

   _____

Case Studies

Dr. Elizabeth King has confirmed that patient Mary O'Keefe is pregnant with her third child.

CASE STUDY REVIEW QUESTIONS

1. Name two minerals that Mary must increase the intake of in her diet.

   _____

   _____

2. Name three reasons why a woman needs to increase her intake of nutrients and calories when she is pregnant.

   _____

   _____

   _____

   _____

   _____

3. What dietary supplement usually needs to be added to a baby's diet?

   _____

   _____

Lourdes Austen, a breast cancer survivor, regularly attends a support group for breast cancer patients and survivors held once a month. Lourdes finds the group a great source of encouragement, information, and support—a safe place to discuss her feelings and concerns about breast cancer. The group is planning a session to talk about nutrition issues, and Lourdes asks clinical medical assistant, Audrey Jones, if she would like to attend the meeting with her to contribute to the group's discussion. With permission from office manager Marilyn Johnson and Lourdes's physician, Dr. Elizabeth King, Audrey attends the meeting. The group members are enthusiastic and ask Audrey many questions, including the following: "Why is good nutition important for cancer patients?" "I don't have much appetite anymore and get nauseous all the time. What can I do?" "I keep hearing about those macrobiotic diets. Are they any good? Should I try them?"

continues

CASE STUDY REVIEW QUESTIONS

1. What information can Audrey give in answer to the question regarding the importance of good nutrition for cancer patients?

_____

_____

_____

_____

_____

_____

_____

2. What suggestion can Audrey offer to patients who have no appetite and have nausea or vomiting?

_____

_____

_____

3. What can Audrey tell the group about macrobiotic diets?

_____

_____

_____

_____

_____

_____

_____

_____

4. What is the role of the medical assistant in attending the breast cancer support group meeting?

_____

_____

_____

_____

CHAPTER POST-TEST

Perform this test without looking at your book. If an answer is "false," rewrite the sentence to make it true.

1. True or False? Homeostasis occurs properly and does not depend on proper nutrients being made available for the body to use.

   _____

   _____

2. True or False? Nutrients provide energy.

   _____

   _____

3. True or False? Fats and carbohydrates provide energy, whereas proteins do not.

   _____

   _____

4. True or False? Fat-soluble vitamins are those vitamins that are stored in the fat of the body.

   _____

   _____

5. True or False? Water-soluble vitamins are not easily depleted, and therefore can build up to dangerous levels.

   _____

   _____

6. True or False? Antioxidants are those substances that help the body's cells overcome the damages of free radicals.

   _____

   _____

7. True or False? Fiber is primarily a carbohydrate and comes only from plant sources.

   _____

   _____

SELF-ASSESSMENT

1. Keep track of your diet for a couple of days. Track everything you eat and drink and the amounts of each item.

   _____

   _____

   _____

   _____

2. Either use the Internet to research the nutritional value of each item or look in a good dietary resource for the information. Figure the number of calories you ate each day, the amount of fiber, the amount and types of fats, how much protein, how many carbohydrates and sugars, and which vitamins and minerals you consumed. Hint: There are specific Web sites that can help you with this project. One example is: http://www.calorie-count.com. This Web site allows you to search through hundreds of different foods and drinks to find the "labels" for them. It is free! You can even create your own personal profile.

A. Now figure in any vitamins and supplements you ingested.

B. Is there any particular part of a nutritious diet that you are lacking?

C. Are there any components that you ate too much of?

1. Use the PDR to locate the pertinent information for each of the following scenarios. Then identify the drug's source or method of production.

   A. Herb Fowler, Dr. Winston Lewis's patient, calls to report he is experiencing nausea, a symptom he believes may be a negative reaction to the Chronulac Syrup® Dr. Lewis recently prescribed for Herb's chronic constipation. Using the PDR, locate the following information:

   Chronulac Syrup's generic name: _____

   The sugar Chronulac Syrup contains is _____

   Identify the drug's source or method of production: _____

   B. Another patient of Dr. Lewis's, Michael Zamboni, has recently been diagnosed with insulin-dependent type II diabetes. Dr. Lewis prescribes Humulin®. Using the PDR, find the following information:

   Humulin's® generic name: _____

   _____

   The source from which Humulin® is derived: _____

   _____

   _____

   Identify the drug's source or method of production: _____

   _____

   C. Susan Marshall, a new patient of Dr. Elizabeth King's, acquired a high-pressure job about 1 month ago. Recently, she has been reporting an upset stomach, which has been attributed to her stressful job and poor eating habits. Dr. King orders prescription-strength Pepcid® for Susan. Using the PDR, locate the following information:

   Pepcid's® generic name: _____

   Pepcid's® active ingredient: _____

   Identify the drug's source or method of production: _____

2. Camille Saunders, another patient of Dr. King's, has been taking Ortho-Tri-Cyclen®, an oral contraceptive, for 6 months. It has just been discovered that Camille has epilepsy. Using the PDR, locate the following information:

   A. Does Ortho-Tri-Cyclen® have any known contraindications to any drugs used in the treatment of epilepsy, and if so, which drugs?

   _____

   _____

   _____

   B. Identify the drug's source or method of production.

   _____

   _____

CASE STUDY

While Anna Preciado, a clinical medical assistant newly hired at the offices of Drs. Lewis and King, is performing her shift duties, she notices a fellow employee exhibiting strange behavior. Audrey Jones, CMA (AAMA), is usually the model of efficiency. Since Anna began working at the Northborough Family Medical Group, she has always known Audrey to be alert, friendly, and able to handle difficult clinical situations with grace under pressure. Lately, however, when Anna asks Audrey questions, Audrey seems irritable and easily confused. Anna also notices Audrey exhibiting a sloppy technique during routine clinical procedures. Anna is disturbed by Audrey's erratic behavior but does not mention anything to anyone. After all, Anna is new to the job. But while counting the contents of the controlled substance cabinet in preparation for the end of her shift, Anna notices that a bottle of phenobarbital is missing. Anna knows that office manager Marilyn Johnson will arrive shortly to verify and record the inventory count. Anna is now worried that perhaps Audrey is to blame for the missing drugs but is afraid of jumping to conclusions and of angering Audrey. Anna knows Audrey is in the staff lounge preparing to leave for a dinner break.

CASE STUDY REVIEW QUESTIONS

1. What is Anna's first action under the circumstances? Should she confront Audrey?

_____

_____

_____

_____

_____

_____

_____

2. What special responsibilities do health care professionals, including medical assistants, have regarding the misuse or abuse of legal or illegal drugs?

_____

_____

_____

_____

_____

_____

_____

_____

_____

C H A P T E R **37**

Electrocardiography

CHAPTER PRE-TEST

Perform this test without looking at your book. If an answer is "false," rewrite the sentence to make it true.

1. True or False? The skin is a great conductor of electricity.

_____

_____

2. True or False? Electrolytes provide moisture, and aid in conduction.

_____

_____

3. True or False? The heart is a two-sided pump that routes blood where it needs to go.

_____

_____

4. True or False? Only certain cells in the heart are able to initiate electricity.

_____

_____

5. True or False? One type of artifact is an electrical interference.

_____

_____

6. True or False? The heart beats approximately 60 times a minute, only resting in-between beats.

_____

_____

VOCABULARY BUILDER

From the following terms, find the misspelled words, circle them, and spell them correctly in the spaces provided.
Then, fill in the blanks in sentences below.

atria	electrocardigraph	sinoatrial node
atrioventrical node	electrocardiography	ventricles
cardiac cycle	oxygenated	
deoxygenated	Purkingi fibers	

_____   _____

_____

1. The lower chambers of the heart are called _____.

2. The upper chambers of the heart are called _____.

3. _____ blood enters the right side of the heart.

4. _____ blood enters the left side of the heart.

5. The _____ is the body's natural pacemaker.

6. From the sinoatrial node, the _____ receives the current of electricity.

7. The fibers that spread the electrical impulses from the bundle branches throughout the ventricles are called the _____.

8. The entire route of the electrical impulses through the heart is referred to as the _____.

9. The _____ is a machine used to perform the ECG procedure.

10. Ultrasonography and _____ are noninvasive diagnostic procedures commonly used in the clinical setting.

LEARNING REVIEW

1. List five reasons why electrocardiography is performed.

_____

_____

_____

_____

_____

_____

2. The first three leads recorded on a standard ECG are Lead I, Lead II, and Lead III. These are called
_____ leads because each of them uses two-limb electrodes that record simultaneously.
For each lead, what electrical activity of the heart is recorded? Draw it on each figure.

Lead I

Lead II

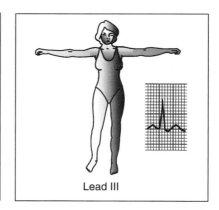

Lead III

3. Fill in the blanks:

   (A) Lead I records electrical activity between the _____ and the _____.

   (B) Lead II records electrical activity between the _____ and the _____.

   (C) Lead III records electrical activity between the _____ and the _____.

4. The next group of leads recorded on a standard ECG are augmented leads, designated aV$_R$, aV$_L$, and aV$_F$.
These are called _____ leads. For each lead, what electrical activity of the heart is recorded?
Draw it on each figure.

Lead aV$_R$

Lead aV$_L$

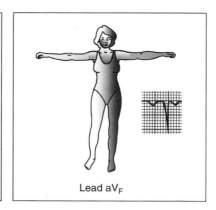

Lead aV$_F$

5. Fill in the blanks:

   (A) Lead aV$_R$ records electrical activity from the _____ and the

   _____.

   (B) Lead aV$_L$ records electrical activity from the _____ and the

   _____.

   (C) Lead aV$_F$ records electrical activity from the _____ and the

   _____.

6. The remaining 6 leads of the standard 12-lead ECG are called the chest leads, or _____
leads. These leads are (*circle the correct one*) unipolar/bipolar. Where are the leads placed on the body?

V1: _____

V2: _____

V3: _____

V4: _____

V5: _____

V6: _____

CERTIFICATION REVIEW

These questions are designed to mimic the certification examination. Select the best response.

1. Repolarization takes place while the heart muscle:

   a. contracts

   b. stops

   c. skips a beat

   d. relaxes

2. Chest leads are also called _____ leads

   a. precordial

   b. limb

   c. augmented

   d. bipolar

3. Augmented leads are also called:

   a. unipolar

   b. bipolar

   c. precordial

   d. standard

4. One millivolt of cardiac electrical activity will deflect the stylus exactly:

   a. 5 mm high

   b. 10 mm high

   c. 25 mm high

   d. 40 mm high

5. A wandering baseline may be caused by:

   a. lotions, creams, or oils on the patient's skin

   b. electrical interference

   c. crossed lead wires

   d. improper grounding

LEARNING APPLICATION

Identifying Artifact Activity

Artifacts are unusual and unwanted activity in the ECG tracing not caused by the electrical activity of the heart. Match each circumstance below to the artifact ECG tracing it would produce and identify the type of artifact in the space provided.

  A. A broken patient cable or lead wire has become detached from an electrode.

  B. The patient sings to himself during the ECG procedure.

  C. The patient uses body lotion.

  D. The lead wires are crossed and do not follow the patient's body contour.

Type of Artifact	Circumstance
_____	____

_____   ____

_____   ____

_____   ____

CASE STUDY

Jim Marshall, a prominent local architect in his late 30s, stays in good physical condition, works out regularly at the gym, and maintains a low-fat, low-cholesterol, low-sodium diet. Aggressive and ambitious, Jim enjoys pushing his mind and body to the limit. His favorite sports are skiing and sailing. At work, Jim is a perfectionist who puts in long hours and demands the same of his employees. Lately, though, Jim is more aware of the high-stress lifestyle he is leading and is worried about his family history of heart failure and diabetes. During periods of high physical exertion, Jim experiences mild chest pain and palpitations. Dr. Lewis prescribes an exercise tolerance test for Jim.

CASE STUDY REVIEW QUESTIONS

1. What is an exercise tolerance test? How is it performed?

   _____

   _____

   _____

   _____

   _____

   _____

   _____

2. Under what conditions would the test be discontinued?

   _____

   _____

   _____

3. At the conclusion of the test, what patient care is given? What special instructions for home care should the patient observe?

   _____

   _____

   _____

   _____

   _____

CHAPTER POST-TEST

Perform this test without looking at your book. If an answer is "false," rewrite the sentence to make it true.

1. True or False? The skin is a poor conductor of electricity.

_____

_____

2. True or False? Electrodes provide moisture and aid in conduction.

_____

_____

3. True or False? The heart is a four-sided pump that routes blood where it needs to go.

_____

_____

_____

4. True or False? All cardiac cells are able to initiate electricity.

_____

_____

_____

5. True or False? Alternating current artifacts are part of the heart's electrical circuitry.

_____

_____

_____

6. True or False? The heart beats approximately 24 times a minute, resting only in-between beats.

_____

_____

_____

SELF-ASSESSMENT

Keep a strict diary of everything you eat and drink for the next three days (a week is better).

1. Count up the total fats you have eaten each day.

_____

_____

_____

_____

2. Separate the types of fats and total each type for each day.

_____

_____

_____

_____

3. Go online and use search words such as "saturated fats" or "trans fats" to learn more about the different fats.

_____

_____

_____

_____

4. Find out about omega-3 fatty acids. Are you eating enough? How could you take in more?

_____

_____

_____

_____

5. What else should you be doing to stay "heart healthy"?

_____

_____

_____

_____

CHAPTER **3 9**

Introduction to the Medical Laboratory

CHAPTER PRE-TEST

Perform this test without looking at your book. If an answer is "false," rewrite the sentence to make it true.

1. True or False? Cytology is the study of cells.

_____

_____

2. A urine culture would be performed in which department of a regional laboratory?

  a. Bacteriology department

  b. Urinalysis department

  c. Culture department

  d. Cytology department

3. Which of the following is a description of a profile?

  a. many tests all billed together at one time

  b. all the tests for one patient during one calendar year

  c. all the tests a doctor orders consistently throughout her or his practice

  d. a related set of tests about an organ, system, or function

4. True or False? Proficiency tests are required by the Occupational Safety and Health Administration (OSHA).

_____

_____

5. True or False? Fasting means that the patient may have water but nothing else by mouth for 12 hours.

_____

_____

VOCABULARY BUILDER

Misspelled Words

Find the words below that are misspelled; circle them, and correctly spell them in the spaces provided. Then insert the proper correct vocabulary terms into the sentences below. Each sentence describes a situation you might find in a POL or in a reference laboratory.

assay	diagnosis	objective
asymptomatic	diaphram	profile
baseline	differential diagnosis	qualitative tests
biopsy	electrolytes	quantative tests
clinical diagnosis	glucose	reagents
condensor	invasive	requisition
control test	normal flora	serum

_____   _____   _____

1. Wanda Slawson, CMA (AAMA), is examining a specimen in the laboratory using a compound microscope. The _____ is the lens system closest to the specimen she is viewing.

2. Dr. Mark Woo orders laboratory tests for a female emergency patient experiencing severe abdominal cramps to make a _____ that will distinguish between a diagnosis of appendicitis and a diagnosis of an ovarian cyst.

3. Richard Butts receives a job offer from a construction company that requires all employees to be tested for misuse or abuse of legal or illegal drugs before they can work on the site. Bruce Goldman, CMA (AAMA), performs Richard's blood test under the direction of Dr. Whitney; his test comes back clean. The results of Richard's test can be used in the future as a _____ measurement, a record of healthy normal results.

4. Dr. King needs a red blood cell (RBC) count, a white blood cell (WBC) count, and a platelet count for Melinda Cool. Joe Guerrero, CMA (AAMA), performs a venipuncture on Melinda and sends a tube of her blood to the laboratory, together with a written _____ containing specific information and instructions about what tests to perform on the specimens.

5. Bruce Goldman, CMA (AAMA), is examining a specimen under a compound microscope. Because he is having difficulty seeing clearly, Bruce opens the microscope's _____ to increase the amount of light on the specimen.

6. Dr. Lewis asks Audrey Jones, CMA (AAMA), to send a tube of Herb Fowler's blood to the laboratory for analysis. Dr. Lewis wants to determine the constituents and relative proportion of each of the enzymes in Herb's serum; this type of analysis is called an _____.

7. Jacquie Cavanaugh comes to see Dr. Lewis and reports that she has been constantly tired for the past two or three months. Because Jacquie's symptoms are so vague, Dr. Lewis orders a blood _____ to help narrow the diagnosis possibilities.

8. Bruce Goldman, CMA (AAMA), always follows Standard Precautions and washes his hands before touching a patient. Although everyone's body contains many natural microorganisms, called _____, aseptic hand washing reduces the potential for exposure to or transmission of pathogens.

9. Hematology laboratories count the WBCs or RBCs in a sample of a patient's blood. In general, these type of counting tests are known as _____.

10. As a method of quality control, a _____ sample is tested together with a patient's sample as a method of ensuring the accuracy of test results.

11. Joe Guerrero, CMA (AAMA), asks Abigail Johnson, who he knows is diagnosed with diabetes mellitus, whether she regularly tests her blood at home to measure her _____ level.

B. Patient Janet Renquiz, a retired homemaker, complies with the treatment plan for her diagnosed case of chronic lymphocytic leukemia by submitting to a regular testing of her blood for the presence of leukemic cells, which monitors the progress of the disease.

_____

_____

C. Anna Ortiz, who is pregnant, has had genital herpes for several years. In the week before her child is to be born, Dr. King takes a culture of Anna's cervical and vaginal mucosa to determine whether her baby is at risk for contracting herpes in the birth canal.

_____

_____

D. Dr. Mark Woo has been treating Edith Leonard, who describes having poor vision and fainting spells. Because Edith's symptoms are vague and he cannot make a firm diagnosis, Dr. Woo orders a complete blood profile to give him additional information about Edith's case.

_____

_____

E. Louise Kipperly comes to Inner City Health Care for her yearly medical checkup. Dr. Esposito orders a series of blood tests to make sure that Louise's cholesterol level is within a normal, healthy range.

_____

_____

F. Fifteen-year-old Hung Chu comes to Inner City Health Care with a severe sore throat. A physical examination detects the presence of fever, headache, difficulty swallowing, and inflamed tonsils. Dr. Whitney orders a complete blood cell count (CBC) and a heterophil antibodies test to confirm a diagnosis of either tonsillitis or infectious mononucleosis. When the results of Hung's blood tests come back from the laboratory, however, atypical lymphocytes in the blood indicate the early onset of infectious mononucleosis.

_____

_____

G. When Naoki Tamura's laboratory tests come back positive for *Herpesvirus hominis*, his girlfriend Eleanor is instructed to come into Inner City Health Care for testing. Eleanor, who has no symptoms, is tested for herpes simplex and nonspecific urethritis.

_____

_____

H. Maria Jover, who was diagnosed with HIV, takes protease inhibitors to help her immune system fight the disease. Dr. King orders blood tests to determine how Maria is responding to the treatment.

_____

_____

5. Name five tests commonly performed in a physician's office laboratory (POL).

_____

_____

_____

6. Name three criteria that would justify using point-of-care testing.

_____

_____

7. Identify each entry that follows as a way an infectious agent leaves the body of a sick person (L), the way an organism may be transmitted (T), or the way an organism enters the body (E).

____   A.   Discharges from infected eyes

____   B.   Contaminated needles and syringes

____   C.   Contaminated water in a river

____   D.   Directly onto mucous membrane

____   E.   Breast milk

____   F.   Towels

____   G.   Health care workers exposed to blood

____   H.   Transplacentally to fetus

____   I.   Contact with blood and body fluids

____   J.   Discharges from respiratory tract

____   K.   Feces and urine

____   L.   Flies

____   M.   Excreta from intestinal tract

____   N.   Directly on the conjunctiva

8. The accuracy of any laboratory test result depends on the performance of quality controls by all health care workers who handle a specimen. Medical assistants must have a thorough knowledge of quality controls and standards. List five factors that can compromise the accuracy of laboratory test results.

_____

_____

_____

_____

9. What is the reason for using a control test sample? Explain in detail.

_____

_____

_____

_____

_____

_____

_____

_____

_____

3. I prefer working in an atmosphere:

   a. that is structured and involves analytic thinking

   b. where the decision-making process is cut-and-dry and the options are well defined

   c. where I do not have to make decisions or interpret anything

4. When preparing a meal or recipe, I:

   a. am very careful to make sure I read the recipe over twice before I start and have each of the ingredients on hand

   b. read the recipe quickly just to make sure I understand the basics

   c. just wing it; I cook by intuition

5. When preparing for a trip or vacation, I:

   a. know exactly where my passport and other important papers are located, make a list of all essential items to bring and check off the list as each is packed, and leave detailed written instructions for the housesitter

   b. know pretty much what I need and where I can find it; but I wait until the day before to get it all together

   c. let someone else do all the packing and handle all the arrangements; too many details for me

6. After a conversation with someone I have just met, I:

   a. remember the exact color of his or her eyes

   b. would be able to make a pretty good guess about what color his or her eyes are

   c. have no idea what color his or her eyes are

7. When giving people driving directions to a destination, I:

   a. make sure to give detailed instructions, using at least two different routes, noting landmarks and the location of gas stations along the way

   b. say basically what area of town they need to head toward and the street address; I know they can figure out the rest on their own

   c. usually give people the wrong directions, so I tell them to ask someone else

8. In regard to friends' birthdays, I:

   a. have them all written down in my calendar, and I send cards out four days before the date

   b. know what month they fall in, and make sure to wish them a happy birthday somewhere around the middle of the month

   c. am usually embarrassed when I find out a friend's birthday has passed; I can never remember dates

Scoring: If most of your answers were A's, you are an extremely detail-oriented and observant person. You are well suited to the tasks performed in the medical laboratory. If your answers were mostly B's, you can be observant, but you do not always pay close attention to details. If your answers were mostly C's, you will need to work on your observation skills.

	Color:
O	Additive:
	Specimen type:
	Tests:

	Color:
O	Additive:
	Specimen type:
	Tests:

	Color:
O	Additive:
	Specimen type:
	Tests:

	Color:
O	Additive:
	Specimen type:
	Tests:

	Color:
O	Additive:
	Specimen type:
	Tests:

	Color:
O	Additive:
	Specimen type:
	Tests:

	Color:
O	Additive:
	Specimen type:
	Tests:

	Color:
O	Additive:
	Specimen type:
	Tests:

CHAPTER **41**

Hematology

CHAPTER PRE-TEST

Perform this test without looking at your book. If an answer is "false," rewrite the sentence to make it true.

1. True or False? Hematology is the study of blood cells and coagulation.

_____

_____

2. True or False? Hematopoiesis is the formation of blood cells.

_____

_____

3. True or False? An increase in neutrophils is indicative of a bacterial infection.

_____

_____

4. True or False? White blood cells (WBCs) are responsible for carrying oxygen to the body's cells.

_____

_____

5. True or False? Platelets assist with clotting.

_____

_____

6. True or False? Red blood cells (RBCs) are the most numerous of all the body's blood cell components.

_____

_____

VOCABULARY BUILDER

Misspelled Words

Find the words in Column A that are misspelled; circle them, and correctly spell them in the spaces provided. Then match each of the vocabulary terms below with the correct definition in Column B.

Column A	Correct Spelling	Column B
1. Complete blood count	_____	A. A hormone triggered by the kidneys that helps produce RBCs
2. Erythrocysts	_____	B. Having less color than normal
3. Esinophil	_____	C. A larger than normal cell
4. Microcytic	_____	D. A WBC without cytoplasmic granules that has a large, convoluted, nonsegmented nucleus
5. Luekocytes	_____	E. A smaller than normal cell
6. Hematacrit	_____	F. WBCs, one of the formed elements of blood
7. Hemaglobin	_____	G. WBC with a dense, nonsegmented nucleus that lacks granules in the cytoplasm
8. Basophil	_____	H. Platelets
9. Thrombocytes	_____	I. Granulocytic WBC with dark purple cytoplasmic granules
10. Lymphocytes	_____	J. Molecule of the RBC that transports oxygen
11. Monocytes	_____	K. Percentage of RBCs within a specimen of anticoagulated whole blood
12. Macrocytic	_____	L. A granulocytic WBC with red-stained granules in the cytoplasm that is increased with allergies
13. Hypochromic	_____	M. RBCs, one of the formed elements of blood
14. Erythropotin	_____	N. Hematologic test consisting of Hct, Hgb, RBC and WBC counts, differential WBC count, and the erythrocyte indices

Handwritten answers in left margin: G J E N A M D H I K B L F

LEARNING REVIEW

Short Answer

1. When Dr. Winston Lewis orders CBCs on his patients, what are the general tests the provider will study to help him make a diagnosis?

_____

_____

_____

2. While Dr. Elizabeth King is reviewing blood tests drawn on one of her patients, she notes the hematocrit is normal, yet the hemoglobin is low. This is an indication of what disease?

_____

_____

3. What two WBC features on a stained differential slide are studied to assist in the identification of the cell?

_____

_____

4. Identify the following erythrocyte indices and list the correct formula for determining each one.

MCH   *27 - 33*   _____

MCHC   *32 - 36 gal*   _____

MCV   _____   _____

5. In Dr. Lewis's office, Larry Dykstra, CMA (AAMA), performs a test of erythrocyte sedimentation rate (ESR) using the Wintrobe method, whereas at Inner City Health Care, Cole Kozloff, CMA (AAMA), uses the Westergren method. Describe the difference between the two procedures.

_____

_____

_____

6. Sedimentation-rate results vary with different states of health. Name two factors that influence the sedimentation rate. Why is the ESR a more accurate tool in diagnosing the onset of a disease than in checking on the progress of treatment?

_____

_____

_____

_____

_____

_____

7. At Inner City Health Care, Mary Kilmer-Tice, CMA (AAMA), uses automated hematology instruments. Automated hematology procedures have many advantages over the manual methods. List five of these advantages.

_____

_____

_____

_____

8. Name three procedures required by CLIA '88 regulations for automated hematology instruments.

_____

_____

_____

_____

_____

Matching

Match the appropriate adult parameters with the following blood tests.

_____   1. 36–55%   A. Hemoglobin

_____   2. 80–100 fl   B. WBC count

_____   3. 4,500–11,000/mm^3 C. Mean corpuscular volume

_____   4. 32–36 g/dL   D. Hematocrit

_____   5. 4.0–6.0 million/mm^3 E. Mean corpuscular hemoglobin concentration

_____   6. 12–18 g/dL   F. RBC count

_____   7. 27–33 pg   G. Mean corpuscular hemoglobin

CERTIFICATION REVIEW

These questions are designed to mimic the certification examination. Select the best response.

1. When a provider collects a bone marrow sample in an adult, the site chosen is the iliac crest or the:

   a. femur

   b. sternum

   c. tibia

   d. scapula

2. The central ion of each heme group is:

   a. magnesium

   b. calcium

   c. potassium

   d. iron

3. A buffy coat contains WBCs and:

   a. RBCs

   b. plasma

   c. platelets

   d. serum

4. When a patient has iron deficiency anemia, the erythrocytes will appear:

   a. hyperchromic

   b. hypochromic

   c. polychromic

   d. bichromic

5. Increased eosinophils may indicate:

   a. hay fever or other allergic conditions

   b. leukemia

   c. appendicitis

   d. tuberculosis

LEARNING APPLICATION

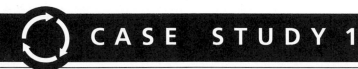

CASE STUDY 1

Wayne Elder is a regular patient at Inner City Health Care. Two days ago, he began to feel fatigued, experiencing development of a cough, fever, and chills. Dr. Ray Rehnolds has examined Mr. Elder and, based on the presented symptoms, makes a clinical diagnosis of influenza.

CASE STUDY REVIEW QUESTIONS

1. What type of blood test will Dr. Reynolds order to confirm his diagnosis?

    _____

    _____

2. What type of results are to be expected based on a diagnosis confirming clinical data?

    _____

    _____

    _____

    _____

CASE STUDY 2

Maria Jover is describing a constant rundown feeling. After examining her, Dr. Elizabeth King has ordered a hemoglobin determination. Also, because of a past history of blood transfusion, she has also ordered an HIV test to be done at an outside reference laboratory. Dr. King asks Ellen Armstrong, CMA (AAMA), to perform the venipuncture procedure on Maria to obtain the blood specimens for analysis.

CASE STUDY REVIEW QUESTIONS

1. What tube will Ellen use to collect the blood sample to be used for the hemoglobin determination test?

    _____

    _____

continues

2. What is Dr. King hoping to learn from the hemoglobin test results?

_____

_____

_____

3. With the fact that HIV infection cannot yet be ruled out, what Standard Precautions should Ellen follow in performing the venipuncture and the automated hemoglobin determination test?

_____

_____

_____

_____

_____

_____

_____

_____

_____

_____

CHAPTER POST-TEST

Perform this test without looking at your book. If an answer is "false," rewrite the sentence to make it true.

1. True or False? Hematology is the study of blood cells, coagulation, and chemistry.

_____

_____

2. True or False? Hematosis is the formation of blood cells.

_____

_____

3. True or False? An increase in lymphocytes is indicative of a bacterial infection.

_____

_____

4. True or False? RBCs are responsible for carrying oxygen to the body's cells.

_____

_____

5. True or False? Thrombocytes assist with clotting.

_____

_____

6. True or False? RBCs are the least numerous of all the body's blood cell components.

_____

_____

SELF-ASSESSMENT

What are your personal feelings about performing venipuncture and testing the blood of individuals who may be infected with HIV?

1. Do you think you will be more cautious than with a non–HIV infected patient?

_____

_____

_____

_____

_____

_____

_____

_____

_____

2. Do you think you should be notified if the blood you are drawing or testing is known to be HIV positive?

_____

_____

_____

_____

3. Do you have the same concerns with hepatitis-infected specimens?

_____

_____

_____

_____

3. When handling urine specimens, Standard Precautions must be followed to ensure that proper infection control standards are observed. In the spaces provided below, list five precautions used when handling urine specimens.

_____

_____

_____

_____

_____

_____

4. List seven regulations of the Clinical Laboratory Improvement Act (CLIA) that apply to the clinical medical assistant performing urine testing.

_____

_____

_____

_____

_____

_____

_____

5. Name the four types of urine specimens frequently ordered by providers.

_____

_____

6. Name the two methods of urine collection.

_____

_____

7. What are the four steps in a physical examination of a urine specimen?

_____

_____

_____

8. What does the specific gravity of urine indicate?

_____

_____

_____

9. Name three methods of measuring the specific gravity of a urine specimen and state the advantages and disadvantages of each. Indicate the method that is available in conjunction with chemical testing.

_____

_____

_____

_____

_____

_____

_____

10. How should reagent test strips be handled and stored?

_____

_____

_____

_____

_____

_____

11. Crystals are the most insignificant part of urinary sediment and are not usually an important element of microscopic analysis, though many laboratories do report them. However, a few crystals may indicate disease states; name three.

_____

_____

12. Casts are formed when protein accumulates and precipitates in the kidney tubules and are then washed into the urine. Identify each cast below and draw an example in the square provided.

Description	Cast Name	Drawing
These casts contain remnants of disintegrated cells that have a fine or coarse appearance.	_____	
These casts contain leukocytes, erythrocytes, or skin cells.	_____	
These casts are difficult to see under the microscope without some light adjustment because of their near transparency.	_____	

13. In the squares below, draw an example of the sediment as seen under a microscope.

Drawing	Sediment
	Spermatoza, cotton fibers, and starch granules
	Yeast
	Squamous epithelial cells
	Bacteria

LEARNING APPLICATION

Labeling Activity

1. One of the most important steps in the collection of urine specimens is to correctly identify the specimen through proper labeling. Make up your own identification number, using Dr. Mark Woo as your provider, and write out complete labeling information for a specimen of your own urine below.

2. What is the proper procedure for testing an unlabeled or incorrectly labeled specimen?

_____

_____

_____

CASE STUDY 1

At Inner City Health Care, Wanda Slawson, CMA (AAMA), gives patient Wendy Janus written directions for a 24-hour urine collection to be performed at home, but Wendy misplaces them. Wanda must give directions to Wendy over the telephone.

CASE STUDY REVIEW QUESTIONS

1. What directions should be given to the patient to correctly perform the urine collection?

_____

_____

_____

_____

_____

_____

_____

_____

_____

continues

2. What communication techniques should Wendy use to make sure the patient understands the collection procedures? What other potential alternatives for communicating the information, besides the telephone, are available?

_____

_____

_____

_____

_____

 # CASE STUDY 2

Wanda Slawson, CMA (AAMA), is asked to give a male adolescent patient the proper procedure for a clean-catch specimen. The 15-year-old boy is visibly embarrassed and will not hold eye contact with Wanda as she relates the instructions for collection to him.

CASE STUDY REVIEW QUESTIONS

1. What instructions are relevant for a clean-catch specimen for this patient?

_____

_____

_____

_____

_____

_____

_____

_____

2. What communication techniques should Wanda use when working with this patient?

_____

_____

_____

_____

_____

C H A P T E R **4 5**

The Medical Assistant as Office Manager

CHAPTER PRE-TEST

Perform this test without looking at your book. If an answer is "false," rewrite the sentence to make it true.

1. True or False? Teamwork results in getting more accomplished with the resources available.

   _____

   _____

2. True or False? Office managers do not need effective communication skills.

   _____

   _____

3. True or False? It is not necessary to update the office procedures manual.

   _____

   _____

4. True or False? Minutes should be sent only to the team members who attended the meeting.

   _____

   _____

5. True or False? When working with an externing student, each step should be explained together with the rationale.

   _____

   _____

6. True or False? Office managers need to be able to accept and offer criticism constructively.

   _____

   _____

7. True or False? The office manager will always serve as the human resources director.

   _____

   _____

VOCABULARY BUILDER

Misspelled Words

Find the words listed below that are misspelled; circle them, and correctly spell them in the spaces provided. Then insert the correct vocabulary terms beside the sentences that follow.

agenda	"going bare"	practicum
ancilliary services	itinerary	procedures manual
benchmarking	liability	professional liability insurance
benefits	marketing	risk management
bond	minutes	teamwork
embezzel	negligance	work statement
externs		

_____   _____   _____

_____

1. Professional occupational companies hired to complete a specific job such as janitorial services, laundry, or disposal of hazardous materials

_____

2. The situation of a provider who does not carry insurance to protect the provider's assets in the event of a liability claim

_____

3. Making a comparison between different organizations relative to how they accomplish tasks, remunerate employees, and so on

_____

4. Designed to protect assets in the event a liability claim is filed and awarded

_____

5. A written record of topics discussed and actions taken during meeting sessions

_____

6. This provides a concise description of the work you plan to accomplish

_____

7. A binding agreement with an employee ensuring recovery of financial loss should funds be stolen or embezzled

_____

8. A printed list of topics to be discussed during a meeting

_____

9. The process by which the provider of services makes the consumer aware of the scope and quality of those services. Examples might include public relations, brochures, patient education seminars, and newsletters.

10. Involves persons synergistically working together

_____

11. A transitional stage providing an opportunity to apply theory learned in the classroom to a health care setting through practical, hands-on experience

_____

12. Remuneration that is in addition to a salary

_____

13. To appropriate fraudulently for one's own use

_____

14. Involves the identification, analysis, and treatment of risks within the medical office or facility

_____ 15. Performing an act that a reasonable and prudent provider would not perform.

_____ 16. Provides detailed information relative to the performance of tasks within the facility in which one is employed

_____ 17. A detailed plan for a proposed trip

LEARNING REVIEW

Short Answer

1. The office manager of a medical office or ambulatory care facility can have many varied responsibilities based on individual facility needs. What are five duties that are the responsibility of the office manager in a health care setting?

_____

_____

_____

_____

_____

_____

_____

_____

_____

_____

2. What are five attributes needed to perform as a quality manager in any office setting?

_____

_____

_____

3. What is the difference between authoritarian and participatory management styles?

_____

_____

_____

_____

4. What does "management by walking around" mean, and why would it be useful in a medical office setting?

_____

_____

_____

5. The table below discusses some of the common risks for medical offices, as well as risk control measures for each one. Fill in any missing information.

Risk	Risk Control Measures
_____	Train various employees to assume other duties and perform them when an employee is ill, on vacation, etc.
Failure of a supplier or contractor	_____ _____ _____ _____ _____
_____	Have protocols in place for handling this situation and make patients aware of the protocols; notify patients immediately if confidential information is disclosed and work with them toward resolution.
Computer failure	_____ _____ _____ _____ _____
_____	Continually review safety procedures; conduct safety surveys; always carry liability insurance; complete an Incident Report to signal risk manager to implement existing protocols to minimize risk

6. Define harassment in the workplace.

_____

_____

_____

_____

7. List the steps that a manager should take if he or she is made aware of harassment in the medical office.

_____

_____

_____

_____

_____

8. Why do some employers put new employees on probation? What is the usual length of an employee's probationary period?

_____

_____

_____

_____

Ordering Activity

All administrative and clinical supplies and equipment in the facility must be inventoried. The following tasks are performed when new supplies and/or equipment are received. Put the tasks steps in the correct order, from 1 to 5.

_____ A. Unpack each item, checking against the packing slip.

_____ B. Write the date the shipment was received and who verified it.

_____ C. Stock each item appropriately.

_____ D. Verify that no items have been substituted or backordered.

_____ E. Find the packing slip listing the items ordered.

Matching

Most marketing tools used in a medical environment provide educational and office services information to patients, potential patients, and the local community. Match the following marketing tools with their potential use in the ambulatory care facility setting.

A. Seminars
B. Brochures
C. Newsletters
D. Press releases
E. Special events

_____ 1. These are used for announcing new equipment, new staff, expanded or remodeled office space, and so on.

_____ 2. These typically come in two types—patient education and office services—and present a professional image of the ambulatory care setting.

_____ 3. These provide an effective way to join with other community organizations to promote wellness.

_____ 4. These can educate patients and provide goodwill in the community. All facility staff can work as a team to organize these.

_____ 5. These can include a wide range of information from health-related topics to staff introductions to insurance updates. They may form the nucleus of a marketing program.

CERTIFICATION REVIEW

These questions are designed to mimic the certification examination. Select the best response.

1. There is a direct correlation between a person's management style and his or her:

   a. technical expertise

   b. educational level

   c. personality

   d. salary

2. Most conflicts occur between employees and supervisors or providers because of:

   a. attitude

   b. poor communication

   c. a misunderstanding

   d. b. and c.

3. The person who applies the team-oriented management style is often comfortable with:

   a. teaching and coaching

   b. building, constructing, and modeling

   c. ideas, information, and data

   d. all of the above

4. A comprehensive safety program is essential to:

   a. marketing functions

   b. team building

   c. risk management

   d. equipment and supply maintenance

5. Leadership for the twenty-first century includes components of flexibility, mentoring, and:

   a. networking

   b. domination

   c. hierarchy

   d. rigidity

6. A rule that defines almost all of the ethical qualities of a manager is:

   a. Murphy's law

   b. the Rule of Nines

   c. the Golden Rule

   d. none of the above

7. The _____ management style is based on the premise that the worker is capable and wants to do a good job.

   a. walking around

   b. participatory

   c. risk

   d. authoritarian

8. The most significant task(s) of the team leader or office manager is (are):

   a. getting the team members to understand and support the specifics of the problem they are asked to solve

   b. enabling the team to develop their own work statement where they will assume ownership of the goals and objectives

   c. establishing a timetable for achieving results and identifying the standards that must be maintained

   d. all of the above

9. The documentation of policies and procedures that make up the office HIPAA manual should be:

   a. filed in a locked cabinet

   b. kept for six years, even though wording has been changed or has been eliminated

   c. made available for all employees

   d. b. and c.

10. If malpractice litigation should occur, the best protocol to follow is to:

    a. be honest with the patients and insurance carriers

    b. let the HR person handle the situation

    c. notify the provider

    d. not get involved

LEARNING APPLICATION

Time Management Activity

To practice your time management skills, make a to-do list for tomorrow or the upcoming weekend. Prioritize the list by importance.

CASE STUDY

Office manager Shirley Brooks is responsible for the preparation and distribution of payroll checks at the offices of Drs. Lewis and King. Because the group practice is in the process of upgrading the computer system to accommodate a recent influx of new patients, Shirley is temporarily preparing the payroll using the manual write-it-once bookkeeping system. She is careful to consult payroll records for each employee, which include the employee's name, address, telephone number, and Social Security number; number of exemptions claimed on the W-4 form; gross salary; deductions withheld for all taxes, including Social Security, federal, state, local unemployment and disability; and date of employment.

CASE STUDY REVIEW QUESTIONS

1. As Shirley writes out the payroll check for Audrey Jones, CMA (AAMA), what information should be included on the paycheck stub?

   _____

   _____

   _____

   _____

   _____

   _____

2. What must the provider's office have to process payroll?

   _____

   _____

   _____

3. What responsibility does the office manager have with regard to the confidentiality of payroll records? How might employees' rights to privacy be maintained?

   _____

   _____

   _____

   _____

   _____

   _____

CHAPTER POST-TEST

Perform this test without looking at your book. If an answer is "false," rewrite the sentence to make it true.

1. True or False? Teamwork results in getting less accomplished with the resources available.

_____

_____

2. True or False? Office managers need effective communication skills.

_____

_____

3. True or False? It is necessary to update the office procedures manual.

_____

_____

4. True or False? Minutes should be sent to all team members, not just those who attended the meeting.

_____

_____

5. True or False? When working with externing students, each step does not need to be explained together with the rationale, because they already have training.

_____

_____

6. True or False? Office managers need to be able to offer criticism constructively, but they should not have to accept criticism.

_____

_____

7. True or False? The person who is the office manager is never the human resources director.

_____

_____

SELF-ASSESSMENT

Put yourself in the place of the office manager.

1. What type of management style do you think you are the most comfortable with?

_____

_____

_____

_____

2. Carefully read about each type of style and explain why you think you are that type.

_____

_____

_____

_____

3. What skills will come naturally to you?

_____

_____

_____

_____

4. What skills will you have to work on the most?

_____

_____

_____

_____

C H A P T E R **4 6**

The Medical Assistant as Human Resources Manager

CHAPTER PRE-TEST

Perform this test without looking at your book. If an answer is "false," rewrite the sentence to make it true.

1. Which of the following is *not* a function of the human resources (HR) manager?

    a. Creating and updating a policy manual

    b. Recruiting and hiring office personnel

    c. Orienting new personnel

    d. Training new personnel

2. True or False? Wage and salary policies should be in writing.

    _____

    _____

3. True or False? A policy manual should contain daily step-by-step instructions.

    _____

    _____

4. True or False? Job descriptions are not always useful because they change so often.

    _____

    _____

5. True or False? All job applicants should be interviewed.

    _____

    _____

6. True or False? It is acceptable to ask job applicants about the last place they worked and a conflict they had there.

    _____

    _____

7. True or False? References are usually checked after the first interview.

_____

_____

8. True or False? The HR manager is responsible for dismissing employees.

_____

_____

9. True or False? Employees have a right to review their personnel files at any time.

_____

_____

10. True or False? Employers have the right to refuse to allow full-time employees to go on jury duty.

_____

_____

VOCABULARY BUILDER

Misspelled Words

Find the words listed below that are misspelled; circle them, and correctly spell them in the spaces provided. Then, insert the correct vocabulary terms into the following sentences.

exit interveiw	letter of referance	overtime
involuntary dismisal	letter of resignation	probation
job desciption	menter	résumés

_____   _____   _____

_____   _____

1. Because of an unexpected staffing shortfall, Audrey Jones, CMA (AAMA), has volunteered to work _____ this week. She will receive 1½ times the regular rate of pay for hours above her regular 40-hour week.

2. An _____ has been scheduled for administrative/clinical medical assistant Liz Corbin before she leaves the clinic to continue her education. This session will give Liz an opportunity to provide her positive and negative opinions of the position and the facility.

3. Office manager Marilyn Johnson has received a _____ from the former instructor of a current job applicant describing the applicant's performance, attitude, and qualifications.

4. The violation of office policies at Inner City Health Care led to the _____ of one of the part-time employees.

5. Liz Corbin, CMA (AAMA), submitted a _____ to her current employer when she decided to leave her present position to return to school to pursue an advanced degree.

6. Office manager Marilyn Johnson will inform all of the job applicants that they will be on _____ for their first three months on the job. During this period, the employee and supervisory personnel can determine if the environment and the position are satisfactory for the employee.

7. Office manager Jane O'Hara, updating the employee manual, includes a _____ for every position in the office, which details tasks, duties, and responsibilities.

8. Administrative medical assistant Ellen Armstrong looks upon office manager Marilyn Johnson as her _____, since Marilyn has been instrumental in Ellen's training, coaching, and guidance in her newly acquired position.

LEARNING REVIEW

Short Answer

1. The manual that identifies clear guidelines and directions required of all employees is known as the policy manual. What are four topics that would be included in a policy manual regardless of the size of the practice identified in this chapter?

_____

_____

_____

2. Office manager Marilyn Johnson has the responsibility of dismissing an employee for a serious violation of office policies. From the list below, select key points to keep in mind when dismissal is necessary by circling the letters of the statements that apply.

   a. Have employee pack his or her belongings from desk.

   b. The dismissal should be made in private.

   c. Take no longer than 20 minutes for the dismissal.

   d. Be direct, firm, and to the point in identifying reasons.

   e. Explain terms of dismissal (keys, clearing out area, final paperwork).

   f. Do not listen to the employee's opinion and emotions.

   g. If he or she insists, allow the employee to finish the work of the day.

   h. Do not engage in an in-depth discussion of performance.

3. Compare and contrast voluntary and involuntary separation.

_____

_____

_____

_____

_____

_____

_____

4. The job description must have enough information to provide both the supervisor and the employee with a clear outline of what the job entails. Name four items that must be included in a job description.

_____

_____

_____

5. The interview worksheet is an excellent tool to make certain that the interviews with each candidate are fair and equitable. Provide six items that should be included on any interview worksheet.

_____

_____

_____

_____

_____

CERTIFICATION REVIEW

These questions are designed to mimic the certification examination. Select the best response.

1. A salary review is:

   a. usually conducted at the beginning of the new year

   b. virtually the same as the performance review

   c. conducted on the anniversary date of hire

   d. normally done every three years

2. Questions regarding drug use, arrest records, and medical history during an interview are:

   a. appropriate

   b. inappropriate

   c. illegal

   d. none of the above

3. Title VII of the Civil Rights Act addresses:

   a. overtime pay

   b. discrimination based on race, age, and sex

   c. hiring and firing practices

   d. sexual harassment

4. When a candidate accepts a position, the HR manager should write a letter outlining the specifics of the job. This letter is called a:

   a. confirmation letter

   b. congratulatory letter

   c. recommendation letter

   d. reference letter

5. A person with AIDS who satisfies the necessary skills for a job and has the experience and education required will be protected from discrimination by:

   a. OSHA

   b. CLIA

   c. AAMA

   d. ADA

6. A job description should be reviewed and updated:

   a. every 2 years

   b. every 90 days

   c. every year

   d. every 5 years

7. Voluntary separation usually occurs when:

    a. advancing to another position

    b. there is a violation of office policies

    c. the employee is relocating

    d. a. and c.

8. Verifying that all employees are authorized to work is done by

    a. asking for verbal clarification

    b. having the candidate complete an I-9 form

    c. having the candidate provide a notarized statement

    d. having the candidate fill out an attestation form

9. What documents should be included in the personnel file? *(circle all that apply)*

    a. Application

    b. Formal review

    c. Awards

    d. Employee handbook

10. What act was established to prevent injuries and illnesses resulting from unsafe and unhealthy working conditions?

    a. Americans with Disabilities Act

    b. Civil Rights Act

    c. OSHA

    d. Equal Pay Act

LEARNING APPLICATION

Since the offices of Drs. Lewis and King have expanded to cover a rapidly growing patient load, including the hiring of a co–office manager and a new clinical medical assistant, the work pace has been hectic, but challenging. At the suggestion of Dr. Lewis, the office managers decide to hold a staff meeting to talk about ways to keep the lines of communication open and to process the many changes occurring at the growing medical practice. Marilyn Johnson and Shirley Brooks encourage staff to be vocal with their feedback, suggestions, and concerns.

CASE STUDY REVIEW QUESTIONS

1. What other techniques can the office managers use to prevent or solve conflicts in the workplace during the period of growth and transition?

   _____

   _____

   _____

   _____

   _____

   _____

   _____

   _____

   _____

2. Why is effective communication one of the most important goals of the HR manager?

   _____

   _____

   _____

CHAPTER POST-TEST

Perform this test without looking at your book. If an answer is "false," rewrite the sentence to make it true.

1. Which of the following are functions of the HR manager? *(Circle all that apply)*

   a. Creating and updating a policy manual

   b. Training new personnel

   c. Recruiting and hiring office personnel

   d. Orienting new personnel

2. True or False? Wage and salary policies need not be in writing as long as both parties agree.

   _____

   _____

3. True or False? A policy manual should contain general policies and practices of the office.

   _____

   _____

4. True or False? Job descriptions are always useful and should be clearly written.

   _____

   _____

5. True or False? Only qualified job applicants should be interviewed.

   _____

   _____

6. True or False? It is good to ask job applicants about conflicts they have had and how they solved them.

   _____

   _____

7. True or False? References are usually checked before the first interview.

   _____

   _____

8. True or False? The HR manager is responsible for the exit interview, but usually not for dismissing employees.

   _____

   _____

9. True or False? Employees do not have the right to review their personnel files unless requested by an attorney.

   _____

   _____

10. True or False? Employers cannot condemn or discriminate against a full-time employee who is on jury duty.

   _____

   _____

SELF-ASSESSMENT

1. If you were put into the position of hiring a new employee, what attributes would you be looking for?

   a. Make a list of the technical skills your new employee would need.

   _____

   _____

   b. Make a list of the affective (behavior) skills your new employee would need, including a positive attitude, a good work ethic, and so forth.

   _____

   _____

   _____

   _____

   c. Determine how you could measure the technical skills you listed.

   _____

   _____

   _____

   d. Determine how you could quantify the affective (behavior) skills you listed in item b. above. How could you determine those qualities?

   _____

   _____

   _____

   e. Which is more difficult to measure: technical or behavioral qualities? Which is more difficult to train?

   _____

   _____

2. When you interview for a job, what technical and behavioral skills on your lists will you need to improve on?

   _____

   _____

Name _____ Date _____ Score _____

CHAPTER **47**

Preparing for Medical Assisting Credentials

CHAPTER PRE-TEST

Perform this test without looking at your book. If an answer is "false," rewrite the sentence to make it true.

1. True or False? A registered medical assistant (RMA) and a certified medical assistant (CMA [AAMA]) have the same bylaws and creed.

   _____

   _____

2. True or False? A CMA (AAMA) may work only in the state in which the credentials were received.

   _____

   _____

3. True or False? Three major areas included in the RMA examination are clinical, administrative, and general medical knowledge.

   _____

   _____

4. True or False? Medical assistants may be trained on the job; however, providers recognize that their offices operate much more efficiently and effectively with professionally trained and formally educated personnel.

   _____

   _____

5. True or False? On meeting CMA recertification requirements, the applicant will receive a new certificate.

   _____

   _____

6. True or False? Once a student has become a member of AAMA, he or she may stay at the student rate for one year after graduation.

   _____

   _____

7. True or False? The National Healthcare Association (NHA) does not offer continuing education programs and does not encourage recertification.

_____

_____

8. True or False? Retaking the RMA examination is not an option for reinstatement or recertification.

_____

_____

VOCABULARY BUILDER

Matching

Match each correct vocabulary term to the aspect of the certification process that best describes it.

_____ 1. Certification examination

_____ 2. Certified medical assistant (CMA [AAMA])

_____ 3. Continuing education units (CEUs)

_____ 4. Certified clinical medical assistant (CCMA)

_____ 5. Recertification

_____ 6. Registered medical assistant (RMA)

_____ 7. Task Force for Test Construction

A. Method for earning points toward recertification

B. A standardized means of evaluating medical assistant competency

C. Maintaining current CMA (AAMA) status

D. Credential awarded for successfully passing the AAMA certification examination

E. Committee of professionals whose responsibility is to update the CMA (AAMA) examination annually to reflect changes in medical assistants' responsibilities and to include new developments in medical knowledge and technology

F. Credential awarded for successfully passing the AMT examination

G. One of the credentials awarded for passing the National Healthcare Association exam

LEARNING REVIEW

Short Answer

1. The AAMA certification examination is a comprehensive test of the knowledge based on tasks performed in today's medical office. The test is updated annually to include the latest changes in medical assistants' daily responsibilities. In addition, the updates include the latest developments in medical knowledge and technology. Name the three major areas tested in the AAMA certification examination and describe what each includes.

_____

_____

_____

_____

_____

_____

_____

_____

2. What are the addresses, telephone numbers, and Web sites for obtaining applications for the certification examinations of the AAMA, AMT, and NHA?

AAMA

_____

_____

_____

AMT

_____

_____

_____

NHA

_____

_____

_____

3. To keep their CMA (AAMA) credentials current, how often are individuals required to recertify? How many continuing education units (CEUs) are necessary to recertify?

_____

_____

_____

4. In addition to the RMA credential, what is the credential that the AMT offers for those who primarily want to be employed in the front office of provider offices, clinics, or hospitals?

_____

_____

5. List the criteria an applicant must possess for taking the NHA certification exam.

_____

_____

_____

_____

_____

CERTIFICATION REVIEW

These questions are designed to mimic the certification examination. Select the best response.

1. General medical assisting knowledge on the AMT certification examination includes anatomy and physiology, medical terminology, and:

   a. insurance and billing

   b. medical ethics

   c. bookkeeping and filing

   d. first aid

2. The AMT registration exam consists of:

   a. 300 multiple choice questions

   b. 250 multiple choice questions

   c. 200–210 four-option multiple choice questions

   d. 500 multiple choice questions

3. A total of how many questions are on the CMA (AAMA) certification examination?

   a. 100

   b. 200

   c. 1,000

   d. It varies year to year.

4. How often does an RMA need to recertify?

   a. Every year

   b. Every 6 years

   c. Every 5 years

   d. Every 3 years

5. A total of how many CEUs are required to recertify the CMA (AAMA) credential?

   a. 45

   b. 60

   c. 100

   d. 120

6. When recertifying through the AAMA, a minimum of _____ points is required in each of the three categories. The remaining _____ points may be accumulated in any of the three content areas or from any combination of the three categories.

   a. 15, 60

   b. 20, 40

   c. 10, 30

   d. 30, 60

7. The purpose of certification is that it:

   a. acknowledges that you are a professional with standard entry-level knowledge and skills

   b. builds your personal self-esteem and confidence in knowing that you can do the job asked of you

   c. helps in your career advancement and compensation

   d. All of the above

LEARNING APPLICATION

CASE STUDY

Michele Lucas is performing her practicum at Inner City Health Care under the direction of office manager Jane O'Hara. Michele has purchased a certification review study guide and has taken the sample 120-question certification examination available from the AAMA. From her studies, she has determined that she needs more work in the area of collections and insurance processing. Part-time administrative medical assistant Karen Ritter is responsible for these duties at Inner City Health Care, under Jane's supervision.

CASE STUDY REVIEW QUESTIONS

1. How can Michele use her practicum experience to help her concentrate on improving her skills in the area of collections and insurance processing?

   _____

   _____

   _____

   _____

   _____

2. What are your own personal strengths and weaknesses in preparing for a certification examination through AAMA, AMT, or NHA? What can you do to improve your areas of weakness?

   _____

   _____

   _____

CHAPTER POST-TEST

Perform this test without looking at your book. If an answer is "false," rewrite the sentence to make it true.

1. True or False? An RMA and a CMA (AAMA) have different bylaws and creeds.

   _____

   _____

2. True or False? A CMA (AAMA) has a national credential, so he or she may work in any state.

   _____

   _____

3. True or False? Three major areas included in the AMT's RMA examination are clinical, administrative, and general.

   _____

   _____

4. True or False? Providers recognize that their offices operate much more efficiently and effectively with professionally trained and formally educated personnel such as medical assistants.

_____

_____

5. True or False? Upon meeting recertification requirements, applicants receive an identification card which will indicate the year of recertification and the expiration date.

_____

_____

6. True or False? Once students have become members of AAMA, they may stay at the student rate for two years after graduation.

_____

_____

7. True or False? The NHA encourages recertification and offers CE programs.

_____

_____

8. True or False? Retaking the RMA examination is an option for reinstatement or recertification.

_____

_____

SELF-ASSESSMENT

1. Think of two different places where you could get continuing education credits.

   a. Investigate each one.

   b. Write a paragraph on the benefits and disadvantages of each method for you in your lifestyle.

2. Find out when and where your local chapter meetings are held.

   a. Attend a meeting with a classmate.

   b. Discuss what you learned from the meeting.

3. What can you do to prepare for the national certification examination?

   a. Write a plan in which you determine how much time you have to prepare and what you will accomplish each week/month in preparation.

   b. Make a calendar showing the steps toward your examination date.

   c. Try to stick with the plan as you progress closer to the examination date.

CHAPTER **4 8**

Employment Strategies

CHAPTER PRE-TEST

Perform this test without looking at your book. If an answer is "false," rewrite the sentence to make it true.

1. True or False? Positive thinking is one of the primary keys to success in planning your career and doing your job search.

   _____

   _____

2. True or False? It would be beneficial to begin your job search by networking with students who have graduated before you and are now successfully employed.

   _____

   _____

3. True or False? Poor appearance is a reason for employers not to hire a job seeker.

   _____

   _____

4. True or False? Employers like it when you know it all. They appreciate it when you do not ask questions.

   _____

   _____

5. True or False? You should never expect to receive a job from an office where you are an extern.

   _____

   _____

6. True or False? When filling out an application, it is acceptable to leave answers blank or write "see résumé."

   _____

   _____

7. True or False? You should always plan ahead and have all your information with you when picking up an application, just in case you are asked to fill it out right there.

   _____

   _____

VOCABULARY BUILDER

Misspelled Words

Find the words listed below that are misspelled; circle them, and correctly spell them in the spaces provided. Then match each correct vocabulary term to the aspect of the job-seeking process that best describes it.

accomplishment statement	cover letter	refrences
application form	cronological résumé	résumé
bullat point	functional résumé	targeted résumé
carreer objective	interview	
contact tracker	power verbs	

_____   _____   _____

_____

_____   1. Expresses your career goal and the position for which you are applying

_____   2. Résumé format used to highlight specialty areas of accomplishments and strengths

_____   3. A form devised by a prospective employer to collect information relative to qualifications, education, and experience in employment

_____   4. Individuals who have known or worked with you long enough to make an honest assessment and recommendation regarding your background history

_____   5. Résumé format used when focusing on a clear, specific job

_____   6. A statement that begins with a power verb and gives a brief description of what you did and the demonstrable results that were produced

_____   7. Asterisk or dot followed by a descriptive phrase

_____   8. A written summary data sheet or brief account of your qualifications and progress in your chosen career

_____   9. Action words used to describe your attributes and strengths

_____   10. A letter used to introduce yourself and your résumé to a prospective employer with the goal of obtaining an interview

_____   11. Résumé format used when you have employment experience

_____   12. A meeting in which you discuss employment opportunities and strengths that you can bring to the organization

_____   13. Form used to keep track of employment contact information, such as name of employer, name of contact person, address and telephone number, date of first contact, résumé sent, interview date, and follow-up information and dates

LEARNING REVIEW

Short Answer

1. List three types of professionals that would make excellent reference choices.

_____

_____

2. Identify an individual you know personally or have contact with who fits each professional reference type listed above and tell why you think they would be an excellent reference for you.

_____

_____

3. Identify the situations in which using a targeted résumé is advantageous by circling the number next to the statements that apply.

   (1) You are just starting your career and have little experience, but you know what you want and you are clear about your capabilities.

   (2) You want to use one résumé for several different applications.

   (3) You are not clear about your abilities and accomplishments.

   (4) You can go in several directions, and you want a different résumé for each.

   (5) You are able to keep your résumé on a computer disk.

4. Identify the situations in which using a chronological résumé is advantageous by circling the number next to the statements that apply.

   (1) The position is in a highly traditional field.

   (2) Your job history shows real growth and development.

   (3) You are changing career goals.

   (4) You are looking for your first job.

   (5) You are staying in the same field as prior jobs.

5. Identify the situations in which using a functional résumé is advantageous by circling the number next to the statements that apply.

   (1) You have extensive specialized experience.

   (2) Your most recent employers have been highly prestigious.

   (3) You have had a variety of different, apparently unconnected, work experiences.

   (4) You want to emphasize a management growth pattern.

   (5) Much of your work has been volunteer, freelance, or temporary.

6. List four guidelines that are essential when preparing an effective cover letter.

_____

_____

_____

_____

_____

_____

_____

_____

_____

_____

_____

7. List four items that are important when completing a job application.

_____

_____

_____

_____

_____

8. Bob Thompson has an interview at Inner City Health Care for a new clinical medical assisting position. He is confident that he has prepared well for the interview. On the way to the interview, Bob reminds himself of three principles he has learned about interviewing.

    (1) _____ before answering questions, and try to provide the information requested in a

    professional manner.

    (2) _____ carefully so that you understand what information the interviewer is requesting.

    (3) _____ if you are uncertain.

9. How would you "dress for success" when preparing for your interview?

_____

_____

_____

_____

_____

_____

CERTIFICATION REVIEW

These questions are designed to mimic the certification examination. Select the best response.

1. Telling your friends, family, personal provider, dentist, and ophthalmologist that you are looking for a position in health care is called:

   a. networking

   b. references

   c. professionalism

   d. critiquing

2. Summarizing employment is acceptable on a résumé if it is prior to how many years ago?

   a. 1 year

   b. 5 years

   c. 10 years

   d. 15 years

3. The type of résumé that should be developed by someone who is just starting a career and has little experience is a(n):

   a. targeted résumé

   b. chronological résumé

   c. functional résumé

   d. objective résumé

4. Poise includes such things as:

   a. skill level

   b. confidence and appearance

   c. a. and b.

   d. none of the above

5. Providing a second opportunity to express your interest in an organization and a position may be done with a:

   a. cover letter

   b. recommendation letter

   c. follow-up letter

   d. strategic letter

6. Your attitude is reflected in how you react to:

   a. taking direction

   b. seeking excellence or doing just enough to get by

   c. assuming responsibility for your actions and considering your problems not to be someone else's fault

   d. all of the above

7. Some examples of transferable skills are *(circle all that apply):*

   a. leadership

   b. communication

   c. keyboarding

   d. drawing blood

8. When using someone as a reference, you should:

   a. always ask permission first before the name is printed on the reference list

   b. use your relatives

   c. verify correct spelling, title, place of employment and position, and telephone number

   d. a. and c.

9. Circle the top errors found with résumés.

   a. Typographical and grammatical errors

   b. Not mentioning jobs having transferable skills

   c. Using the same résumé for all job applications

   d. Listing your credentials

10. During the interview, it is *not* appropriate to ask:

    a. if this is a newly created position

    b. if there are opportunities for advancement

    c. about salary, sick leave, benefits, or vacation

    d. what the interviewer considers to be the most difficult task on the job

LEARNING APPLICATION

CASE STUDY

CASE STUDY REVIEW QUESTIONS

1. You are the subject of this case study. Complete the Self-Evaluation Worksheet that follows. Use your answers to help you determine the working environment you are most interested in and that best suits you. The worksheet can become a useful tool when researching prospective employers to target for your exciting first job in the medical assisting profession.

SELF-EVALUATION WORKSHEET

Respond to the following questions honestly and sincerely. They are meant to assist you in self-assessment.

1. List your strongest attributes as related to people, data, or things.

   i.e., Interpersonal skills related to people

   Accuracy related to data

   Mechanical ability related to things

   _____ related to _____

   _____ related to _____

   _____ related to _____

2. List your three weakest attributes related to people, data, or things.

   _____ related to _____

   _____ related to _____

   _____ related to _____

3. How do you express yourself? excellent, good, fair, poor

   Orally_____ In writing _____

4. Do you work well as a leader of a group or team? Yes _____ No_____

5. Do you prefer to work alone and on your own? Yes _____ No_____

6. Can you work under stress/pressure? Yes_____ No_____

7. Do you enjoy new ideas and situations? Yes_____ No_____

8. Are you comfortable with routines/schedules? Yes_____ No_____

9. Which work setting do you prefer?

   Single-physician setting _____Multiphysician setting _____

   Small clinic setting _____Large clinic setting_____

   Single-specialty setting?_____Multispecialty setting _____

10. Are you willing to relocate? _____ Willing to travel?_____

Application Activities

1. In the Case Study, you completed a self-assessment form to help you find the type of working environment you are most interested in and best suits you. Create a contact tracker file for yourself, based on the one shown in Figure 48-2 in your textbook. Compile a list from the Yellow Pages, the Internet, want ads in your local paper, your program director, and other sources (hint: other sources are listed in the textbook).

2. Refer to Figure 48-10 in your textbook, which lists typical questions asked during an interview. Write what you would say to a potential employer in response to all of these questions. Then role play with another student, acting as interviewer and interviewee, with these questions and answers to gain confidence for an interview.

3. Recall that the interview process is a "two-way street." You, as the interviewee, should interview the employer. The text lists several example questions you might ask the interviewer during an interview. Develop a list of at least two additional questions that are important to you during the interview process.

CHAPTER POST-TEST

Perform this test without looking at your book. If an answer is "false," rewrite the sentence to make it true.

1. True or False? Positive thinking is a good thing, but it is not all that important to success in planning your career and doing your job search.

   _____

   _____

2. True or False? When beginning your job search, it would be beneficial to network with students who have graduated before you and are now successfully employed in the field.

   _____

   _____

3. True or False? Professional appearance is one reason for employers to want to hire a job seeker.

   _____

   _____

4. True or False? Employers do not expect that you will know it all. They appreciate it when you ask questions.

   _____

   _____

5. True or False? Students often receive job offers from the office where they extern.

   _____

   _____

6. True or False? When filling out an application, it is never acceptable to leave answers blank or to write "see résumé."

   _____

   _____

7. True or False? Plan ahead and have all your information with you when you pick up an application, just in case you are asked to fill it out right there.

   _____

   _____

SELF-ASSESSMENT

Imagine you are interviewing a recent graduate for a medical assisting position.

1. What questions might you ask during the interviewing process?

_____

_____

_____

_____

2. Do you think you could determine the best person for the job by meeting him or her just once? What else might you do to get to know the person better or get to know his or her work style better?

_____

_____

_____

_____

3. Did the applicant use power verbs effectively? Did they pique your interest?

_____

_____

_____

Competency Assessment Tracking Sheet

Student Name: _____

Procedure Number and Title	Date Assessment Completed and Competency Achieved			
	Date/Initials	Date/Initials	Date/Initials	Date/Initials
EXAMPLE: 22-1 Medical Asepsis Hand Wash (Hand Hygiene)	**2/23/XX DF**	**3/15/XX SL**	**4/20/XX SP**	**5/1/XX JP**
4-1 Identifying Community Resources				
9-1 Control of Bleeding				
9-2 Applying an Arm Splint				
11-1 Booting Up and Shutting Down the Computer				
11-2 Software Installation				
11-3 Hardware Installation				
12-1 Answering and Screening Incoming Calls				
12-2 Transferring a Call				
12-3 Taking a Telephone Message				
12-4 Calling a Pharmacy to Refill an Authorized Prescription				
12-5 Handling Problem Calls				
12-6 Placing Outgoing Calls				
12-7 Recording a Telephone Message on an Answering Device or Voice Mail System				
12-8 Preparing, Sending, and Receiving a Fax				
13-1 Establishing the Appointment Matrix in a Paper System				
13-2 Establishing the Appointment Matrix Using Medical Office Simulation Software (MOSS)				
13-3 Making an Appointment on the Telephone Using a Paper System				
13-4 Making an Appointment on the Telephone Using Medical Office Simulation Software (MOSS)				
13-5 Checking In Patients in a Paper System				

Procedure Number and Title	Date Assessment Completed and Competency Achieved			
	Date/Initials	Date/Initials	Date/Initials	Date/Initials
13-6 Checking In Patients Using Medical Office Simulation Software (MOSS)				
13-7 Cancellation and Rescheduling Procedures Using Paper Scheduling				
13-8 Cancellation and Rescheduling in Medical Office Simulation Software (MOSS)				
13-9 Scheduling of Inpatient and Outpatient Admissions and Procedures				
14-1 Establishing a Paper Medical Chart for a New Patient				
14-2 Establishing an Electronic Medical Record for a New Patient Using Medical Office Simulation Software (MOSS)				
14-3 Correcting a Paper Medical Record				
14-4 Correcting an Electronic Medical Record				
14-5 Steps for Manual Filing with an Alphabetic System				
14-6 Steps for Manual Filing with a Numeric System				
14-7 Steps for Manual Filing with a Subject Filing System				
15-1 Preparing and Composing Business Correspondence Using All Components (Computerized Approach)				
15-2 Addressing Envelopes According to United States Postal Regulations				
15-3 Folding Letters for Standard Envelopes				
15-4 Creating a Mass Mailing Using Mail Merge				
15-5 Preparing Outgoing Mail According to United States Postal Regulations				
17-1 Applying Managed Care Policies and Procedures				
17-2 Screening for Insurance				

Procedure Number and Title	Date Assessment Completed and Competency Achieved			
	Date/Initials	Date/Initials	Date/Initials	Date/Initials
17-3 Obtaining Referrals and Authorizations				
17-4 Computing the Medicare Fee Schedule				
18-1 Current Procedural Terminology Coding				
18-2 International Classification of Diseases, 9th Revision, Clinical Modification Coding				
18-3 Applying Third-Party Guidelines				
18-4 Completing a Medicare CMS-1500 (08-05) Claim Form				
19-1 Recording/Posting Patient Charges, Payments, and Adjustments in a Manual System				
19-2 Balancing Day Sheets in a Manual System				
19-3 Posting Patient Charges Using Medical Office Simulation Software (MOSS)				
19-4 Insurance Billing Using Medical Office Simulation Software (MOSS)				
19-5 Posting Patient and Adjustments Using Medical Office Simulation Software (MOSS)				
19-6 Processing Credit Balances and Refunds Using Medical Office Simulation Software (MOSS)				
19-7 Preparing a Deposit				
19-8 Recording a Nonsufficient Funds Check in a Manual System				
19-9 Writing a Check				
19-10 Reconciling a Bank Statement				
19-11 Establishing and Maintaining a Petty Cash Fund				
20-1 Explaining Fees in the First Telephone Interview				
20-2 Prepare Itemized Patient Accounts for Billing in a Manual System				

Procedure Number and Title	Date Assessment Completed and Competency Achieved			
	Date/Initials	Date/Initials	Date/Initials	Date/Initials
20-3 Identify Accounts Receivable Using Medical Office Simulation Software (MOSS)				
20-4 Preparing Itemized Patient Accounts for Billing Using Medical Office Simulation Software (MOSS)				
20-5 Post/Record Collection Agency Adjustments in a Manual System				
20-6 Post/Record Adjustments Using Medical Office Simulation Software (MOSS)				
21-1 Preparing Accounts Receivable Trial Balance in a Manual System				
21-2 Preparing Accounts Receivable Trial Balance Using Medical Office Simulation Software (MOSS)				
22-1 Medical Asepsis Hand Wash (Hand Hygiene)				
22-2 Removing Contaminated Gloves				
22-3 Transmission-Based Precautions: Donning a Gown, Mask, Gloves, and Cap (Isolation Technique)				
22-4 Sanitization of Instruments				
23-1 Taking a Medical History for a Paper Record				
24-1 Measuring an Oral Temperature Using an Electronic Thermometer				
24-2 Measuring an Aural Temperature Using a Tympanic Thermometer				
24-3 Measuring a Temperature Using a Temporal Artery (TA) Thermometer				
24-4 Measuring a Rectal Temperature Using a Digital Thermometer				
24-5 Measuring an Axillary Temperature				
24-6 Measuring an Oral Temperature Using a Disposable Oral Strip Thermometer				
24-7 Measuring a Radial Pulse				
24-8 Taking an Apical Pulse				

Procedure Number and Title	Date Assessment Completed and Competency Achieved			
	Date/Initials	Date/Initials	Date/Initials	Date/Initials
24-9 Measuring the Respiration Rate				
24-10 Measuring Blood Pressure				
24-11 Measuring Height				
24-12 Measuring Adult Weight				
25-1 Assisting with a Complete Physical Examination				
26-1 Assisting with Routine Prenatal Visits				
26-2 Assisting with Pelvic Examination and Pap Test (Conventional and ThinPrep® Methods)				
26-3 Assisting with Insertion of an Intrauterine Device (IUD)				
26-4 Wet Prep/Wet Mount and Potassium Hydroxide (KOH) Prep				
26-5 Amplified DNA ProbeTec Test for Chlamydia and Gonorrhea				
27-1 Administration of a Vaccine				
27-2 Maintaining Immunization Records				
27-3 Measuring the Infant: Weight, Length, and Head and Chest Circumference				
27-4 Taking an Infant's Rectal Temperature with a Digital Thermometer				
27-5 Taking an Apical Pulse on an Infant				
27-6 Measuring Infant's Respiratory Rate				
27-7 Obtaining a Urine Specimen from an Infant or Young Child				
28-1 Instructing Patient in Testicular Self-Examination				
30-1 Urinary Catheterization of a Female Patient				
30-2 Urinary Catheterization of a Male Patient				
30-3 Fecal Occult Blood Test				

Procedure Number and Title	Date Assessment Completed and Competency Achieved			
	Date/Initials	Date/Initials	Date/Initials	Date/Initials
30-4 Performing Visual Acuity Testing Using a Snellen Chart				
30-5 Measuring Near Visual Acuity				
30-6 Testing Color Vision Using the Ishihara Plates				
30-7 Performing Eye Instillation				
30-8 Performing Eye Patch Dressing Application				
30-9 Performing Eye Irrigation				
30-10 Assisting with Audiometry				
30-11 Performing Ear Irrigation				
30-12 Performing Ear Instillation				
30-13 Assisting with Nasal Examination				
30-14 Cautery Treatment of Epistaxis				
30-15 Performing Nasal Instillation				
30-16 Administer Oxygen by Nasal Cannula for Minor Respiratory Distress				
30-17 Instructing Patient in Use of Metered Dose Inhaler				
30-18 Spirometry				
30-19 Pulse Oximetry				
30-20 Assisting with Plaster Cast Application				
30-21 Assisting with Cast Removal				
30-22 Assisting the Physician during a Lumbar Puncture or Cerebrospinal Fluid Aspiration				
30-23 Assisting the Provider with a Neurologic Screening Examination				
31-1 Applying Sterile Gloves				
31-2 Chemical "Cold" Sterilization of Endoscopes				
31-3 Preparing Instruments for Sterilization in Autoclave				
31-4 Sterilization of Instruments (Autoclave)				

Procedure Number and Title	Date Assessment Completed and Competency Achieved			
	Date/Initials	Date/Initials	Date/Initials	Date/Initials
31-5 Setting Up and Covering a Sterile Field				
31-6 Opening Sterile Packages of Instruments and Supplies and Applying Them to a Sterile Field				
31-7 Pouring a Sterile Solution into a Cup on a Sterile Field				
31-8 Assisting with Office/Ambulatory Surgery				
31-9 Dressing Change				
31-10 Wound Irrigation				
31-11 Preparation of a Patient's Skin before Surgery				
31-12 Suturing of Laceration or Incision Repair				
31-13 Sebaceous Cyst Excision				
31-14 Incision and Drainage of Localized Infection				
31-15 Aspiration of Joint Fluid				
31-16 Hemorrhoid Thrombectomy				
31-17 Suture/Staple Removal				
31-18 Application of Sterile Adhesive Skin Closure Strips				
33-1 Transferring Patient from Wheelchair to Examination Table				
33-2 Transferring Patient from Examination Table to Wheelchair				
33-3 Assisting the Patient to Stand and Walk				
33-4 Care of the Falling Patient				
33-5 Assisting a Patient to Ambulate with a Walker				
33-6 Teaching the Patient to Ambulate with Crutches				
33-7 Assisting a Patient to Ambulate with a Cane				
34-1 Provide Instruction for Health Maintenance and Disease Prevention				

Procedure Number and Title	Date Assessment Completed and Competency Achieved			
	Date/Initials	Date/Initials	Date/Initials	Date/Initials
35-1 Proper Disposal of Drugs				
36-1 Administration of Oral Medications				
36-2 Withdrawing Medication from a Vial				
36-3 Withdrawing Medication from an Ampule				
36-4 Administration of Subcutaneous, Intramuscular, and Intradermal Injections				
36-5 Administering a Subcutaneous Injection				
36-6 Administering an Intramuscular Injection				
36-7 Administering an Intradermal Injection of Purified Protein Derivative (PPD)				
36-8 Reconstituting a Powder Medication for Administration				
36-9 Z-Track Intramuscular Injection Technique				
37-1 Perform Single-Channel or Multichannel Electrocardiogram				
37-2 Holter Monitor Application (Cassette and Digital)				
39-1 Using the Microscope				
40-1 Palpating a Vein and Preparing a Patient for Venipuncture				
40-2 Venipuncture by Syringe				
40-3 Venipuncture by Vacuum Tube System				
40-4 Venipuncture by Butterfly Needle System				
40-5 Capillary Puncture				
40-6 Obtaining a Capillary Specimen for Transport Using a Microtainer Transport Unit				
40-7 Obtaining Blood for Blood Culture				
41-1 Hemoglobin Determination Using a CLIA Waived Hemoglobin Analyzer				
41-2 Microhematocrit Determination				

Procedure Number and Title	Date Assessment Completed and Competency Achieved			
	Date/Initials	Date/Initials	Date/Initials	Date/Initials
41-3 Erythrocyte Sedimentation Rate				
41-4 Prothrombin Time (Using a CLIA Waived ProTime Analyzer)				
42-1 Assessing Urine Volume, Color, and Clarity				
42-2 Using the Refractometer to Measure Specific Gravity				
42-3 Performing a Urinalysis Chemical Examination				
42-4 Preparing Slide for Microscopic Examination of Urine Sediment				
42-5 Performing a Complete Urinalysis				
42-6 Utilizing a Urine Transport System for C&S				
42-7 Instructing a Patient in the Collection of a Clean-Catch, Midstream Urine Specimen				
43-1 Procedure for Obtaining a Throat Specimen for Culture				
43-2 Wet Mount and Hanging Drop Slide Preparations				
43-3 Performing Strep Throat Testing				
43-4 Instructing a Patient on Obtaining a Fecal Specimen				
44-1 Pregnancy Test				
44-2 Performing Infectious Mononucleosis Test				
44-3 Obtaining Blood Specimen for Phenylkctonuria (PKU) Test				
44-4 Screening Test for PKU				
44-5 Measurement of Blood Glucose Using an Automated Analyzer				
44-6 Cholesterol Testing				
45-1 Completing a Medical Incident Report				
45-2 Preparing a Meeting Agenda				
45-3 Supervising a Student Practicum				
45-4 Developing and Maintaining a Procedure Manual				
45-5 Making Travel Arrangements with a Travel Agent				

Procedure Number and Title	Date Assessment Completed and Competency Achieved			
	Date/Initials	**Date/Initials**	**Date/Initials**	**Date/Initials**
45-6 Making Travel Arrangements via the Internet				
45-7 Processing Employee Payroll				
45-8 Perform an Inventory of Equipment and Supplies				
45-9 Perform Routine Maintenance or Calibration of Administrative and Clinical Equipment				
46-1 Develop and Maintain a Policy Manual				
46-2 Prepare a Job Description				
46-3 Conduct Interviews				
46-4 Orient Personnel				

Competency Assessment Checklists

Name _____ Date _____ Score _____

COMPETENCY ASSESSMENT

Procedure 9-1   Control of Bleeding

Task: To control bleeding caused by an open wound.

Conditions: Sterile dressings, sterile gloves, mask, eye protection, a gown, biohazard waste container

Standards: Perform the Task within 15 minutes with a minimum score of _____ points.

***Work
Documentation:***   Simulated entry in Patient's Chart in Work Documentation area

No.	Step	Points	Check #1	Check #2	Check #3
1	Wash hands and gather equipment quickly.				
2	Apply gloves and other PPE; eye mask, gown if splashing likely.				
3	Apply pressure bandages and apply pressure for 10 minutes. If bleeding continues, elevate arm above heart. If continues, press adjacent artery against bone.				
4	Throughout procedure, demonstrate professional behavior in manner, organization and attire, including: • Recognize the effects of stress on all persons involved in emergency situations. • Demonstrate self-awareness in responding to emergency situations.				
5	Dispose of waste in biohazard container and wash hands.				
6	Document procedure.				
Student's Total Points					
Points Possible					
Final Score (Student's Total Points/ Possible Points)					

Name _____   **Date** _____   **Score** _____

WORK DOCUMENTATION

_____

Instructor's/Evaluator's Comments and Suggestions:

_____
_____
_____
_____
_____

CHECK #1	
Evaluator's Signature:	Date:

CHECK #2	
Evaluator's Signature:	Date:

CHECK #3	
Evaluator's Signature:	Date:

ABHES Competency: VI.A.1.a(4)(f) Perform first aid and CPR; VI.A.1.a.4.e Recognize emergencies

CAAHEP Curriculum: XI.P.XI.11 Perform first aid procedures

Name _____ Date _____ Score _____

COMPETENCY ASSESSMENT

Procedure 9-2   Applying an Arm Splint

Task: To immobilize the area above and below the injured part of the arm to reduce pain and prevent further injury.

Conditions: Thin piece of rigid board and gauze roller bandage

Standards: Perform the Task within 15 minutes with a minimum score of _____ points.

Work Documentation: Simulated entry in Patient's Chart in Work Documentation area

No.	Step	Points	Check #1	Check #2	Check #3
1	Place a padded splint under the injured area. Hold the splint in place with roller gauze.				
2	Check circulation (note color and temperature of skin and nails, and check pulse).				
3	Apply sling to keep arm elevated.				
4	Throughout procedure, demonstrate professional behavior in manner, organization, and attire, including: • Recognize the effects of stress on all persons involved in emergency situations. • Demonstrate self awareness in responding to emergency situations.				
5	Wash hands.				
6	Document procedure.				
Student's Total Points					
Points Possible					
Final Score (Student's Total Points/ Possible Points)					

Name _____ **Date** _____ **Score** _____

WORK DOCUMENTATION

_____

Instructor's/Evaluator's Comments and Suggestions:

_____

_____

_____

_____

_____

CHECK #1 Evaluator's Signature:	Date:

CHECK #2 Evaluator's Signature:	Date:

CHECK #3 Evaluator's Signature:	Date:

ABHES Competency: VI.A.1.a(4)(f) Perform first aid and CPR

CAAHEP Curriculum: XI.P.XI.11 Perform first aid procedures

Name _____ Date _____ Score _____

COMPETENCY ASSESSMENT

Procedure 11-1   Booting Up and Shutting Down the Computer

Task: To properly turn on and shut down the computer.

Conditions: Computer, portable media device (such as a flash drive or CD)

Standards: Perform the Task within 10 minutes with a minimum score of _____ points.

No.	Step	Points	Check #1	Check #2	Check #3
1	Turn on the computer and monitor. Log in using a username and password, if applicable.				
2	When work has been completed, save all open files and close all open software programs.				
3	Remove and store all portable media devices (CD, flash drive, etc.) appropriately.				
4	Close out of the operating system, shut down the computer, and power the computer and monitor off.				
Student's Total Points					
Points Possible					
Final Score (Student's Total Points/ Possible Points)					

Name _____ **Date** _____ **Score** _____

Instructor's/Evaluator's Comments and Suggestions:

_____

_____

_____

_____

_____

CHECK #1

Evaluator's Signature: _____   Date:

CHECK #2

Evaluator's Signature: _____   Date:

CHECK #3

Evaluator's Signature: _____   Date:

ABHES Competency: VI.A.1.a.2.n Application of electronic technology

Name _____ Date _____ Score _____

COMPETENCY ASSESSMENT

Procedure 11-2   Software Installation

Task: To add software to the computer system for later call up and use.

Conditions: Computer, StudyWARE Software CD in back of the textbook (*Note:* students may install any software program as directed by the instructor)

Standards: Perform the Task within 10 minutes with a minimum score of _____ points.

No.	Step	Points	Check #1	Check #2	Check #3
Automatic Installation					
1	Close all open programs.				
2	Insert the CD into the CD drive.				
3	Follow the prompts in the Installation Wizard screens that appear, choosing an appropriate location for the program.				
4	Click Finish and launch the StudyWARE program.				
Manual Installation					
1	Close all open programs.				
2	Insert CD into the CD drive.				
3	From My Computer, double click the icon for the CD drive. Follow the prompts in the Installation Wizard screens that appear, choosing an appropriate location for the program.				
4	Click Finish and launch the StudyWARE program.				
Student's Total Points					
Points Possible					
Final Score (Student's Total Points/ Possible Points)					

Name _____   **Date** _____   **Score** _____

Instructor's/Evaluator's Comments and Suggestions:

_____

_____

_____

_____

_____

CHECK #1

Evaluator's Signature: _____   Date:

CHECK #2

Evaluator's Signature: _____   Date:

CHECK #3

Evaluator's Signature: _____   Date:

ABHES Competency: VI.A.1.a.2.n Application of electronic technology; VI.A.1.a.3.d Apply computer concepts for office procedures

CAAHEP Curriculum: V.P.6 Use office hardware and software to maintain office systems

Name _____ Date _____ Score _____

COMPETENCY ASSESSMENT

Procedure 11-3   Hardware Installation

Task: To add hardware to the computer system for later use.

Conditions: Computer, hardware to be installed

Standards: Perform the Task within 15 minutes with a minimum score of _____ points.

No.	Step	Points	Check #1	Check #2	Check #3
Using Automatic Initiation from Microsoft Windows® Installation Wizard					
1	Close all open programs.				
2	Answer questions appropriately such as: Manufacturer, Model Number, etc.				
3	Follow onscreen directions.				
Using Manual Initiation of Microsoft Windows® Installation Wizard					
1	Close all open programs.				
2	Go to START, SETTINGS, CONTROL PANEL, and double click ADD HARDWARE.				
3	Find the Hardware you wish to install and follow onscreen instructions.				
Student's Total Points					
Points Possible					
Final Score (Student's Total Points/ Possible Points)					

Name _____   **Date** _____   **Score** _____

Instructor's/Evaluator's Comments and Suggestions:

_____

_____

_____

_____

_____

CHECK #1

Evaluator's Signature: _____   Date:

CHECK #2

Evaluator's Signature: _____   Date:

CHECK #3

Evaluator's Signature: _____   Date:

ABHES Competency: VI.A.1.a.2.n Application of electronic technology; VI.A.1.a.3.d Apply computer concepts for office procedures

CAAHEP Curriculum: V.P.6 Use office hardware and software to maintain office systems

Name _____   Date _____   Score _____

COMPETENCY ASSESSMENT

Procedure 13-2   Establishing the Appointment Matrix Using Medical Office Simulation Software (MOSS)

Task: To have a current and accurate record of appointment times available for scheduling patient visits, in an electronic system.

Condition: MOSS, computer, Scenario information

Standards: Perform the Task within 15 minutes with a minimum score of _____ points.

Work Documentation: Screen shots of completed block calendar window or screen shots of the appointment schedule showing calendar blocks

No.	Step	Points	Check #1	Check #2	Check #3
1	Open MOSS, select the Appointment Scheduling module.				
2	Find the appropriate date; select Block Calendar option.				
3	Enter correct information for the type of block, the start and end dates, the start and end times, the frequency, and the providers to whom the blocks apply. (Take screen shots of the complete block calendar window.)				
4	Save each calendar block, and review the schedule to ensure that each block has been properly applied. (Take screen shots of the appointment schedule showing the calendar blocks.)				
Student's Total Points					
Points Possible					
Final Score (Student's Total Points/ Possible Points)					

Name _____   **Date** _____   **Score** _____

WORK DOCUMENTATION

*Attach screen shots of completed block calendar window or screen shots of the appointment schedule showing calendar blocks.

Instructor's/Evaluator's Comments and Suggestions:

_____

_____

_____

_____

CHECK #1

Evaluator's Signature: _____   Date:

CHECK #2

Evaluator's Signature: _____   Date:

CHECK #3

Evaluator's Signature: _____   Date:

ABHES Competency: VI.A.1.a.2.n Application of electronic technology; VI.A.1.a.3.c Schedule and monitor appointments; VI.A.1.a.3.d Apply computer concepts for office procedures

CAAHEP Curriculum: V.P.1 Manage appointment schedule, using established priorities; V.P.6 Use office hardware and software to maintain office systems

Name _____ **Date** _____ **Score** _____

COMPETENCY ASSESSMENT

Procedure 13-4   Making an Appointment on the Telephone Using Medical Office Simulation Software (MOSS)

Task: To schedule an appointment entering information in the appointment schedule according to office policy.

Condition: Telephone, MOSS, computer, Scenario information

Standards: Perform the Task within 15 minutes with a minimum score of _____ points.

Work Documentation: Screen shot of the completed Patient Appointment Form

No.	Step	Points	Check #1	Check #2	Check #3
1	Answer phone professionally and appropriately.				
2	Open MOSS, select the Appointment Scheduling module. Find and select the appropriate date for the appointment, and the appropriate patient.				
3	During call, demonstrate professional behavior, including: • Demonstrate empathy in communicating with patients, family, and staff • Apply active listening skills • Demonstrate recognition of the patient's level of understanding in communications • Analyze communications in providing appropriate responses/feedback				
4	Populate the fields on the Patient Appointment Form with the correct information. (Take a screen shot of the completed Patient Appointment Form.)				
5	Save the appointment, and review the schedule to ensure that the appointment was properly applied.				
6	Repeat the date and time to the patient, provide any necessary instructions; end the call politely.				
Student's Total Points					
Points Possible					
Final Score (Student's Total Points/ Possible Points)					

Name _____ **Date** _____ **Score** _____

WORK DOCUMENTATION

*Attach screen shot of completed Patient Appointment Form.

_____

Instructor's/Evaluator's Comments and Suggestions:

_____

_____

_____

_____

_____

CHECK #1	
Evaluator's Signature:	Date:

CHECK #2	
Evaluator's Signature:	Date:

CHECK #3	
Evaluator's Signature:	Date:

ABHES Competency: VI.A.1.a.2.e Use proper telephone techniques; VI.A.1.a.2.n Application of electronic technology; VI.A.1.a.3.c Schedule and monitor appointments; VI.A.1.a.3.d Apply computer concepts for office procedures

CAAHEP Curriculum: IV.P.7 Demonstrate telephone techniques; V.P.1 Manage appointment schedule, using established priorities; V.P.6 Use office hardware and software to maintain office systems

Name _____   Date _____   Score _____

COMPETENCY ASSESSMENT

Procedure 13-6   Checking in Patients Using Medical Office Simulation Software (MOSS)

Task: To ensure the patient is given prompt and proper care; to meet legal safeguards for documentation.

Condition: MOSS, computer, Scenario information

Standards: Perform the Task within 5 minutes with a minimum score of _____ points.

Work Documentation: Screen shot of completed Patient Appointment Form

No.	Step	Points	Check #1	Check #2	Check #3
1	Open MOSS, select the Appointment Scheduling module. Find and select the appropriate date for the appointment, and the appropriate patient.				
2	Check in the patient on the Patient Appointment Form with the correct information in the correct field. (Take a screen shot of the completed Patient Appointment Form.)				
3	During exchange with patient: • Review vital information, protect privacy • Recognize and protect personal boundaries in communicating with others				
4	Save the appointment. Ask patient to be seated and indicate wait time.				
Student's Total Points					
Points Possible					
Final Score (Student's Total Points/ Possible Points)					

Name _____ Date _____ Score _____

WORK DOCUMENTATION

*Attach screen shot of completed Patient Appointment Form.

Instructor's/Evaluator's Comments and Suggestions:

_____

_____

_____

_____

_____

CHECK #1

Evaluator's Signature: Date:

CHECK #2

Evaluator's Signature: Date:

CHECK #3

Evaluator's Signature: Date:

ABHES Competency: VI.A.1.a.3.c Schedule and monitor appointments

CAAHEP Curriculum: IV.P.2 Report relevant information to others succinctly and accurately; V.P.1 Manage appointment schedule, using established priorities

Name _____ Date _____ Score _____

COMPETENCY ASSESSMENT

Procedure 13-8   Cancellation and Rescheduling in Medical Office Simulation Software (MOSS)

Task: To protect the provider from legal complications; to free up care time for other patients; and to assure quality patient care.

Condition: MOSS, computer, Scenario information

Standards: Perform the Task within 15 minutes with a minimum score of _____ points.

Work Documentation: Screen shot of Patient Appointment Form

No.	Step	Points	Check #1	Check #2	Check #3
1	Open MOSS, select the Appointment Scheduling module. Using the Scenario information, find and select the appropriate date, and the appropriate patient.				
2	*Rescheduling:* Choose "Rescheduled" on the Patient Appointment Form, select the reason and find a new time to reschedule the patient. (Take a screen shot of the completed Patient Appointment Form.) *Cancellations:* Choose "Cancelled," select the reason. (Take a screen shot of the completed Patient Appointment Form.)				
3	During interaction with patient, demonstrate professional behavior, including: • Demonstrate empathy in communicating with patients, family, and staff • Apply active listening skills • Demonstrate recognition of the patient's level of understanding in communications • Analyze communications in providing appropriate responses/feedback				
4	Save the appointment changes.				
Student's Total Points					
Points Possible					
Final Score (Student's Total Points/ Possible Points)					

Name _____ **Date** _____ **Score** _____

WORK DOCUMENTATION

*Attach screen shot of completed Patient Appointment Form.

_____

Instructor's/Evaluator's Comments and Suggestions:

_____

_____

_____

_____

_____

CHECK #1

Evaluator's Signature: _____ Date: _____

CHECK #2

Evaluator's Signature: _____ Date: _____

CHECK #3

Evaluator's Signature: _____ Date: _____

ABHES Competency: VI.A.1.a.2.n Application of electronic technology; VI.A.1.a.3.c Schedule and monitor appointments; VI.A.1.a.3.d Apply computer concepts for office procedures

CAAHEP Curriculum: IV.P.8 Document patient care; V.P.1 Manage appointment schedule, using established priorities; V.P.6 Use office hardware and software to maintain office systems

Name _____ Date _____ Score _____

COMPETENCY ASSESSMENT

Procedure 14-2   Establishing an Electronic Medical Record for a New Patient Using Medical Office Simulation Software (MOSS)

Task: To demonstrate an understanding of the principles for establishing a paper medical chart.

Condition: Supplies listed in Procedure 14-7

Standards: Perform the Task within 15 minutes with a minimum score of _____ points.

Work Documentation: Screen shots of completed tabs in the Patient Registration screen

No.	Step	Points	Check #1	Check #2	Check #3
1	Open MOSS and select the Patient Registration module. Select Add on the Patient Registration dialog box.				
2	Complete the Patient Information tab with correct information (take a screen shot). Click Save.				
3	Complete the Primary Insurance tab with correct information (take a screen shot). Click Save.				
4	Complete the HIPAA tab with correct information (take a screen shot). Click Save.				
5	During procedure, demonstrate time management principles to maintain effective office function.				
Student's Total Points					
Points Possible					
Final Score (Student's Total Points/ Possible Points)					

Name _____   **Date** _____   **Score** _____

WORK DOCUMENTATION

*Attach screen shots of completed tabs in Registration section: Patient Information, Insurance Information, HIPAA.

Instructor's/Evaluator's Comments and Suggestions:

_____

_____

_____

_____

_____

CHECK #1

Evaluator's Signature: _____   Date: _____

CHECK #2

Evaluator's Signature: _____   Date: _____

CHECK #3

Evaluator's Signature: _____   Date: _____

ABHES Competency: VI.A.1.a.3.a Perform basic secretarial skills; VI.A.1.a.3.b Prepare and maintain medical records

CAAHEP Curriculum: V.P.3 Organize a patient's medical record; V.P.5 Execute data management using electronic healthcare records such as the EMR

Name _____ **Date** _____ **Score** _____

COMPETENCY ASSESSMENT

Procedure 14-4   Correcting an Electronic Medical Record

Task: To demonstrate the appropriate method of correction errors in electronic medical records.

Condition: Computer with screen open to document containing error, document containing correction

Standards: Perform the Task within 3 minutes with a minimum score of _____ points.

No.	Step	Points	Check #1	Check #2	Check #3
1	Set the software to track the area to be corrected.				
2	Line out the error using the dash key.				
3	Key in the correction to be made beside the error.				
4	Follow standard clinic protocol in making the correction: *(options: make "error" or "correction" notation above error or corrected information):* • Demonstrate awareness of the consequences of not working within the legal scope of practice • Recognize the importance of local, state, and federal legislation and regulations in the practice setting				
5	Initial and date the correction.				
Student's Total Points					
Points Possible					
Final Score (Student's Total Points/ Possible Points)					

Name _____ **Date** _____ **Score** _____

Instructor's/Evaluator's Comments and Suggestions:

_____

_____

_____

_____

_____

CHECK #1

Evaluator's Signature: _____ Date:

CHECK #2

Evaluator's Signature: _____ Date:

CHECK #3

Evaluator's Signature: _____ Date:

ABHES Competency: VI.A.1.a.3.b Prepare and maintain medical records

CAAHEP Curriculum: IX.P.7 Document accurately in the patient record

Name _____   Date _____   Score _____

COMPETENCY ASSESSMENT

Procedure 15-2   Addressing Envelopes According to United States Postal Regulations

Task: To address envelopes according to U.S. Postal Service regulations to ensure timely delivery.

Condition: Supplies listed in Procedure 15-2

Standards: Perform the Task within 5 minutes with a minimum score of _____ points.

Work Documentation: Completed envelope

No.	Step	Points	Check #1	Check #2	Check #3
1	Select the envelope format from the software program, or use labels.				
2	Place the address within the proper area as directed by the U.S. postal regulations.				
3	Key the address correctly. If not using preprinted envelopes, key the return address correctly.				
4	Proofread the envelope; make corrections as necessary.				
Student's Total Points					
Points Possible					
Final Score (Student's Total Points/ Possible Points)					

Name _____ **Date** _____ **Score** _____

WORK DOCUMENTATION
*Attach completed envelope.

_____

Instructor's/Evaluator's Comments and Suggestions:

_____

_____

_____

_____

_____

CHECK #1	
Evaluator's Signature:	Date:

CHECK #2	
Evaluator's Signature:	Date:

CHECK #3	
Evaluator's Signature:	Date:

ABHES Competency: VI.A.1.a.3.a Perform basic secretarial skills

Name _____ **Date** _____ **Score** _____

COMPETENCY ASSESSMENT

Procedure 15-4   Creating a Mass Mailing Using Mail Merge

Task: To create a mass mailing using the computer's Mail Merge Helper feature contained within Microsoft® Word.

Condition: Supplies listed in Procedure 15-4

Standards: Perform the Task within 15 minutes with a minimum score of _____ points.

No.	Step	Points	Check #1	Check #2	Check #3
1	Compose and type the document.				
2	Develop a data source.				
3	Insert merge fields into the main document.				
4	Send the merged document to the printer.				
Student's Total Points					
Points Possible					
Final Score (Student's Total Points/ Possible Points)					

Name _____ **Date** _____ **Score** _____

Instructor's/Evaluator's Comments and Suggestions:

_____

_____

_____

_____

_____

CHECK #1

Evaluator's Signature: Date:

CHECK #2

Evaluator's Signature: Date:

CHECK #3

Evaluator's Signature: Date:

ABHES Competency: VI.A.1.a.3.a Perform basic secretarial skills; VI.A.1.a.3.d Apply computer concepts for office procedures

Name _____ Date _____ Score _____

COMPETENCY ASSESSMENT

Procedure 17-1   Applying Managed Care Policies and Procedures

Task: To apply managed care policies and procedures that the provider and/or medical facility has partnership agreements with.

Condition: Managed care contracts, managed care policies and procedures manuals, patient record, authorized forms from managed care organizations, clerical supplies

Standards: Perform the Task within 15 minutes with a minimum score of _____ points.

Work Documentation: Entry in patient's medical record

No.	Step	Points	Check #1	Check #2	Check #3
1	Called insurance company and obtained the correct information, including: • Verified patient has insurance in effect and was eligible for benefits • Confirmed exclusions and noncovered services • Determined deductibles, copayments or other payments the patient is responsible for • Inquired about preauthorizations • Used appropriate telephone techniques during call • Documented the name, title, and extension of person contacted				
2	Collected information from patient, and correctly documented the information collected.				
3	During procedure, demonstrated professional behavior in manner, organization, and attire.				
	Student's Total Points				
	Points Possible				
	Final Score (Student's Total Points/ Possible Points)				

Name _____   Date _____   Score _____

WORK DOCUMENTATION

_____

Instructor's/Evaluator's Comments and Suggestions:

_____

_____

_____

_____

_____

CHECK #1

Evaluator's Signature: _____   Date:

CHECK #2

Evaluator's Signature: _____   Date:

CHECK #3

Evaluator's Signature: _____   Date:

ABHES Competency: VI.A.1.a.3.t Apply managed care policies and procedures; VI.A.1.a.8.c Analyze and use current third-party guidelines for reimbursement

CAAHEP Curriculum: VII.P.1 Apply both managed care policies and procedures; VII.P.2 Apply third party guidelines; VII.P.6 Verify eligibility for managed care services

Name _____ **Date** _____ **Score** _____

COMPETENCY ASSESSMENT

Procedure 17-2   Screening for Insurance

Task: To verify insurance coverage and obtain vital information required for processing and billing insurance claim forms.

Condition: Patient registration forms, clipboard and black ink pen, patient's chart

Standards: Perform the Task within 15 minutes with a minimum score of _____ points.

No.	Step	Points	Check #1	Check #2	Check #3
1	Ask patients to bring their insurance cards and arrive 15–20 minutes before appointment time.				
2	Review completed patient registration form for legibility and completeness. Verify address and insurance coverage; check insurance card; determine that primary care provider is performing the procedure and that the procedure is covered; determine if referral is needed.				
3	Make front and back photocopies of patient's insurance card and attach to patient's chart. Verify proof of eligibility for Medicaid patients.				
4	During interaction with patient, demonstrate professional behavior, including: • Demonstrate sensitivity in communicating with patient • Communicate in language the patient can understand regarding managed care and insurance plans				
Student's Total Points					
Points Possible					
Final Score (Student's Total Points/ Possible Points)					

Name _____ **Date** _____ **Score** _____

Instructor's/Evaluator's Comments and Suggestions:

_____

_____

_____

_____

_____

CHECK #1 Evaluator's Signature: Date:

CHECK #2 Evaluator's Signature: Date:

CHECK #3 Evaluator's Signature: Date:

ABHES Competency: VI.A.1.a.3.t Apply managed care policies and procedures; VI.A.1.a.8.c Analyze and use current third-party guidelines for reimbursement

CAAHEP Curriculum: VII.P.1 Apply both managed care policies and procedures; VII.P.2 Apply third party guidelines; VII.P.6 Verify eligibility for managed care services

Name _____   Date _____   Score _____

COMPETENCY ASSESSMENT

Procedure 17-3   Obtaining Referrals and Authorizations

Task: To ascertain coverage by the insurance carrier for specific medical services, hospital admissions, inpatient or outpatient surgeries, elective procedures, or when the primary care provider elects to refer the patient to another provider.

Condition: Patient's medical chart and copy of the patient's insurance card, name of the carrier contact person and telephone number, completed referral form, telephone/fax machine, pen/pencil

Standards: Perform the Task within 15 minutes with a minimum score of _____ points.

*Work
Documentation:*   Completed copy of the referral form

No.	Step	Points	Check #1	Check #2	Check #3
1	Collect all necessary documents and equipment. Determine the service or procedure requiring preauthorization.				
2	Complete and proofread the referral form. Use language that demonstrates assertive communication with managed care and/or insurance providers.				
3	Fax the completed form to the insurance carrier. Maintain a completed copy of the referral form in the patient's chart.				
4	Maintain a completed copy of the authorization number/code in the patient's chart.				
Student's Total Points					
Points Possible					
Final Score (Student's Total Points/ Possible Points)					

Name _____ **Date** _____ **Score** _____

WORK DOCUMENTATION
*Attach completed referral form.

_____

Instructor's/Evaluator's Comments and Suggestions:

_____

_____

_____

_____

_____

CHECK #1	
Evaluator's Signature:	Date:

CHECK #2	
Evaluator's Signature:	Date:

CHECK #3	
Evaluator's Signature:	Date:

ABHES Competency: VI.A.1.a.3.t Apply managed care policies and procedures; VI.A.1.a.3.u Obtain managed care referrals and pre-certification; VI.A.1.a.8.c Analyze and use current third-party guidelines for reimbursement

CAAHEP Curriculum: VII.P.4 Obtain precertification, including documentation; VII.P.5 Obtain preauthorization, including documentation

Name _____ Date _____ Score _____

COMPETENCY ASSESSMENT

Procedure 17-4   Computing the Medicare Fee Schedule

Task: To compute the Medicare allowable (MA) payment for services.

Condition: CPT book, computer, calculator

Standards: Perform the Task within 15 minutes with a minimum score of _____ points.

Work
Documentation: Calculation and correct answer in the Work Documentation area

No.	Step	Points	Check #1	Check #2	Check #3
1	Obtained the correct CPT code for the procedure or service performed.				
2	Used the Medicare Fee Schedule and correctly determined the Medicare allowable fee: • Determined each value of the allowable formula • Used the formula correctly to calculate the fee • Correctly rounded, if appropriate				
Student's Total Points					
Points Possible					
Final Score (Student's Total Points/ Possible Points)					

Name _____   Date _____   Score _____

WORK DOCUMENTATION

_____

Instructor's/Evaluator's Comments and Suggestions:

_____

_____

_____

_____

_____

CHECK #1

Evaluator's Signature: _____

Date:

CHECK #2

Evaluator's Signature: _____

Date:

CHECK #3

Evaluator's Signature: _____

Date:

ABHES Competency: VI.A.1.a.3.t Apply managed care policies and procedures

CAAHEP Curriculum: VII.P.1 Apply both managed care policies and procedures

Name _____   **Date** _____   **Score** _____

COMPETENCY ASSESSMENT

Procedure 18-1   Current Procedural Terminology Coding

Task: To convert commonly accepted descriptions of medical procedures (services) and for visits of all kinds—office, hospital, nursing facility, home services—into a five-digit numeric code with two-digit numeric modifiers when required.

Condition: CPT code book for the current year; copy of the encounter form and access to the patient's chart, pencil and paper; Scenario information

Standards: Perform the Task within 15 minutes with a minimum score of _____ points.

Work Documentation: Correct code selection in Work Documentation section

No.	Step	Points	Check #1	Check #2	Check #3
1	Using the CPT code book and the Scenario information, find the correct E&M service code.				
2	In the Index, find the correct code for the procedure.				
3	Now locate the code you have found in Step 2 in the Pathology and Laboratory section; ensure the description provided matches what the provider has documented in the patient's chart.				
Student's Total Points					
Points Possible					
Final Score (Student's Total Points/ Possible Points)					

Name _____   **Date** _____   **Score** _____

WORK DOCUMENTATION

Enter correct code:

_____

Instructor's/Evaluator's Comments and Suggestions:

_____

_____

_____

_____

_____

CHECK #1

Evaluator's Signature: _____   Date:

CHECK #2

Evaluator's Signature: _____   Date:

CHECK #3

Evaluator's Signature: _____   Date:

ABHES Competency: VI.A.1.a.8.b Implement current procedural terminology and ICD-9 coding

CAAHEP Curriculum: VIII.P.1 Perform procedural coding

Name _____   **Date** _____   **Score** _____

COMPETENCY ASSESSMENT

Procedure 18-2   International Classification of Diseases, 9th Revision, Clinical Modification Coding

Task: The ICD-9-CM code books provide a diagnostic coding system for the compilation and reporting of morbidity and mortality statistics for reimbursement purposes.

Condition: Volumes 1 and 2 of the ICD-9-CM code books for the current year, copy of the encounter form and access to the patient's chart, pencil and paper

Standards: Perform the Task within 15 minutes with a minimum score of _____ points.

Work Documentation: Correct code selection in Work Documentation section

No.	Step	Points	Check #1	Check #2	Check #3
1	Using Volume II of the ICD-9-CM code books, look up the main reason or condition that brought the patient to the facility, or the specific diagnosis confirmed by test results.				
2	Using Volume I, look up the code you found in Step 1. Read all listings and determine the appropriate code having the greatest level of specificity.				
Student's Total Points					
Points Possible					
Final Score (Student's Total Points/ Possible Points)					

Name _____   **Date** _____   **Score** _____

WORK DOCUMENTATION

Enter correct code:

_____

Instructor's/Evaluator's Comments and Suggestions:

_____

_____

_____

_____

_____

CHECK #1

Evaluator's Signature: _____   Date:

CHECK #2

Evaluator's Signature: _____   Date:

CHECK #3

Evaluator's Signature: _____   Date:

ABHES Competency: VI.A.1.a.3.v Perform diagnostic coding; VI.A.1.a.8.b Implement current procedural terminology and ICD-9 coding

CAAHEP Curriculum: VIII.P.2 Perform diagnostic coding

Name _____ Date _____ Score _____

COMPETENCY ASSESSMENT

Procedure 18-3   Applying Third-Party Guidelines

Task: To obtain written authorization to release necessary medical information to third-party payers.

Condition: Patient chart, CMS-1500 claim form

Standards: Perform the Task within 5 minutes with a minimum score of _____ points.

Work Documentation: Completed CMS-1500 claim form in Work Documentation section

No.	Step	Points	Check #1	Check #2	Check #3
1	When patient signs in, check her/his chart to ascertain if an "Authorization to Release Medical Information" has been signed and is currently valid.				
2	During interaction with patient, demonstrate professional behavior, including: • Communicating in language the patient can understand regarding managed care and insurance plans				
3	If there is no record of signature on file, have the patient sign Block 12 of the CMS-1500 form.				
Student's Total Points					
Points Possible					
Final Score (Student's Total Points/ Possible Points)					

Name _____ **Date** _____ **Score** _____

WORK DOCUMENTATION
*Attach Block 12 of CMS-1500 form.

Instructor's/Evaluator's Comments and Suggestions:

_____

_____

_____

_____

_____

CHECK #1

Evaluator's Signature: Date:

CHECK #2

Evaluator's Signature: Date:

CHECK #3

Evaluator's Signature: Date:

ABHES Competency: VI.A.1.a.3.v Perform diagnostic coding; VI.A.1.a.8.b Implement current procedural terminology and ICD-9 coding

CAAHEP Curriculum: VII.P.2 Apply third party guidelines

Name _____ **Date** _____ **Score** _____

COMPETENCY ASSESSMENT

Procedure 18-4 Completing a Medicare CMS-1500 (08-05) Claim Form

Task: To complete the CMS-1500 insurance claim form for reimbursement.

Condition: Patient information, patient account or ledger card, copy of patient's insurance card, insurance claim form, computer and printer

Standards: Perform the Task within 30 minutes with a minimum score of _____ points.

Work Documentation: Completed CMS-1500 form

No.	Step	Points	Check #1	Check #2	Check #3
1	Correctly complete the Carrier section, in the upper portion of the form.				
2	Correctly complete the Patient and Insured section of the form, Blocks 1–13.				
3	Correctly complete the Physician or Supplier section of the form, Blocks 14–33.				
4	Proofread the form to ensure information is correct.				
Student's Total Points					
Points Possible					
Final Score (Student's Total Points/ Possible Points)					

Name _____ **Date** _____ **Score** _____

WORK DOCUMENTATION
*Attach completed CMS-1500 form.

_____

Instructor's/Evaluator's Comments and Suggestions:

_____

_____

_____

_____

_____

CHECK #1

Evaluator's Signature: Date:

CHECK #2

Evaluator's Signature: Date:

CHECK #3

Evaluator's Signature: Date:

ABHES Competency: VI.A.1.a.3.v Perform diagnostic coding; VI.A.1.a.3.w Complete insurance claim forms; VI.A.1.a.8.b Implement current procedural terminology and ICD-9 coding

CAAHEP Curriculum: VIII.P.2 Perform diagnostic coding

Name _____   Date _____   Score _____

COMPETENCY ASSESSMENT

Procedure 19-3   Posting Patient Charges Using Medical Office Simulation Software (MOSS)

Task: To electronically post charges to a patient's account.

Condition: Computer, MOSS, Scenario information

Standards: Perform the Task within 15 minutes with a minimum score of _____ points.

Work Documentation: Screen shot of completed Procedure Posting screens

No.	Step	Points	Check #1	Check #2	Check #3
1	Open MOSS and select Procedure Posting from the Main Menu.				
2	Find Jordan Connell in the patient menu and correctly Post all of the charges from his visit (take a screen shot of the completed Procedure Posting screen after all the procedures have been entered).				
3	Find Edward Gormann in the patient menu and correctly Post all of the charges from his visit (take a screen shot of the completed Procedure Posting screen after all the procedures have been entered).				
4	Find Elane Ybarra in the patient menu and correctly Post all of the charges from her visit (take a screen shot of the completed Procedure Posting screen after all the procedures have been entered).				
Student's Total Points					
Points Possible					
Final Score (Student's Total Points/ Possible Points)					

Name _____ **Date** _____ **Score** _____

WORK DOCUMENTATION

*Attach screen shots of completed Procedure Posting screens.

Instructor's/Evaluator's Comments and Suggestions:

_____

_____

_____

_____

_____

CHECK #1

Evaluator's Signature: _____ Date:

CHECK #2

Evaluator's Signature: _____ Date:

CHECK #3

Evaluator's Signature: _____ Date:

ABHES Competency: VI.A.1.a.3.d Apply computer concepts for office procedures; VI.A.1.a.3.l Perform billing and collection procedures; VI.A.1.a.8.a Use manual and computerized bookkeeping systems

CAAHEP Curriculum: VI.P.2.b Perform billing procedures; VI.P.3 Utilize computerized office billing systems

Name _____ Date _____ Score _____

COMPETENCY ASSESSMENT

Procedure 19-4 Insurance Billing Using Medical Office Simulation Software (MOSS)

Task: To complete the CMS-1500 insurance claim form for reimbursement using a computerized system.

Condition: MOSS, computer, printer, Scenario information

Standards: Perform the Task within 15 minutes with a minimum score of _____ points.

Work Documentation: Printed pre-billing worksheet; printed transmission report

No.	Step	Points	Check #1	Check #2	Check #3
1	Open MOSS and select the Insurance Billing module from the Main Menu.				
2	Correctly complete the Claims Preparation screen for Jordan Connell.				
3	Click on the Prebilling Worksheet button and verify information is correct; print this report for Jordan Connell and close.				
4	Select Generate Claims and verify CMS-1500 form is correct; select transmit EMC to send the report to the payer. Print the transmission status report for Jordan Connell and close.				
5	Following the same steps, transmit a claim for Edward Gormann. Print prebilling worksheet and transmission report.				
6	Following the same steps, transmit a claim for Elane Ybarra. Print prebilling worksheet and transmission report.				
Student's Total Points					
Points Possible					
Final Score (Student's Total Points/ Possible Points)					

Name _____ **Date** _____ **Score** _____

WORK DOCUMENTATION

*Attach pre-billing worksheets and transmission reports.

Instructor's/Evaluator's Comments and Suggestions:

_____

_____

_____

_____

_____

CHECK #1	
Evaluator's Signature:	Date:

CHECK #2	
Evaluator's Signature:	Date:

CHECK #3	
Evaluator's Signature:	Date:

ABHES Competency: VI.A.1.a.3.d Apply computer concepts for office procedures; VI.A.1.a.3.w Complete insurance claim forms

CAAHEP Curriculum: VI.P.3 Utilize computerized office billing systems; VII.P.3 Complete insurance claim forms

Name _____   Date _____   Score _____

COMPETENCY ASSESSMENT

Procedure 19-5   Posting Payments and Adjustments Using Medical Office Simulation Software (MOSS)

Task: To post insurance payments and adjustments electronically.

Condition: Computer, MOSS, Scenario information

Standards: Perform the Task within 15 minutes with a minimum score of _____ points.

Work Documentation: Screen shot of completed Payment Posting screens

No.	Step	Points	Check #1	Check #2	Check #3
1	Open MOSS and select Posting Payments from the Main Menu.				
2	Find Edward Gormann in the patient menu and correctly Post all insurance payments and adjustments (take a screen shot of the completed Payment Posting screen after all the payments and adjustments have been entered).				
3	Find Jordan Connell in the patient menu and correctly Post all insurance payments and adjustments (take a screen shot of the completed Payment Posting screen after all the payments and adjustments have been entered).				
4	Find Elane Ybarra in the patient menu and correctly Post all insurance payments and adjustments (take a screen shot of the completed Payment Posting screen after all the payments and adjustments have been entered).				
Student's Total Points					
Points Possible					
Final Score (Student's Total Points/ Possible Points)					

Name _____   **Date** _____   **Score** _____

WORK DOCUMENTATION
*Attach screen shots of completed Payment Posting screens.

_____

Instructor's/Evaluator's Comments and Suggestions:

_____

_____

_____

_____

_____

CHECK #1	
Evaluator's Signature:	Date:

CHECK #2	
Evaluator's Signature:	Date:

CHECK #3	
Evaluator's Signature:	Date:

ABHES Competency: VI.A.1.a.3.d Apply computer concepts for office procedures; VI.A.1.a.3.l Perform billing and collection procedures; VI.A.1.a.3.o Post adjustments; VI.A.1.a.8.a Use manual and computerized bookkeeping systems

CAAHEP Curriculum: VI.P.2.c Perform collection procedures; VI.P.2.d Post adjustments; VI.P.3 Utilize computerized office billing systems

Name _____ Date _____ Score _____

COMPETENCY ASSESSMENT

Procedure 19-6   Processing Credit Balances and Refunds Using Medical Office Simulation Software (MOSS)

Task: To process credit balances and refunds electronically.

Condition: Computer, MOSS, Scenario information

Standards: Perform the Task within 15 minutes with a minimum score of _____ points.

Work Documentation: Screen shot of completed Payment Posting screens

No.	Step	Points	Check #1	Check #2	Check #3
1	Open MOSS and select Posting Payments from the Main Menu.				
2	Find Josephine Albertson in the patient menu and correctly process her refund and click Post (take a screen shot of the completed Payment Posting screen).				
3	Find Andrew Jefferson in the patient menu and select correctly process his overpayment and click Post (take a screen shot of the completed Payment Posting screen).				
4	Find Alice Maxwell in the patient menu and correctly process her refund and click Post (take a screen shot of the completed Payment Posting screen).				
Student's Total Points					
Points Possible					
Final Score (Student's Total Points/ Possible Points)					

Name _____   **Date** _____   **Score** _____

WORK DOCUMENTATION
*Attach screen shots of completed Payment Posting screens.

_____

Instructor's/Evaluator's Comments and Suggestions:

_____

_____

_____

_____

_____

CHECK #1

Evaluator's Signature: Date:

CHECK #2

Evaluator's Signature: Date:

CHECK #3

Evaluator's Signature: Date:

ABHES Competency: VI.A.1.a.3.d Apply computer concepts for office procedures; VI.A.1.a.3.p Process credit balance; VI.A.1.a.3.p Process refunds; VI.A.1.a.8.a Use manual and computerized bookkeeping systems

CAAHEP Curriculum: VI.P.2.e Process a credit balance; VI.P.2.f Process refunds; VI.P.3 Utilize computerized office billing systems

Name _____   Date _____   Score _____

COMPETENCY ASSESSMENT

Procedure 20-3   Identify Accounts Receivable Using Medical Office Simulation Software (MOSS)

Task: To determine credit balances for patient billing.

Condition: Computer, MOSS, printer

Standards: Perform the Task within 15 minutes with a minimum score of _____ points.

Work Documentation: Printed Billing and Payment report

No.	Step	Points	Check #1	Check #2	Check #3
1	Open MOSS and select Report Generation from the Main Menu.				
2	Select the "Billing and Payment Report" and print it out.				
3	Go through the printed report and correctly determine which patients have outstanding balances. Circle those patients with balances.				
4	Confirm that each patient has a balance by reviewing the patient's ledger.				
Student's Total Points					
Points Possible					
Final Score (Student's Total Points/ Possible Points)					

Name _____ **Date** _____ **Score** _____

WORK DOCUMENTATION
*Attach printed Billing and Payment report.

_____

Instructor's/Evaluator's Comments and Suggestions:

_____
_____
_____
_____

CHECK #1

Evaluator's Signature: _____   Date:

CHECK #2

Evaluator's Signature: _____   Date:

CHECK #3

Evaluator's Signature: _____   Date:

ABHES Competency: VI.A.1.a.3.d Apply computer concepts for office procedures; VI.A.1.a.3.l Perform billing and collection procedures; VI.A.1.a.8.d Manage accounts payable and receivable

CAAHEP Curriculum: VI.P.3.c Perform collections procedures; VI.P.3 Utilize computerized office billing systems

Name _____   **Date** _____   **Score** _____

COMPETENCY ASSESSMENT

Procedure 20-4   Preparing Itemized Patient Accounts for Billing Using Medical Office Simulation Software (MOSS)

Task: To notify patients of the fees for services rendered and collect on those accounts.

Condition: Computer, MOSS, Billing and Payments report generated in Procedure 20-3

Standards: Perform the Task within 15 minutes with a minimum score of _____ points.

Work Documentation: Printed Remainder Statements

No.	Step	Points	Check #1	Check #2	Check #3
1	Open MOSS and select Patient Billing from the Main Menu.				
2	Correctly populate the Patient Billing screen, selecting Remainder Statement, date range, all patients and all providers.				
3	In field 6, type "Your insurance has been billed. The balance shown is your responsibility," and in field 7, select the patients who are to receive this message.				
4	Click the Process button and review the statements on screen, comparing them with the Billing and Payment report. Print the statements.				
Student's Total Points					
Points Possible					
Final Score (Student's Total Points/ Possible Points)					

Name _____ **Date** _____ **Score** _____

WORK DOCUMENTATION

*Attached printed Remainder Statements.

Instructor's/Evaluator's Comments and Suggestions:

_____

_____

_____

_____

_____

CHECK #1

Evaluator's Signature: _____   Date:

CHECK #2

Evaluator's Signature: _____   Date:

CHECK #3

Evaluator's Signature: _____   Date:

ABHES Competency: VI.A.1.a.3.d Apply computer concepts for office procedures; VI.A.1.a.3.l Perform billing and collection procedures; VI.A.1.a.8.d Manage accounts payable and receivable

CAAHEP Curriculum: VI.P.3.c Perform collections procedures; VI.P.3 Utilize computerized office billing systems

Name _____   **Date** _____   **Score** _____

COMPETENCY ASSESSMENT

Procedure 20-6   Post/Record Adjustments Using Medical Office Simulation Software (MOSS)

Task: To keep track of financial adjustments.

Condition: Computer, MOSS, Post/Record Adjustments Exercises in Procedure 20-6

Standards: Perform the Task within 15 minutes with a minimum score of _____ points.

*Work
Documentation:*   Screen shot of the completed Payment Posting screen

No.	Step	Points	Check #1	Check #2	Check #3
1	Open MOSS and select Payment Posting from the Main Menu.				
2	Find Megan Caldwell in the patient menu and select Apply Payment. Correctly Post the adjustment to her account (take a screen shot of the completed screen after the adjustment has been entered). Close out of patient account.				
3	Find Justin McNamara in the patient menu and select Apply Payment. Correctly Post the adjustment to his account (take a screen shot of the completed screen after the adjustment has been entered). Close out of patient account.				
4	Find Evan Lagasse in the patient menu and select Apply Payment. Correctly Post the adjustment to his account (take a screen shot of the completed screen after the adjustment has been entered). Close out of patient account.				
Student's Total Points					
Points Possible					
Final Score (Student's Total Points/ Possible Points)					

Name _____ **Date** _____ **Score** _____

WORK DOCUMENTATION

*Attach screen shot of the completed Payment Posting screens.

_____

Instructor's/Evaluator's Comments and Suggestions:

_____

_____

_____

_____

_____

CHECK #1

Evaluator's Signature: Date:

CHECK #2

Evaluator's Signature: Date:

CHECK #3

Evaluator's Signature: Date:

ABHES Competency: VI.A.1.a.3.d Apply computer concepts for office procedures; VI.A.1.a.3.o Post adjustments

CAAHEP Curriculum: VI.P.2.d Post adjustments; VI.P.3 Utilize computerized office billing systems

Name _____ **Date** _____ **Score** _____

COMPETENCY ASSESSMENT

Procedure 21-2 Preparing Accounts Receivable Trial Balance Using Medical Office Simulation Software (MOSS)

Task: A trial balance will determine if there is any problem between the daily journal and the ledger or patient accounts.

Condition: Computer, MOSS, printer

Standards: Perform the Task within 15 minutes with a minimum score of _____ points.

Work Documentation: Printed Monthly Summary report

No.	Step	Points	Check #1	Check #2	Check #3
1	Open MOSS and select Report Generation from the Main Menu.				
2	Select the "Monthly Summary." Review the report for errors.				
3	Print the report.				
Student's Total Points					
Points Possible					
Final Score (Student's Total Points/ Possible Points)					

Name _____ **Date** _____ **Score** _____

WORK DOCUMENTATION
*Attach printed Monthly Summary report.

_____

Instructor's/Evaluator's Comments and Suggestions:

_____
_____
_____
_____
_____

CHECK #1

Evaluator's Signature: _____ Date: _____

CHECK #2

Evaluator's Signature: _____ Date: _____

CHECK #3

Evaluator's Signature: _____ Date: _____

ABHES Competency: VI.A.1.a.3.d Apply computer concepts for office procedures; VI.A.1.a.8.d Manage accounts payable and receivable

CAAHEP Curriculum: VI.P.3 Utilize computerized office billing systems

Name _____ **Date** _____ **Score** _____

COMPETENCY ASSESSMENT

Procedure 22-1 Medical Asepsis Hand Wash (Hand Hygiene)

Task: To reduce pathogens on hands and wrists, thereby decreasing transmission of disease.

Condition: Sink with running warm water, liquid soap in dispenser, paper towels, hand lotion

Standards: Perform the Task within 3 minutes with a minimum score of _____ points.

No.	Step	Points	Check #1	Check #2	Check #3
1	Organized supplies, removed jewelry.				
2	Turned on faucet, set water temperature.				
3	Performed the procedure correctly and safely, including: • Did not touch inside of sink. • Did not lean against sink or counter. • Performed hand washing for proper amount of time. • Cleaned fingernails. • Rinsed well. • Repeated if appropriate (directed by instructor). • Dried hands well and disposed of towel without contaminating hands.				
4	Turned off faucet using barrier towel.				
5	Applied lotion.				
6	During procedure, demonstrated professional behavior in manner, organization, and attire.				
Student's Total Points					
Points Possible					
Final Score (Student's Total Points/ Possible Points)					

Name _____ **Date** _____ **Score** _____

Instructor's/Evaluator's Comments and Suggestions:

_____

_____

_____

_____

_____

CHECK #1

Evaluator's Signature: Date:

CHECK #2

Evaluator's Signature: Date:

CHECK #3

Evaluator's Signature: Date:

ABHES Competency: VI.A.1.a.4.c Apply principles of aseptic techniques and infection control

CAAHEP Curriculum: III.P.4. Perform handwashing

Name _____   **Date** _____   **Score** _____

COMPETENCY ASSESSMENT

Procedure 22-2   Removing Contaminated Gloves

Task: To remove and dispose of contaminated gloves without exposing surroundings to contamination.

Condition: Biohazard waste container, contaminated gloves, hand washing equipment

Standards: Perform the Task within 3 minutes with a minimum score of _____ points.

No.	Step	Points	Check #1	Check #2	Check #3
1	Performed the procedure professionally and safely: • Held hands down and away from body, made a fist with the left hand. • Grasped the left glove with the right hand and carefully turned it inside out over left hand. • Dropped the removed glove into the right hand without contaminating the uncovered left hand. • Fisted the right hand over the left glove, turned the right hand over and carefully grasped the back inner edge of the cuff with the fingers of the left hand. • Inverted the right glove over the right hand and the left glove. • Disposed of gloves into biohazard waste container.				
2	Cleaned hands thoroughly and applied lotion.				
3	During procedure, demonstrated professional behavior in manner, organization, and attire.				
Student's Total Points					
Points Possible					
Final Score (Student's Total Points/ Possible Points)					

Name _____ **Date** _____ **Score** _____

Instructor's/Evaluator's Comments and Suggestions:

_____

_____

_____

_____

_____

CHECK #1

Evaluator's Signature: _____   Date:

CHECK #2

Evaluator's Signature: _____   Date:

CHECK #3

Evaluator's Signature: _____   Date:

ABHES Competency: VI.A.1.a.4.c Apply principles of aseptic techniques and infection control; VI.A.1.a.4.q Dispose of biohazardous materials; VI.A.1.a.4.r Practice standard precautions

CAAHEP Curriculum: III.P.2. Practice Standard Precautions

Name _____   Date _____   Score _____

COMPETENCY ASSESSMENT

Procedure 22-3   Transmission-Based Precautions: Donning a Gown, Mask, Gloves, and Cap (Isolation Technique)

Task: To provide protection from infectious diseases while in an inpatient setting.

Condition: Disposable gown, cap, mask, gloves. Hand washing equipment, biohazard waste bag, labeling pen, and writing pen

Standards: Perform the Task within 20 minutes with a minimum score of _____ points.

No.	Step	Points	Check #1	Check #2	Check #3
1	Reviewed physician orders, institutional protocol and policies, and specific isolation precautions.				
2	Organized supplies and reviewed patient's type of isolation.				
3	Removed jewelry and all unnecessary items.				
4	Performed the procedure correctly and safely: • Washed hands. • Applied barrier clothing, cap, gown, gloves, mask. • Entered patient's room with needed supplies. • Performed needed patient care, assessment, and documentation • Discarded contaminated articles into biohazard bag and labeled it. • Removed contaminated gloves, washed hands, untied waist of gown. • Removed mask, discarded properly, washed hands. • Untied neck of gown, washed hands. • Removed gown using proper technique, discarded properly. • Washed hands thoroughly, applied lotion.				
5	Demonstrated professional behavior in manner, organization, and attire.				
Student's Total Points					
Points Possible					
Final Score (Student's Total Points/ Possible Points)					

Name _____   **Date** _____   **Score** _____

Instructor's/Evaluator's Comments and Suggestions:

_____

_____

_____

_____

_____

CHECK #1

Evaluator's Signature: _____   Date:

CHECK #2

Evaluator's Signature: _____   Date:

CHECK #3

Evaluator's Signature: _____   Date:

ABHES Competency: VI.A.1.a.4.c Apply principles of aseptic techniques and infection control; VI.A.1.a.4.q Dispose of biohazardous materials; VI.A.1.a.4.r Practice standard precautions

CAAHEP Curriculum: III.P.2. Practice Standard Precautions; III.P.3. Select appropriate barrier/personal protective equipment (PPE) for potentially infectious situations

Name _____ **Date** _____ **Score** _____

COMPETENCY ASSESSMENT

Procedure 22-4   Sanitization of Instruments

Task: To properly clean instruments to remove all tissues and fluids.

Condition: Sink with running water, sanitizing agent with enzymatic action, soft brush, towels, protective plastic apron, heavy duty gloves

Standards: Perform the Task within 15 minutes with a minimum score of _____ points.

No.	Step	Points	Check #1	Check #2	Check #3
1	Organized supplies.				
2	Applied PPE.				
3	Performed the procedure correctly and safely: • Rinsed instruments in cool water. • Scrubbed each instrument well. • Rinsed in hot water. • Placed instruments on soft absorbent toweling. • Dried instruments thoroughly. • Removed gloves, washed hands.				
4	Demonstrated professional behavior in manner, organization, and attire.				
Student's Total Points					
Points Possible					
Final Score (Student's Total Points/ Possible Points)					

Name _____   **Date** _____   **Score** _____

Instructor's/Evaluator's Comments and Suggestions:

_____

_____

_____

_____

_____

CHECK #1

Evaluator's Signature: Date:

CHECK #2

Evaluator's Signature: Date:

CHECK #3

Evaluator's Signature: Date:

ABHES Competency: VI.A.1.a.4.c Apply principles of aseptic techniques and infection control

Name _____ **Date** _____ **Score** _____

COMPETENCY ASSESSMENT

Procedure 23-1   Taking a Medical History for a Paper Medical Record

Task: To obtain and record a medical history for a new patient.

Condition: Patient history forms, clipboard, pen

Standards: Perform the Task within 25 minutes with a minimum score of _____ points.

Work Documentation: Completed patient history form

No.	Step	Points	Check #1	Check #2	Check #3
1	Introduced self to the patient, confirmed the patient's identity, and escorted her/him to the exam room.				
2	Made eye contact with the patient, established a professional and caring relationship.				
3	Performed the procedure correctly and safely: • Positioned the patient safely and comfortably, made eye contact while establishing a professional yet caring relationship. • Washed hands. • Began the interview with simple questions, spoke clearly. • Documented accurately and completely.				
4	Demonstrated professional behavior in manner, organization, and attire.				
Student's Total Points					
Points Possible					
Final Score (Student's Total Points/ Possible Points)					

Name _____   **Date** _____   **Score** _____

WORK DOCUMENTATION

*Attach completed patient history form

_____

Instructor's/Evaluator's Comments and Suggestions:

_____

_____

_____

_____

CHECK #1	
Evaluator's Signature:	Date:

CHECK #2	
Evaluator's Signature:	Date:

CHECK #3	
Evaluator's Signature:	Date:

ABHES Competency: VI.A.1.a.2.f Interview effectively; VI.A.1.a.2.g Use appropriate medical terminology; VI.A.1.a.4.a Interview and record patient history

CAAHEP Curriculum: I.P.6. Perform patient screening using established protocols; IV.P.1. Use reflection, restatement and clarification techniques to obtain a patient history; IV.P.3. Use medical terminology, pronouncing medical terms correctly, to communicate information, patient history, data and observations; IV.P.8. Document patient care

Name _____ Date _____ Score _____

COMPETENCY ASSESSMENT

Procedure 24-1   Measuring an Oral Temperature Using an Electronic Thermometer

Task: Obtain an accurate oral temperature.

Condition: Electronic thermometer, probe cover, biohazard waste container, patient chart

Standards: Perform the Task within 3 minutes with a minimum score of _____ points.

*Work
Documentation:*   Patient chart entry

No.	Step	Points	Check #1	Check #2	Check #3
1	Organized supplies and room.				
2	Greeted the patient correctly and appropriately.				
3	Washed hands and used proper PPE.				
4	Performed the procedure correctly and safely: • Ensured the thermometer was calibrated. • Placed thermometer gently and correctly. • Ensured patient comfort. • Removed thermometer gently when it beeped.				
5	Obtained accurate temperature.				
6	Demonstrated professional behavior in manner, organization, and attire, including: • Communicated appropriately and comfortably with the patient.				
7	Cleaned/disposed of supplies and equipment appropriately and washed hands.				
8	Documented correctly.				
Student's Total Points					
Points Possible					
Final Score (Student's Total Points/ Possible Points)					

Name _____   **Date** _____   **Score** _____

WORK DOCUMENTATION

_____

Instructor's/Evaluator's Comments and Suggestions:

_____

_____

_____

_____

_____

CHECK #1	
Evaluator's Signature:	Date:

CHECK #2	
Evaluator's Signature:	Date:

CHECK #3	
Evaluator's Signature:	Date:

ABHES Competency: VI.A.1.a.4.d Take vital signs

CAAHEP Curriculum: I.P.1 Obtain vital signs

Name _____ **Date** _____ **Score** _____

COMPETENCY ASSESSMENT

Procedure 24-2   Measuring an Aural Temperature Using a Tympanic Thermometer

Task: Obtain an accurate aural temperature.

Condition: Tympanic thermometer, probe cover, biohazard waste container, patient chart

Standards: Perform the Task within 3 minutes with a minimum score of _____ points.

Work Documentation: Patient chart entry

No.	Step	Points	Check #1	Check #2	Check #3
1	Organized supplies and room.				
2	Greeted the patient correctly and appropriately.				
3	Washed hands and used proper PPE.				
4	Performed the procedure correctly and safely: • Ensured the thermometer was calibrated. • Placed thermometer gently and correctly. • Ensured patient comfort. • Removed thermometer gently when it beeped.				
5	Obtained accurate temperature.				
6	Demonstrated professional behavior in manner, organization, and attire, including: • Communicated appropriately and comfortably with the patient.				
7	Cleaned/disposed of supplies and equipment appropriately and washed hands.				
8	Documented correctly.				
Student's Total Points					
Points Possible					
Final Score (Student's Total Points/ Possible Points)					

Name _____   **Date** _____   **Score** _____

WORK DOCUMENTATION

Instructor's/Evaluator's Comments and Suggestions:

_____

_____

_____

_____

_____

CHECK #1

Evaluator's Signature: _____   Date:

CHECK #2

Evaluator's Signature: _____   Date:

CHECK #3

Evaluator's Signature: _____   Date:

ABHES Competency: VI.A.1.a.4.d Take vital signs

CAAHEP Curriculum: I.P.1 Obtain vital signs

Name _____ Date _____ Score _____

COMPETENCY ASSESSMENT

Procedure 24-3   Measuring a Temperature Using a Temporal Artery (TA) Thermometer

Task: Obtain an accurate temporal artery temperature.

Condition: Temporal artery thermometer, probe cap or cover, alcohol wipes, patient chart

Standards: Perform the Task within 3 minutes with a minimum score of _____ points.

**Work
Documentation:**   Patient chart entry

No.	Step	Points	Check #1	Check #2	Check #3
1	Organized supplies and room.				
2	Greeted the patient correctly and appropriately.				
3	Washed hands and used proper PPE.				
4	Performed the procedure correctly and safely: • Ensured the thermometer was calibrated. • Cleared patient's forehead of perspiration, hair. • Placed thermometer gently and correctly. • Slid thermometer gently and correctly over the forehead. • Ensured patient comfort.				
5	Obtained accurate temperature.				
6	Demonstrated professional behavior in manner, organization, and attire, including: • Communicated appropriately and comfortably with the patient.				
7	Cleaned/disposed of supplies and equipment appropriately and washed hands.				
8	Documented correctly.				
Student's Total Points					
Points Possible					
Final Score (Student's Total Points/ Possible Points)					

Name _____ **Date** _____ **Score** _____

WORK DOCUMENTATION

_____

Instructor's/Evaluator's Comments and Suggestions:

_____

_____

_____

_____

_____

CHECK #1

Evaluator's Signature: _____ Date: _____

CHECK #2

Evaluator's Signature: _____ Date: _____

CHECK #3

Evaluator's Signature: _____ Date: _____

ABHES Competency: VI.A.1.a.4.d Take vital signs

CAAHEP Curriculum: I.P.1 Obtain vital signs

Name _____   Date _____   Score _____

COMPETENCY ASSESSMENT

Procedure 24-4   Measuring a Rectal Temperature Using a Digital Thermometer

Task: Obtain an accurate rectal temperature.

Conditions: Digital rectal thermometer, probe cover, lubricating jelly, biohazard waste container, patient chart

Standards: Perform the Task within 3 minutes with a minimum score of _____ points.

Work Documentation: Patient chart entry

No.	Step	Points	Check #1	Check #2	Check #3
1	Organized supplies and room.				
2	Greeted the patient correctly and appropriately.				
3	Washed hands and used proper PPE.				
4	Performed the procedure correctly and safely: • Ensured the thermometer was calibrated. • Placed thermometer gently and correctly. • Ensured patient comfort. • Removed thermometer gently when it beeped.				
5	Obtained accurate temperature.				
6	Demonstrated professional behavior in manner, organization, and attire, including: • Communicated appropriately and comfortably with the patient.				
7	Cleaned/disposed of supplies and equipment appropriately and washed hands.				
8	Documented correctly.				
Student's Total Points					
Points Possible					
Final Score (Student's Total Points/ Possible Points)					

Name _____ **Date** _____ **Score** _____

WORK DOCUMENTATION

_____

Instructor's/Evaluator's Comments and Suggestions:

_____

_____

_____

_____

CHECK #1	
Evaluator's Signature:	Date:

CHECK #2	
Evaluator's Signature:	Date:

CHECK #3	
Evaluator's Signature:	Date:

ABHES Competency: VI.A.1.a.4.d Take vital signs

CAAHEP Curriculum: I.P.1 Obtain vital signs

Name _____   Date _____   Score _____

COMPETENCY ASSESSMENT

Procedure 24-5   Measuring an Axillary Temperature

Task: Obtain an accurate axillary temperature.

Conditions: Digital thermometer, probe cover, tissues, biohazard waste container, patient chart

Standards: Perform the Task within 3 minutes with a minimum score of _____ points.

Work Documentation: Patient chart entry

No.	Step	Points	Check #1	Check #2	Check #3
1	Organized supplies and room.				
2	Greeted the patient correctly and appropriately.				
3	Washed hands and used proper PPE.				
4	Performed the procedure correctly and safely: • Ensured the thermometer was calibrated. • Dried the axillary space if needed. • Placed thermometer gently and correctly. • Ensured patient comfort. • Removed thermometer gently when it beeped.				
5	Obtained accurate temperature.				
6	Demonstrated professional behavior in manner, organization, and attire, including: • Communicated appropriately and comfortably with the patient.				
7	Cleaned/disposed of supplies and equipment appropriately and washed hands.				
8	Documented correctly.				
Student's Total Points					
Points Possible					
Final Score (Student's Total Points/ Possible Points)					

Name _____ **Date** _____ **Score** _____

WORK DOCUMENTATION

_____

Instructor's/Evaluator's Comments and Suggestions:

_____

_____

_____

_____

_____

CHECK #1

Evaluator's Signature: _____ Date:

CHECK #2

Evaluator's Signature: _____ Date:

CHECK #3

Evaluator's Signature: _____ Date:

ABHES Competency: VI.A.1.a.4.d Take vital signs

CAAHEP Curriculum: I.P.1 Obtain vital signs

Name _____   Date _____   Score _____

COMPETENCY ASSESSMENT

Procedure 24-6   Measuring an Oral Temperature Using a Disposable Oral Strip Thermometer

Task: Obtain an accurate oral temperature.

Conditions: Disposable oral strip thermometer, biohazard waste container, patient chart

Standards: Perform the Task within 3 minutes with a minimum score of _____ points.

Work Documentation: Patient chart entry

No.	Step	Points	Check #1	Check #2	Check #3
1	Organized supplies and room.				
2	Greeted the patient correctly and appropriately.				
3	Washed hands and used proper PPE.				
4	Performed the procedure correctly and safely: • Checked the package expiration date. • Placed thermometer gently and correctly. • Ensured patient comfort. • Removed thermometer gently at the appropriate time.				
5	Obtained accurate temperature.				
6	Demonstrated professional behavior in manner, organization, and attire, including: • Communicated appropriately and comfortably with the patient.				
7	Cleaned/disposed of supplies and equipment appropriately and washed hands.				
8	Documented correctly.				
Student's Total Points					
Points Possible					
Final Score (Student's Total Points/ Possible Points)					

Name _____   **Date** _____   **Score** _____

WORK DOCUMENTATION

_____

Instructor's/Evaluator's Comments and Suggestions:

_____

_____

_____

_____

_____

CHECK #1

Evaluator's Signature: _____   Date:

CHECK #2

Evaluator's Signature: _____   Date:

CHECK #3

Evaluator's Signature: _____   Date:

ABHES Competency: VI.A.1.a.4.d Take vital signs

CAAHEP Curriculum: I.P.1 Obtain vital signs

Name _____   Date _____   Score _____

COMPETENCY ASSESSMENT

Procedure 24-7   Measuring a Radial Pulse

Task: Obtain an accurate radial pulse.

Conditions: Watch or clock with a second hand, patient chart

Standards: Perform the Task within 3 minutes with a minimum score of _____ points.

Work Documentation: Patient chart entry

No.	Step	Points	Check #1	Check #2	Check #3
1	Organized supplies and room and washed hands.				
2	Greeted the patient correctly and appropriately.				
3	Performed the procedure correctly and safely: • Counted the pulse for 30 seconds or a full minute if irregularities noted. • Assessed the pulse for irregularities in rate, rhythm, force/volume. • Ensured patient comfort and safety.				
4	Obtained accurate pulse rate.				
5	Demonstrated professional behavior in manner, organization, and attire, including: • Communicated appropriately and comfortably with the patient.				
6	Washed hands.				
7	Documented correctly.				
Student's Total Points					
Points Possible					
Final Score (Student's Total Points/ Possible Points)					

Name _____ **Date** _____ **Score** _____

WORK DOCUMENTATION

_____

Instructor's/Evaluator's Comments and Suggestions:

_____

_____

_____

_____

_____

CHECK #1

Evaluator's Signature: _____ Date:

CHECK #2

Evaluator's Signature: _____ Date:

CHECK #3

Evaluator's Signature: _____ Date:

ABHES Competency: VI.A.1.a.4.d Take vital signs

CAAHEP Curriculum: I.P.1 Obtain vital signs

Name _____   Date _____   Score _____

COMPETENCY ASSESSMENT

Procedure 24-8   Taking an Apical Pulse

Task: Obtain an accurate apical pulse rate.

Conditions: Watch or clock with a second hand, patient chart

Standards: Perform the Task within 3 minutes with a minimum score of _____ points.

Work Documentation: Patient chart entry

No.	Step	Points	Check #1	Check #2	Check #3
1	Organized supplies and room and washed hands.				
2	Greeted the patient correctly and appropriately.				
3	Performed the procedure correctly and safely: • Prepared patient properly, assisting if needed. • Draped patient appropriately. • Determined correct location of apical pulse site. • Counted the pulse rate for respirations for full minute. • Assessed the pulse for irregularities in rate, rhythm, and sounds. • Assisted patient while ensuring his/her comfort and safety.				
4	Obtained accurate pulse rate.				
5	Demonstrated professional behavior in manner, organization, and attire, including: • Communicated appropriately and comfortably with the patient.				
6	Washed hands.				
7	Documented correctly.				
Student's Total Points					
Points Possible					
Final Score (Student's Total Points/ Possible Points)					

Name _____   **Date** _____   **Score** _____

WORK DOCUMENTATION

_____

Instructor's/Evaluator's Comments and Suggestions:

_____

_____

_____

_____

_____

CHECK #1

Evaluator's Signature: _____   Date:

CHECK #2

Evaluator's Signature: _____   Date:

CHECK #3

Evaluator's Signature: _____   Date:

ABHES Competency: VI.A.1.a.4.d Take vital signs

CAAHEP Curriculum: I.P.1 Obtain vital signs

Name _____   **Date** _____   **Score** _____

COMPETENCY ASSESSMENT

Procedure 24-9   Measuring the Respiration Rate

Task: Obtain an accurate respiratory rate.

Conditions: Watch or clock with a second hand, patient chart

Standards: Perform the Task within 3 minutes with a minimum score of _____ points.

Work Documentation: Patient chart entry

No.	Step	Points	Check #1	Check #2	Check #3
1	Organized supplies and room and washed hands.				
2	Greeted the patient correctly and appropriately.				
3	Performed the procedure correctly and safely: • Counted the respirations for 30 seconds or a full minute if irregularities noted. • Assessed the breathing for irregularities in rate, rhythm, and breath sounds. • Ensured patient comfort and safety.				
4	Obtained accurate respiratory rate.				
5	Demonstrated professional behavior in manner, organization, and attire, including: • Communicated appropriately and comfortably with the patient.				
6	Washed hands.				
7	Documented correctly.				
Student's Total Points					
Points Possible					
Final Score (Student's Total Points/ Possible Points)					

Name _____   **Date** _____   **Score** _____

WORK DOCUMENTATION

_____

Instructor's/Evaluator's Comments and Suggestions:

_____

_____

_____

_____

_____

CHECK #1

Evaluator's Signature: Date:

CHECK #2

Evaluator's Signature: Date:

CHECK #3

Evaluator's Signature: Date:

ABHES Competency: VI.A.1.a.4.d Take vital signs

CAAHEP Curriculum: I.P.1 Obtain vital signs

Name _____ **Date** _____ **Score** _____

COMPETENCY ASSESSMENT

Procedure 24-10   Measuring Blood Pressure

Task: Obtain an accurate blood pressure.

Conditions: Stethoscope, sphygmomanometer/BP cuff, patient chart

Standards: Perform the Task within 3 minutes with a minimum score of _____ points.

Work
Documentation: Patient chart entry

No.	Step	Points	Check #1	Check #2	Check #3
1	Organized supplies and room and washed hands.				
2	Greeted the patient correctly and appropriately.				
3	Performed the procedure correctly and safely using proper body mechanics: • Positioned the patient properly. • Exposed arm appropriately. • Determined proper cuff size. • Positioned cuff correctly. • Held patient arm at proper level in relaxed position. • Positioned stethoscope ear buds at proper angle, positioned diaphragm correctly. • Released pressure at appropriate speed.				
4	Obtained accurate blood pressure reading.				
5	Demonstrated professional behavior in manner, organization, and attire, including: • Communicated appropriately and comfortably with the patient.				
6	Washed hands.				
7	Documented correctly.				
Student's Total Points					
Points Possible					
Final Score (Student's Total Points/ Possible Points)					

Name _____ **Date** _____ **Score** _____

WORK DOCUMENTATION

_____

Instructor's/Evaluator's Comments and Suggestions:

_____

_____

_____

_____

_____

CHECK #1

Evaluator's Signature: _____ Date: _____

CHECK #2

Evaluator's Signature: _____ Date: _____

CHECK #3

Evaluator's Signature: _____ Date: _____

ABHES Competency: VI.A.1.a.4.d Take vital signs

CAAHEP Curriculum: I.P.1 Obtain vital signs

Name _____ Date _____ Score _____

COMPETENCY ASSESSMENT

Procedure 24-11   Measuring Height

Task: Obtain an accurate patient height.

Conditions: Height scale, patient chart

Standards: Perform the Task within 3 minutes with a minimum score of _____ points.

Work Documentation: Patient chart entry

No.	Step	Points	Check #1	Check #2	Check #3
1	Prepared scale and area around scale: • Arranged for a place for patient to sit to remove shoes and hang coat. • Ensured that height scale was properly calibrated and functioning.				
2	Washed hands.				
3	Greeted the patient correctly and appropriately.				
4	Performed the procedure correctly and safely: • Assisted patient with removal of coat and shoes as needed. • Assisted patient in storing coat, shoes, and other property. • Positioned patient correctly and safely for proper height measurement. • Measured properly. • Returned height scale to original position.				
5	Obtained accurate height measurement.				
6	Demonstrated professional behavior in manner, organization, and attire, including: • Communicated appropriately and comfortably with the patient.				
7	Washed hands.				
8	Documented correctly.				
Student's Total Points					
Points Possible					
Final Score (Student's Total Points/ Possible Points)					

Name _____ **Date** _____ **Score** _____

WORK DOCUMENTATION

_____

Instructor's/Evaluator's Comments and Suggestions:

_____

_____

_____

_____

_____

CHECK #1

Evaluator's Signature: _____ Date:

CHECK #2

Evaluator's Signature: _____ Date:

CHECK #3

Evaluator's Signature: _____ Date:

ABHES Competency: VI.A.1.a.4.d Take vital signs

CAAHEP Curriculum: I.P.1 Obtain vital signs

Name _____ Date _____ Score _____

COMPETENCY ASSESSMENT

Procedure 24-12   Measuring Adult Weight

Task: Obtain an accurate patient weight.

Conditions: Weight scale, patient chart

Standards: Perform the Task within 3 minutes with a minimum score of _____ points.

Work Documentation: Patient chart entry

No.	Step	Points	Check #1	Check #2	Check #3
1	Prepared scale and area around scale: • Arranged for a place for patient to sit to remove shoes and hang coat. • Ensured that height scale was properly calibrated and functioning.				
2	Washed hands.				
3	Greeted the patient correctly and appropriately.				
4	Performed the procedure correctly and safely: • Assisted patient with removal of coat and shoes as needed. • Assisted patient in storing coat, shoes, and other property. • Positioned patient correctly and safely for proper weight measurement. • Measured weight properly. • Returned weight balance to original position.				
5	Obtained accurate weight measurement.				
6	Demonstrated professional behavior in manner, organization, and attire, including: • Communicated appropriately and comfortably with the patient.				
7	Washed hands.				
8	Documented correctly.				
Student's Total Points					
Points Possible					
Final Score (Student's Total Points/ Possible Points)					

Name _____   **Date** _____   **Score** _____

WORK DOCUMENTATION

_____

Instructor's/Evaluator's Comments and Suggestions:

_____

_____

_____

_____

_____

CHECK #1

Evaluator's Signature: Date:

CHECK #2

Evaluator's Signature: Date:

CHECK #3

Evaluator's Signature: Date:

ABHES Competency: VI.A.1.a.4.d Take vital signs

CAAHEP Curriculum: I.P.1 Obtain vital signs

Name _____ Date _____ Score _____

COMPETENCY ASSESSMENT

Procedure 25-1   Assisting with a Complete Physical Examination

Task: To assist the physician with a complete examination.

Conditions: Scale for height and weight, patient gown, drape, thermometer, stethoscope, sphygmomanometer, alcohol wipes, examination light, otoscope, ophthalmoscope, penlight, nasal
speculum, tongue depressor, percussion hammer, tape measure, cotton balls, safety pin or
sensory wheel, gloves, tissues, lubricant, emesis basin, gauze sponges, specimen bottle,
slides and requisition form, biohazard waste container, and specific test kits as needed

Standards: Perform the Task within 25 minutes with a minimum score of _____ points.

Work
Documentation: Patient chart entry

No.	Step	Points	Check #1	Check #2	Check #3
1	Washed hands, organized equipment and exam room.				
2	Introduced self to the patient, confirmed the patient's identity. Made eye contact with the patient.				
3	Performed the procedure correctly and safely: • Positioned the patient safely and comfortably. • Washed hands in front of the patient. • Interviewed the patient for current medications, tetanus status, update of medical history, determination of chief complaint. • Obtained and recorded vital signs. • Obtained lab work if previously ordered. • Performed diagnostic tests if previously ordered (EKG or spirometry). • Assisted the patient to prepare for examination. • Assisted the physician during and after the examination as needed. • Escorted the patient to the next phase (such as to the front desk for rescheduling, to the laboratory for testing).				
4	Demonstrated professional behavior in manner, organization, and attire.				
5	Washed hands and cleaned, sanitized, and disinfected the exam room for the next patient.				
6	Documented accurately and completely.				
Student's Total Points					
Points Possible					
Final Score (Student's Total Points/ Possible Points)					

Name _____   **Date** _____   **Score** _____

WORK DOCUMENTATION

_____

Instructor's/Evaluator's Comments and Suggestions:

_____

_____

_____

_____

_____

CHECK #1	
Evaluator's Signature:	Date:

CHECK #2	
Evaluator's Signature:	Date:

CHECK #3	
Evaluator's Signature:	Date:

ABHES Competency: VI.A.1.a.4.b Prepare patients for procedures; VI.A.1.a.4.d Take vital signs; VI.A.1.a.4.g Prepare and maintain examination and treatment area; VI.A.1.a.4.h Prepare patient for and assist physician with routine and specialty examinations and treatments and minor office surgeries

CAAHEP Curriculum: I.P.1 Obtain vital signs; I.P.10 Assist physician with patient care; IV.P.6 Prepare a patient for procedures and/or treatments

Name _____ Date _____ Score _____

COMPETENCY ASSESSMENT

Procedure 26-1   Assisting with Routine Prenatal Visits

Task: To assist in routine examination to monitor the progress of a pregnancy.

Conditions: Disposable gloves, patient gown, scale, tape measure, sphygmomanometer, stethoscope, Doppler fetoscope and accessories, urine specimen container, urinalysis supplies, thermometer, patient chart

Standards: Perform the Task within 10 minutes with a minimum score of _____ points.

Work Documentation: Patient chart entry

No.	Step	Points	Check #1	Check #2	Check #3
1	Organized supplies and room.				
2	Greeted the patient correctly and appropriately.				
3	Washed hands and used proper PPE.				
4	Performed the procedure correctly and safely: • Obtained accurate weight. • Obtained accurate blood pressure and pulse. • Performed chemical examination of urine accurately and safely. • Assisted the provider as needed. • Assisted the patient as needed.				
5	Demonstrated professional behavior in manner, organization, and attire, including: • Communicating appropriately and comfortably with the patient.				
6	Cleaned/disposed of supplies and equipment appropriately and washed hands.				
7	Documented correctly.				
	Student's Total Points				
	Points Possible				
	Final Score (Student's Total Points/ Possible Points)				

Name _____ Date _____ Score _____

WORK DOCUMENTATION

_____

Instructor's/Evaluator's Comments and Suggestions:

_____

_____

_____

_____

_____

CHECK #1

Evaluator's Signature: _____ Date:

CHECK #2

Evaluator's Signature: _____ Date:

CHECK #3

Evaluator's Signature: _____ Date:

ABHES Competency: VI.A.1.a.4.b Prepare patients for procedures; VI.A.1.a.4.d Take vital signs; VI.A.1.a.4.h Prepare patient for and assist physician with routine and specialty examinations and treatments and minor office surgeries

CAAHEP Curriculum: I.P.1 Obtain vital signs; I.P.10 Assist physician with patient care; IV.P.6 Prepare a patient for procedures and/or treatments

Name _____   Date _____   Score _____

COMPETENCY ASSESSMENT

Procedure 26-2   Assisting with Pelvic Examination and Pap Test (Conventional and ThinPrep® Methods)

Task: To assist the provider in collection of cervical cells for laboratory analysis for early detection of abnormal cells of the cervix, including cancer, to assess the health of the patient's reproductive organs, to detect disease, leading to diagnosis and treatment.

Conditions: Patient chart, patient gown, patient drape, disposable gloves, tissues, lubricant, 4 × 4, vaginal speculum, tissues, urine cup and testing supplies, warm water or warming light, light for viewing, adjustable stool for provider, supplies for Pap test according to method used (see Procedure 26-2)

Standards: Perform the Task within 25 minutes with a minimum score of _____ points.

Work Documentation: Patient chart entry, lab requisition

No.	Step	Points	Check #1	Check #2	Check #3
1	Organized supplies and room.				
2	Prepared patient for pelvic examination: • Greeted patient correctly and appropriately. • Had patient empty bladder, saving the specimen for testing if needed. • Instructed patient to undress and put on a gown. • Explained procedure to patient. • Asked patient to sit at end of table. • Draped patient for privacy.				
3	Labeled the Pap bottles and completed the requisition as required for method used.				
4	Assisted the physician as needed through examination: • Assisted patient into lithotomy position safely and correctly, and draped patient. • Applied gloves. • Warmed the speculum. • Handed supplies to the physician as needed. • Prepared the specimen for the laboratory properly. • Disposed of waste into proper containers. • Removed gloves, washed hands.				

No.	Step	Points	Check #1	Check #2	Check #3
5	Assisted the patient as needed after the examination: • Helped her to a sitting position, using safe and correct body mechanics. • Helped her dress as needed. • Answered any questions she had. • Informed her of when the results would be available. • Scheduled her next regular examination or set up a reminder at a later date.				
6	Demonstrated professional behavior in manner, organization, and attire, including: • Communicated appropriately and comfortably with the patient throughout.				
7	Prepared the specimen for transport to the laboratory and completed the requisition properly.				
8	Documented correctly.				
9	Cleaned and prepared room for next patient; took instruments to the cleaning area for sanitization and sterilization.				
Student's Total Points					
Points Possible					
Final Score (Student's Total Points/ Possible Points)					

Name _____ **Date** _____ **Score** _____

WORK DOCUMENTATION

*Also attach lab requisition.

_____

Instructor's/Evaluator's Comments and Suggestions:

_____

_____

_____

_____

_____

CHECK #1	
Evaluator's Signature:	Date:

CHECK #2	
Evaluator's Signature:	Date:

CHECK #3	
Evaluator's Signature:	Date:

ABHES Competency: VI.A.1.a.4.b Prepare patients for procedures; VI.A.1.a.4.h Prepare patient for and assist physician with routine and specialty examinations and treatments and minor office surgeries

CAAHEP Curriculum: I.P.10 Assist physician with patient care; IV.P.6 Prepare a patient for procedures and/or treatments

Name _____   **Date** _____   **Score** _____

COMPETENCY ASSESSMENT

Procedure 26-3   Assisting with Insertion of an Intrauterine Device (IUD)

Task: To assist the provider with the insertion of an intrauterine device.

Condition: Nonsterile gloves, sterile gloves, vaginal speculum, light source and stool for provider, drape and gown, tissue, lubricant, prepackaged IUD, biohazard waste container, local anesthetic, syringe and needle, antiseptic such as Betadine® solution or swabs, emesis basin for used items such as speculum

Standards: Perform the Task within 25 minutes with a minimum score of _____ points.

Work Documentation: Patient chart entry

No.	Step	Points	Check #1	Check #2	Check #3
1	Washed hands and organized supplies and room, including drawing up anesthetic into syringe as directed by the provider.				
2	Prepared patient for pelvic examination.				
3	Assisted the provider as needed through procedure: • Applied gloves. • Warmed the speculum. • Handed supplies to the physician as needed. • Prepared the specimen for the laboratory properly. • Disposed of waste into proper containers. • Removed gloves, washed hands.				
4	Assisted the patient as needed after the procedure: • Checked vital signs. • Helped her to a sitting position, using safe and correct body mechanics. • Helped her dress as needed. • Answered any questions she had. • Scheduled a follow-up appointment.				
5	Demonstrated professional behavior in manner, organization, and attire, including: • Communicated appropriately and comfortably with the patient throughout.				
6	Documented correctly.				
7	Cleaned and prepared room for next patient; took instruments to the cleaning area for sanitization and sterilization.				
Student's Total Points					
Points Possible					
Final Score (Student's Total Points/ Possible Points)					

Name _____ **Date** _____ **Score** _____

WORK DOCUMENTATION

_____

Instructor's/Evaluator's Comments and Suggestions:

_____

_____

_____

_____

_____

CHECK #1	
Evaluator's Signature:	Date:

CHECK #2	
Evaluator's Signature:	Date:

CHECK #3	
Evaluator's Signature:	Date:

ABHES Competency: VI.A.1.a.4.b Prepare patients for procedures; VI.A.1.a.4.h Prepare patient for and assist physician with routine and specialty examinations and treatments and minor office surgeries

CAAHEP Curriculum: I.P.10 Assist physician with patient care; IV.P.6 Prepare a patient for procedures and/or treatments

Name _____ Date _____ Score _____

COMPETENCY ASSESSMENT

Procedure 26-4   Wet Prep/Wet Mount and Potassium Hydroxide (KOH) Prep

Task: To test the vaginal area for the determination and diagnosis of vaginitis. The wet prep mount test for ycast, bacteria, and trichomonas; the KOH prep tests for fungi.

Conditions: Patient chart, patient gown, patient drape, urine cup, disposable gloves, tissues, lubricant, 4 × 4, vaginal speculum and other supplies as needed for the vaginal examination. For wet prep: Cotton-tipped applicators, small test tubes, normal saline (0.5 mL, or a few drops), two microscope slides and cover slips. For KOH: 10% potassium hydrochloride solution (0.5 mL or a few drops), two microscope slides and cover slips, microscope

Standards: Perform the Task within 25 minutes with a minimum score of _____ points.

**Work
Documentation:**   Patient chart entry, lab report

No.	Step	Points	Check #1	Check #2	Check #3
1	Organized supplies and room.				
2	Prepared patient for pelvic examination.				
3	Assisted the physician as needed through examination.				
4	Prepared the specimen for the laboratory properly: • Placed several drops of normal saline in small test tube. • After physician obtained vaginal discharge sample, rinsed the swab in the saline solution, pressing the cotton tip against the inside of the tube to express the specimen. • Disposed of the applicator into sharps container. • Applied a drop of sample/solution onto a microscope slide and covered with cover slip.				
5	Assisted the patient as needed after the examination: • Helped her to a sitting position, using safe and correct body mechanics. • Helped her dress as needed. • Informed her that you and the provider would return when lab testing was finished.				
6	Removed gloves and washed hands.				

No.	Step	Points	Check #1	Check #2	Check #3
7	Took sample to laboratory, set up for physician to perform the microscopic examination.				
8	While the physician was examining the slide, prepared the sample for KOH examination: • Applied a few drops of KOH into the remaining solution in the test tube. • Mixed well. • Applied a drop onto a fresh slide, covered with a cover slip. • Set up for the provider to perform the microscopic examination.				
9	After the microscopy was performed, cleaned and disinfected the laboratory, disposing of supplies into proper receptacles.				
10	Went back to assist patient as needed.				
11	Demonstrated professional behavior in manner, organization, and attire, including: • Communicated appropriately and comfortably with the patient throughout.				
12	Documented correctly.				
13	Cleaned and prepared room for next patient; took instruments to the cleaning area for sanitization and sterilization.				
Student's Total Points					
Points Possible					
Final Score (Student's Total Points/ Possible Points)					

Name _____ **Date** _____ **Score** _____

WORK DOCUMENTATION

*Also attach lab report.

Instructor's/Evaluator's Comments and Suggestions:

_____

_____

_____

_____

_____

| **CHECK #1** |
| Evaluator's Signature: Date: |

| **CHECK #2** |
| Evaluator's Signature: Date: |

| **CHECK #3** |
| Evaluator's Signature: Date: |

ABHES Competency: VI.A.1.a.4.b Prepare patients for procedures; VI.A.1.a.4.h Prepare patient for and assist physician with routine and specialty examinations and treatments and minor office surgeries

CAAHEP Curriculum: I.P.10 Assist physician with patient care; IV.P.6 Prepare a patient for procedures and/or treatments

Name _____   **Date** _____   **Score** _____

COMPETENCY ASSESSMENT

Procedure 26-5   Amplified DNA ProbeTec Test for Chlamydia and Gonorrhea

Task: To test the vaginal area for diagnosis of chlamydia and gonorrhea and to use as a screening for pregnant women.

Conditions: Patient chart, patient gown, patient drape, urine cup, disposable gloves, tissues, lubricant, 4×4, vaginal speculum and other supplies as needed for the vaginal examination; Amplified DNA ProbeTec Kit (pink), laboratory requisition, biohazard transport bag

Standards: Perform the Task within 25 minutes with a minimum score of _____ points.

Work Documentation: Patient chart entry, lab requisition

No.	Step	Points	Check #1	Check #2	Check #3
1	Organized supplies and room.				
2	Prepared patient for pelvic examination.				
3	Assisted the physician as needed through examination: • First handed the large swab to provider. • Discarded it into biohazard. • Handed the Mini-tip Culturette Swab to provider.				
4	Prepared the specimen for the laboratory properly: • After the physician obtained a sample of the vaginal secretion on the mini-tip swab, immediately placed the swab into the transport tube and recapped it (per ProbeTec Wet Transport tube directions: broke off the tip of the swab into the liquid and recapped). • Placed specimen into biohazard specimen transport bag.				
5	Removed gloves and washed hands.				
6	Assisted the patient as needed after the examination: • Helped her to a sitting position, using safe and correct body mechanics. • Helped her dress as needed.				
7	Completed lab requisition, placed it into the outer pocket of the transport bag.				

No.	Step	Points	Check #1	Check #2	Check #3
8	Demonstrated professional behavior in manner, organization, and attire, including: • Communicated appropriately and comfortably with the patient throughout.				
9	Documented correctly.				
10	Cleaned and prepared room for next patient; took instruments to the cleaning area for sanitization and sterilization.				
Student's Total Points					
Points Possible					
Final Score (Student's Total Points/ Possible Points)					

Name _____   **Date** _____   **Score** _____

WORK DOCUMENTATION

*Also attach lab requisition.

_____

Instructor's/Evaluator's Comments and Suggestions:

_____

_____

_____

_____

_____

CHECK #1
Evaluator's Signature: _____   Date: _____

CHECK #2
Evaluator's Signature: _____   Date: _____

CHECK #3
Evaluator's Signature: _____   Date: _____

ABHES Competency: VI.A.1.a.4.b Prepare patients for procedures; VI.A.1.a.4.h Prepare patient for and assist physician with routine and specialty examinations and treatments and minor office surgeries

CAAHEP Curriculum: I.P.10 Assist physician with patient care; IV.P.6 Prepare a patient for procedures and/or treatments

Name _____ **Date** _____ **Score** _____

COMPETENCY ASSESSMENT

Procedure 27-1   Administration of a Vaccine

Task: To administer a vaccine.

Conditions: Vaccination order, vaccine, child's vaccination record, patient chart, pen or electronic chart, current VIS (Vaccine Information Statement); if administering by injection: syringe/needle as appropriate, alcohol wipe, sharps container

Standards: Perform the Task within 15 minutes with a minimum score of _____ points.

Work
Documentation: Patient chart entry, vaccine administration record

No.	Step	Points	Check #1	Check #2	Check #3
1	Gave the parent the most recent copy of the Vaccine Information Statement (VIS).				
2	Followed the proper steps for selecting and drawing up medication, including checking the order with the medication three times and checking expiration date.				
3	Administered the medication properly: • Used correct route. • If injecting, used proper technique and site.				
4	After administering the vaccine, documented the procedure in the patient's medical chart and in his/her vaccine record: • Used the medication note and the vaccine vial to fill out the vaccine record. • Noted the type of vaccine, the date given, dose, site, route, vaccine lot number, and manufacturer. • Documented which VIS was given to the patient.				
5	Filed the clinic copy and gave the parent the patient copy.				
6	Demonstrated professional behavior in manner, organization, and attire.				
Student's Total Points					
Points Possible					
Final Score (Student's Total Points/ Possible Points)					

Name _____   **Date** _____   **Score** _____

WORK DOCUMENTATION

*Also attach vaccination administration record.

_____

Instructor's/Evaluator's Comments and Suggestions:

_____

_____

_____

_____

_____

CHECK #1

Evaluator's Signature: _____   Date:

CHECK #2

Evaluator's Signature: _____   Date:

CHECK #3

Evaluator's Signature: _____   Date:

ABHES Competency: VI.A.1.a.4.m Prepare and administer oral and parenteral medications as directed by physician; VI.A.1.a.4.n Maintain medication and immunization records

CAAHEP Curriculum: I.P.7 Select proper sites for administering parenteral medication; I.P.9 Administer parenteral (excluding IV) medications; IV.P.8 Document patient care

Name _____ Date _____ Score _____

COMPETENCY ASSESSMENT

Procedure 27-2 Maintaining Immunization Records

Task: To establish and maintain a record of childhood immunizations.

Conditions: Medication order, vial of vaccination administered, child's vaccination record, patient chart, pen or electronic chart

Standards: Perform the Task within 15 minutes with a minimum score of _____ points.

Work Documentation: Patient chart entry, vaccine administration record

No.	Step	Points	Check #1	Check #2	Check #3
1	Gave the parent the most recent copy of the Vaccine Information Statement (VIS).				
2	After administering the vaccine, documented the procedure in the patient's medical chart and in his/her vaccine record: • Used the medication note and the vaccine vial to fill out the vaccine record. • Noted the type of vaccine, the date given, dose, site, route, vaccine lot number, and manufacturer. • Documented which VIS was given to the patient.				
3	Filed the clinic copy and gave the parent the patient copy.				
4	Demonstrated professional behavior in manner, organization, and attire.				
Student's Total Points					
Points Possible					
Final Score (Student's Total Points/ Possible Points)					

Name _____   **Date** _____   **Score** _____

WORK DOCUMENTATION
*Also attach vaccine administration record.

Instructor's/Evaluator's Comments and Suggestions:

_____

_____

_____

_____

_____

CHECK #1

Evaluator's Signature: Date:

CHECK #2

Evaluator's Signature: Date:

CHECK #3

Evaluator's Signature: Date:

ABHES Competency: VI.A.1.a.4.m Prepare and administer oral and parenteral medications as directed by physician; VI.A.1.a.4.n Maintain medication and immunization records

CAAHEP Curriculum: I.P.7 Select proper sites for administering parenteral medication; I.P.9 Administer parenteral (excluding IV) medications; IV.P.8 Document patient care

Name _____   Date _____   Score _____

COMPETENCY ASSESSMENT

Procedure 27-3   Measuring the Infant: Weight, Length, and Head and Chest Circumference

Task: To obtain an accurate measurement of an infant's weight, length, and head and chest circumferences.

Conditions: Patient chart including a growth grid, infant scale with protector, measuring tape or calibrated measuring mat, patient drape or blanket

Standards: Perform the Task within 30 minutes with a minimum score of _____ points.

Work Documentation: Patient chart entry, growth chart

No.	Step	Points	Check #1	Check #2	Check #3
1	Assembled equipment and arranged the room.				
2	Identified patient and explained the procedure to the parents; washed hands.				
3	Correctly weighed the infant: • Undressed the infant and/or assisted the parents as needed. • Placed protective sheet on scale and calibrated scale. • Gently placed infant on scale and ensured patient safety while on scale. • Adjusted the scale until weight was determined, while infant was lying still. • Noted infant's weight. • Returned scale weights to original position. • Removed protective sheet, disposed of it properly, and disinfected the scale. • Assisted parents to re-dress infant as needed.				
4	Correctly measured infant's length: If using a calibrated measuring mat: • Placed the infant on the mat with head touching the headboard. • Adjusted the foot board so the infant's heel and foot were flat against it and infant was lying straight; noted the length.				

No.	Step	Points	Check #1	Check #2	Check #3
	If using tape measure on examination table: • Laid the infant on the examination table, noted head position on the table paper. • Straightened the infant gently and marked the heel position on the table paper. • Lifted infant carefully and gave to parent. • Measured the distance between the head and heel marks, and noted the length.				
5	Correctly measured the head circumference: • Placed measuring tape around the largest part of the head, keeping the tape straight. • Noted head circumference in centimeters.				
6	Correctly measured the chest circumference: • Placed the measuring tape around the infant's chest, under the arms, just above the nipples, keeping the tape straight. • Noted chest circumference in centimeters.				
7	Correctly documented all measurements in the patient's record and on the growth chart.				
8	Demonstrated professional behavior in manner, organization, and attire, including communicating professionally with the patient and parents.				
Student's Total Points					
Points Possible					
Final Score (Student's Total Points/ Possible Points)					

Name _____ **Date** _____ **Score** _____

WORK DOCUMENTATION

*Also attach growth chart.

_____

Instructor's/Evaluator's Comments and Suggestions:

_____

_____

_____

_____

_____

| **CHECK #1** |
| Evaluator's Signature: |
| Date: |

| **CHECK #2** |
| Evaluator's Signature: |
| Date: |

| **CHECK #3** |
| Evaluator's Signature: |
| Date: |

CAAHEP Curriculum: II.P.3 Maintain growth charts; IV.P.8 Document patient care

Name _____ **Date** _____ **Score** _____

COMPETENCY ASSESSMENT

Procedure 27-4 Taking an Infant's Rectal Temperature with a Digital Thermometer

Task: To obtain an accurate rectal temperature.

Conditions: Digital thermometer and probe cover, lubricating jelly, 4 × 4 gauze square, spare diaper, gloves, patient chart, pen or electronic chart

Standards: Perform the Task within 15 minutes with a minimum score of _____ points.

Work Documentation: Patient chart entry

No.	Step	Points	Check #1	Check #2	Check #3
1	Assembled equipment and supplies.				
2	Identified patient and explained the procedure to the parents.				
3	Used proper technique to obtain rectal temperature: • Removed the infant's diaper or assisted the parents as needed. • Applied gloves. • Positioned infant properly and safely. • Attached the probe cover to thermometer. • Lubricated the tip. • Inserted thermometer properly (0.5 inch). • Restrained infant as needed for safety. • When thermometer beeped, removed it and noted temperature. • Discarded probe cover into biohazard waste, removed gloves, washed hands. • Assisted parents in dressing the infant as needed.				
4	Disinfected thermometer and area.				
5	Correctly documented temperature.				
6	Demonstrated professional behavior in manner, organization, and attire, including communicating clearly with parents.				
Student's Total Points					
Points Possible					
Final Score (Student's Total Points/ Possible Points)					

Name _____   **Date** _____   **Score** _____

WORK DOCUMENTATION

Instructor's/Evaluator's Comments and Suggestions:

_____

_____

_____

_____

_____

CHECK #1

Evaluator's Signature: _____   Date:

CHECK #2

Evaluator's Signature: _____   Date:

CHECK #3

Evaluator's Signature: _____   Date:

ABHES Competency: VI.A.1.a.4.d Take vital signs

CAAHEP Curriculum: I.P.1 Obtain vital signs

Name _____   **Date** _____   **Score** _____

COMPETENCY ASSESSMENT

Procedure 27-5 Taking an Apical Pulse on an Infant

Task: To obtain an accurate apical pulse rate of an infant.

Conditions: Stethoscope, watch with second hand, alcohol wipes, patient drape, patient chart, pen or electronic chart

Standards: Perform the Task within 15 minutes with a minimum score of _____ points.

Work Documentation: Patient chart entry

No.	Step	Points	Check #1	Check #2	Check #3
1	Assembled equipment and supplies.				
2	Identified patient and explained the procedure to the parents; washed hands.				
3	Prepared the infant for the procedure: • Undressed the infant and/or assisted the parent(s) as needed. • Provided a drape sheet for comfort if appropriate. • Positioned the patient in supine position.				
4	Took the apical pulse rate: • Located the 5th intercostal space at the midclavicular line on the left side of the chest. • Placed the warmed stethoscope bell on the space and listened for the heartbeat. • Counted the pulse for one full minute. • Noted the rate.				
5	Correctly documented apical pulse rate.				
6	Demonstrated professional behavior in manner, organization, and attire, including communicating clearly with parents.				
Student's Total Points					
Points Possible					
Final Score (Student's Total Points/ Possible Points)					

Name _____ **Date** _____ **Score** _____

WORK DOCUMENTATION

Instructor's/Evaluator's Comments and Suggestions:

_____

_____

_____

_____

_____

CHECK #1
Evaluator's Signature:
Date:

CHECK #2
Evaluator's Signature:
Date:

CHECK #3
Evaluator's Signature:
Date:

ABHES Competency: VI.A.1.a.4.d Take vital signs

CAAHEP Curriculum: I.P.1 Obtain vital signs

Name _____ Date _____ Score _____

COMPETENCY ASSESSMENT

Procedure 27-6   Measuring Infant's Respiration Rate

Task: To obtain an accurate respiratory rate of an infant.

Conditions: Watch with second hand, patient chart, pen or electronic chart

Standards: Perform the Task within 15 minutes with a minimum score of _____ points.

Work
Documentation: Patient chart entry

No.	Step	Points	Check #1	Check #2	Check #3
1	Assembled equipment and supplies.				
2	Identified patient and explained the procedure to the parents; washed hands.				
3	Took the respiratory rate: • Positioned the patient in supine position. • Placed hand on infant's chest to feel the respirations. • Counted the respirations for one full minute. • Noted the rate, depth, rhythm, and breath sounds. • Returned infant to parents.				
4	Correctly documented the respiration rate.				
5	Demonstrated professional behavior in manner, organization, and attire, including communicating clearly with parents.				
Student's Total Points					
Points Possible					
Final Score (Student's Total Points/ Possible Points)					

Name _____   **Date** _____   **Score** _____

WORK DOCUMENTATION

_____

Instructor's/Evaluator's Comments and Suggestions:

_____

_____

_____

_____

_____

CHECK #1

Evaluator's Signature: _____   Date:

CHECK #2

Evaluator's Signature: _____   Date:

CHECK #3

Evaluator's Signature: _____   Date:

ABHES Competency: VI.A.1.a.4.d Take vital signs

CAAHEP Curriculum: I.P.1 Obtain vital signs

Name _____   **Date** _____   **Score** _____

COMPETENCY ASSESSMENT

Procedure 27-7   Obtaining a Urine Specimen from an Infant or Young Child

Task: To obtain a specimen of urine from an infant or young child.

Conditions: Urine collection bag, laboratory request form, urine cup, urinalysis supplies, gloves, cleansing cloth, drying pad, patient chart, pen or electronic chart

Standards: Perform the Task within 15 minutes with a minimum score of _____ points.

Work Documentation: Patient chart entry, urinalysis report form, lab requisition

No.	Step	Points	Check #1	Check #2	Check #3
1	Assembled equipment and supplies.				
2	Identified patient and explained the procedure to the parents; washed hands.				
3	Prepared the patient for the procedure: • Positioned patient in supine position. • Removed diaper or assisted parent(s) as needed.				
4	Obtained the urine specimen: • Applied the bag to the patient properly. • Replaced the diaper. • Checked frequently or instructed parents • When specimen was collected, carefully removed bag and returned infant to parents. • Transported specimen to urine cup. • Prepared for transport or test in POL.				
5	Correctly documented the procedure.				
6	Demonstrated professional behavior in manner, organization, and attire, including communicating clearly with parents.				
Student's Total Points					
Points Possible					
Final Score (Student's Total Points/ Possible Points)					

Name _____ Date _____ Score _____

WORK DOCUMENTATION

*Also attach urinalysis report form and lab requisition.

Instructor's/Evaluator's Comments and Suggestions:

_____

_____

_____

_____

CHECK #1

Evaluator's Signature: Date:

CHECK #2

Evaluator's Signature: Date:

CHECK #3

Evaluator's Signature: Date:

ABHES Competency: VI.A.1.a.4.j Collect and process specimens

CAAHEP Curriculum: III.P.7 Obtain specimens for microbiological testing

Name _____ **Date** _____ **Score** _____

COMPETENCY ASSESSMENT

Procedure 28-1 Instructing Patient in Testicular Self-Examination

Task: To provide the patient with the correct procedure for performing monthly testicular self-examination.

Conditions: Patient chart, testicular model, testicular self-examination brochure and/or DVD

Standards: Perform the Task within 15 minutes with a minimum score of _____ points.

Work Documentation: Patient chart entry

No.	Step	Points	Check #1	Check #2	Check #3
1	Organized supplies and room.				
2	Identified and greeted patient appropriately.				
3	Performed the instruction correctly and professionally: • Using a DVD and/or patient brochure, instructed the patient on the proper method to perform the self-examination. • Discussed ideal positioning, frequency, and method to follow while examining the testicles, as well as what the patient is to be aware of during the self-examination. • Answered any questions from the patient. • Provided additional educational resources as approved by the provider.				
4	Instructed patient to notify the provider immediately if any abnormalities are found.				
5	Demonstrated professional behavior in manner, organization, and attire, including communicating clearly and comfortably with patient.				
6	Washed hands.				
7	Correctly documented the procedure.				
Student's Total Points					
Points Possible					
Final Score (Student's Total Points/ Possible Points)					

Name _____ **Date** _____ **Score** _____

WORK DOCUMENTATION

Instructor's/Evaluator's Comments and Suggestions:

_____

_____

_____

_____

_____

CHECK #1

Evaluator's Signature: _____   Date: _____

CHECK #2

Evaluator's Signature: _____   Date: _____

CHECK #3

Evaluator's Signature: _____   Date: _____

ABHES Competency: VI.A.1.a.2.m Adaptation for individualized needs; VI.A.1.a.7.c Teach patients methods of health promotion and disease prevention

CAAHEP Curriculum: IV.P.5 Instruct patients according to their needs to promote health maintenance and disease prevention; IV.P.9 Document patient education

Name _____ Date _____ Score _____

COMPETENCY ASSESSMENT

Procedure 30-1 Urinary Catheterization of a Female Patient

Task: To obtain a sterile urine specimen for analysis, to measure post-void residual, or to relieve urinary retention.

Conditions: Catheter kit containing needed supplies, sterile gloves, antiseptic cleansing solution, waxed bag or nearby biohazard bag, lubricant, sterile cotton balls, sterile forceps and Betadine® or Betadine® swabs, sterile urine cup, sterile 2 × 2 gauze, sterile absorbent pad, sterile fenestrated drape, tissue, sterile catheter as ordered, laboratory requisition, biohazard specimen transfer bag if needed

Standards: Perform the Task within 20 minutes with a minimum score of _____ points.

Work Documentation: Patient chart entry

No.	Step	Points	Check #1	Check #2	Check #3
1	Organized supplies and room.				
2	Identified and greeted patient appropriately; washed hands.				
3	Prepared the patient for the procedure: • Directed the patient to undress from the waist down and provided a drape. • Helped the patient onto the examination table. • Positioned the patient on back with feet together and knees apart.				
4	Set up the catheter tray, using sterile technique: • Opened the catheter kit using sterile technique on Mayo tray. • Placed the non-fenestrated drape under the patient's buttocks. • Emptied the kit onto the sterile field. • Placed the container into position without compromising sterility. • Applied sterile gloves. • Prepared Betadine cleansers and lubricant within sterile field.				

No.	Step	Points	Check #1	Check #2	Check #3
5	Performed catheterization properly without compromising sterility: • Placed fenestrated drape over patient's genitalia to create a sterile field. • Used nondominant hand to hold labia apart. • Cleansed area with three Betadine wipes using sterile dominant hand. • Dipped catheter tip into lubricant, placed other end into the container between patient's legs, and gently inserted the lubricated tip into the urethra. • Inserted catheter about 4 inches or until urine flowed. • When urine ceased, removed the catheter gently and slowly.				
6	Cared for the patient and the urine sample after catheterization: • Moved the urine container to the tray. • Transferred the urine to a capped sterile urine cup. • Disposed of contents of tray into biohazard bag. • Removed gloves, washed hands. • Assisted the patient to sit up and get dressed as needed.				
7	Demonstrated professional behavior in manner, organization, and attire, including communicating clearly and comfortably with patient.				
8	Correctly documented the procedure.				
Student's Total Points					
Points Possible					
Final Score (Student's Total Points/ Possible Points)					

Name _____   **Date** _____   **Score** _____

WORK DOCUMENTATION

Instructor's/Evaluator's Comments and Suggestions:

_____

_____

_____

_____

_____

CHECK #1	
Evaluator's Signature:	Date:

CHECK #2	
Evaluator's Signature:	Date:

CHECK #3	
Evaluator's Signature:	Date:

ABHES Competency: VI.A.1.a.4.h Prepare patient for and assist physician with routine and specialty examinations and treatments and minor office surgeries

Name _____ Date _____ Score _____

COMPETENCY ASSESSMENT

Procedure 30-2   Urinary Catheterization of a Male Patient

Task: To obtain a sterile urine specimen for analysis, to measure post-void residual, or to relieve urinary retention.

Conditions: Catheter kit containing needed supplies, sterile gloves, antiseptic cleansing solution, waxed bag or nearby biohazard bag, lubricant, sterile cotton balls, sterile forceps and Betadine® or Betadine® swabs, sterile urine cup, sterile 2×2 gauze, sterile absorbent pad, sterile fenestrated drape, tissue, sterile catheter as ordered, laboratory requisition, biohazard specimen transfer bag if needed

Standards: Perform the Task within 15 minutes with a minimum score of _____ points.

Work Documentation: Patient chart entry

No.	Step	Points	Check #1	Check #2	Check #3
1	Organized supplies and room.				
2	Identified and greeted patient appropriately; washed hands.				
3	Prepared the patient for the procedure: • Directed the patient to undress from the waist down and provided a drape. • Helped the patient onto the examination table. • Positioned the patient on his back with legs straight.				
4	Set up the catheter tray, using sterile technique: • Opened the catheter kit using sterile technique on Mayo tray. • Placed the non-fenestrated drape on the patient's thighs. • Emptied the kit onto the sterile field. • Placed the container into position without compromising sterility. • Applied sterile gloves. • Prepared Betadine cleansers and lubricant within sterile field.				

No.	Step	Points	Check #1	Check #2	Check #3
5	Performed catheterization properly without compromising sterility: • Placed non-fenestrated drape over patient's thighs and fenestrated drape over penis to create a sterile field. • Used nondominant hand to hold penis taut, pulled back foreskin if necessary. • Cleansed area with three Betadine wipes using sterile dominant hand. • Dipped catheter tip into lubricant, placed other end into the container between patient's legs, and gently inserted the lubricated tip into the urethra. • Inserted catheter about 6 inches or until urine flowed. • When urine ceased, removed the catheter gently and slowly.				
6	Cared for the patient and the urine sample after catheterization: • Moved the urine container to the tray. • Transferred the urine to a capped sterile urine cup. • Disposed of contents of tray into biohazard bag. • Removed gloves, washed hands. • Assisted the patient to sit up and get dressed as needed.				
7	Demonstrated professional behavior in manner, organization, and attire, including communicating clearly and comfortably with patient.				
8	Correctly documented the procedure.				
Student's Total Points					
Points Possible					
Final Score (Student's Total Points/ Possible Points)					

Name _____   **Date** _____   **Score** _____

WORK DOCUMENTATION

_____

Instructor's/Evaluator's Comments and Suggestions:

_____
_____
_____
_____
_____

CHECK #1
Evaluator's Signature: _____   Date: _____

CHECK #2
Evaluator's Signature: _____   Date: _____

CHECK #3
Evaluator's Signature: _____   Date: _____

ABHES Competency: VI.A.1.a.4.h Prepare patient for and assist physician with routine and specialty examinations and treatments and minor office surgeries

Name _____   **Date** _____   **Score** _____

COMPETENCY ASSESSMENT

Procedure 30-3   Fecal Occult Blood Test

Task: To teach the patient how to properly obtain a fecal specimen and then return it to the office for testing. To test feces for occult blood in the provider's office laboratory (POL).

Conditions: *Obtaining the specimen:* An occult slide test kit containing three slides, six applicators, envelope, and instructions. *Testing the specimen:* Prepared slides from the patient, occult blood developer from same manufacturer, gloves, biohazard waste container

Standards: Perform the Task within 15 minutes with a minimum score of _____ points.

Work Documentation: Two patient chart entries

No.	Step	Points	Check #1	Check #2	Check #3
1	Organized supplies and room.				
2	Identified and greeted patient appropriately; washed hands.				
3	Explained the procedure to the patient. Directed the patient to: • Follow the instructions on the slides. • Keep slides away from moisture, heat, and direct sunlight. • Label slide prior to obtaining the specimen. • Take a specimen each day for three days or three separate bowel movements. • Return the specimen to the office for testing. • Ingest no red meat, vitamin C, or aspirin products for three days prior to testing.				
4	Provided the patient with a biohazard envelope for the completed slides.				
5	Correctly documented the procedure.				
6	Demonstrated professional behavior in manner, organization, and attire, including communicating clearly and comfortably with patient.				

No.	Step	Points	Check #1	Check #2	Check #3
7	Tested for occult fecal blood by developing the slides: • Applied gloves. • Checked the dates and name on the slides. • Checked expiration date and label for the developing reagent. • Opened the back of each slide and, following instructions, applied drops of reagent onto the specimens and the controls. • Read the slides immediately for any evidence of blue color.				
8	Disposed of slides into biohazard waste container.				
9	Disinfected area, removed gloves, washed hands.				
10	Correctly documented the procedure.				
Student's Total Points					
Points Possible					
Final Score (Student's Total Points/ Possible Points)					

Name _____   **Date** _____   **Score** _____

WORK DOCUMENTATION

_____

Instructor's/Evaluator's Comments and Suggestions:

_____
_____
_____
_____
_____

CHECK #1

Evaluator's Signature: Date:

CHECK #2

Evaluator's Signature: Date:

CHECK #3

Evaluator's Signature: Date:

ABHES Competency: VI.A.1.a.4.j Collect and process specimens; VI.A.1.a.4.l Screen and follow up patient test results; VI.A.1.a.4.x Instruct patient in the collection of fecal specimen

CAAHEP Curriculum: I.P.6 Screen test results; IV.P.9 Document patient education

Name _____   **Date** _____   **Score** _____

COMPETENCY ASSESSMENT

Procedure 30-4   Performing Visual Acuity Testing Using a Snellen Charting

Task: To perform a visual screening test to determine a patient's distance visual acuity.

Conditions: Snellen eye chart (appropriate for age and language ability) placed at eye level without glare on it, occluder, pointer, disinfectant wipes

Standards: Perform the Task within 15 minutes with a minimum score of _____ points.

Work Documentation: Patient chart entry

No.	Step	Points	Check #1	Check #2	Check #3
1	Organized supplies and area for testing, ensured good lighting with no glare at a distance of 20 feet.				
2	Identified and greeted patient appropriately; washed hands.				
3	Explained the procedure to the patient.				
4	Performed the procedure, directing the patient to: • Stand back at 20 feet, cover one eye with the occluder, and read the chart as directed. • Cover the other eye and read the chart again as directed. • Point to each line on the chart, starting large and going smaller while noting the patient's accuracy, reactions, and comfort. • Perform the same test with both eyes.				
5	Demonstrated professional behavior in manner, organization, and attire, including communicating clearly and comfortably with patient.				
6	Disinfected the occluder, washed hands.				
7	Correctly documented the procedure.				
Student's Total Points					
Points Possible					
Final Score (Student's Total Points/ Possible Points)					

Name _____ **Date** _____ **Score** _____

WORK DOCUMENTATION

_____

Instructor's/Evaluator's Comments and Suggestions:

_____

_____

_____

_____

_____

CHECK #1

Evaluator's Signature: _____ Date:

CHECK #2

Evaluator's Signature: _____ Date:

CHECK #3

Evaluator's Signature: _____ Date:

ABHES Competency: VI.A.1.a.4.h Prepare patient for and assist physician with routine and specialty examinations and treatments and minor office surgeries

Name _____   Date _____   Score _____

COMPETENCY ASSESSMENT

Procedure 30-5   Measuring Near Visual Acuity

Task:　　　　　　To measure the near vision of a patient.

Conditions:　　　Visual acuity eye chart, occluder, disinfectant wipes

Standards:　　　Perform the Task within 15 minutes with a minimum score of _____ points.

Work
Documentation:　Patient chart entry

No.	Step	Points	Check #1	Check #2	Check #3
1	Organized supplies and area for testing, ensured good lighting with no glare.				
2	Identified and greeted patient appropriately; washed hands.				
3	Explained the procedure to the patient.				
4	Performed the procedure: • Instructed patient to cover one eye with occluder and hold vision card 14 inches from bridge of nose. • Instructed patient to read the paragraphs on the card. • Noted the acuity measurement number. • Instructed the patient to cover the other eye and read the chart again as before. • Noted the number for the second eye. • Performed the same test with both eyes and noted the number.				
5	Demonstrated professional behavior in manner, organization, and attire, including communicating clearly and comfortably with patient.				
6	Disinfected the occluder, washed hands.				
7	Correctly documented the procedure.				
Student's Total Points					
Points Possible					
Final Score (Student's Total Points/ Possible Points)					

Name _____ **Date** _____ **Score** _____

WORK DOCUMENTATION

_____

Instructor's/Evaluator's Comments and Suggestions:

_____

_____

_____

_____

_____

CHECK #1
Evaluator's Signature: _____ Date: _____

CHECK #2
Evaluator's Signature: _____ Date: _____

CHECK #3
Evaluator's Signature: _____ Date: _____

ABHES Competency: VI.A.1.a.4.h Prepare patient for and assist physician with routine and specialty examinations and treatments and minor office surgeries

Name _____   Date _____   Score _____

COMPETENCY ASSESSMENT

Procedure 30-6   Testing Color Vision Using the Ishihara Plates

Task: To assess a patient's ability to distinguish between the colors red and green.

Conditions: Ishihara color plates

Standards: Perform the Task within 15 minutes with a minimum score of _____ points.

**Work
Documentation:** Patient chart entry

No.	Step	Points	Check #1	Check #2	Check #3
1	Organized supplies and area for testing, ensured good lighting with no glare.				
2	Identified and greeted patient appropriately; washed hands.				
3	Explained the procedure to the patient.				
4	Tested the patient's color vision: • Held each plate 30 inches and directly within the patient's line of vision. • Recorded the number the patient saw on each plate. • Assessed the accuracy and noted the correctly read plates.				
5	Demonstrated professional behavior in manner, organization, and attire, including communicating clearly and comfortably with patient.				
6	Disinfected the occluder, washed hands.				
7	Correctly documented the procedure.				
Student's Total Points					
Points Possible					
Final Score (Student's Total Points/ Possible Points)					

Name _____   **Date** _____   **Score** _____

WORK DOCUMENTATION

Instructor's/Evaluator's Comments and Suggestions:

_____

_____

_____

_____

_____

CHECK #1

Evaluator's Signature: _____   Date:

CHECK #2

Evaluator's Signature: _____   Date:

CHECK #3

Evaluator's Signature: _____   Date:

ABHES Competency: VI.A.1.a.4.h Prepare patient for and assist physician with routine and specialty examinations and treatments and minor office surgeries

Name _____ **Date** _____ **Score** _____

COMPETENCY ASSESSMENT

Procedure 30-7   Performing Eye Instillation

Task: To treat eye infections, soothe irritations, anesthetize the eye, or dilate the pupils.

Conditions: Sterile eye dropper, sterile ophthalmic medication as ordered by the physician, sterile cotton balls, sterile gloves, tissue or gauze

Standards: Perform the Task within 10 minutes with a minimum score of _____ points.

Work
Documentation: Patient chart entry

No.	Step	Points	Check #1	Check #2	Check #3
1	Organized supplies and room. Selected the ordered medication properly, checked order, dose, and expiration date.				
2	Identified and greeted patient appropriately; washed hands.				
3	Set the sterile field.				
4	Checked the medication order carefully again, including the order, the dose, and the expiration date.				
5	Explained the procedure to the patient, including that medication may blur vision temporarily.				
6	Instilled the eye medication: • Positioned the patient properly. • Applied gloves. • Instructed the patient to look up at a fixed spot and exposed the lower conjunctiva by using the gauze. • Applied the amount of medication ordered without touching the applicator to the eye or surrounding area. • Instructed the patient to close the eye and roll the eyeball gently to distribute the medication. • Blotted the excess medication or tears from the skin with tissue without rubbing or wiping the eye.				
7	Disposed of all supplies according to OSHA regulations; removed gloves, washed hands.				

No.	Step	Points	Check #1	Check #2	Check #3
8	Demonstrated professional behavior in manner, organization, and attire, including communicating clearly and comfortably with patient.				
9	Correctly documented the procedure.				
Student's Total Points					
Points Possible					
Final Score (Student's Total Points/ Possible Points)					

Name _____   **Date** _____   **Score** _____

WORK DOCUMENTATION

_____

Instructor's/Evaluator's Comments and Suggestions:

_____

_____

_____

_____

_____

CHECK #1   Evaluator's Signature: Date:

CHECK #2   Evaluator's Signature: Date:

CHECK #3   Evaluator's Signature: Date:

ABHES Competency: VI.A.1.a.4.h Prepare patient for and assist physician with routine and specialty examinations and treatments and minor office surgeries

CAAHEP Curriculum: I.P.10 Assisting physician with patient care

Name _____ Date _____ Score _____

COMPETENCY ASSESSMENT

Procedure 30-8 Performing Eye Patch Dressing Application

Task: To apply a sterile eye patch.

Conditions: Sterile eye patch(es) (some physicians request double layer), tape

Standards: Perform the Task within 10 minutes with a minimum score of _____ points

Work Documentation: Patient chart entry

No.	Step	Points	Check #1	Check #2	Check #3
1	Organized supplies and room.				
2	Identified and greeted patient appropriately; washed hands.				
3	Prepared the patient for procedure: • Explained the procedure. • Determined if patient had a ride home. • Positioned the patient in supine position. • Instructed patient to close both eyes during procedure.				
4	Performed the dressing application: • Opened eye patch using sterile technique. • Applied the eye patch, keeping inside sterile. • Correctly secured patch(es) in place with tape.				
5	Washed hands.				
6	Demonstrated professional behavior in manner, organization, and attire, including communicating clearly and comfortably with patient.				
7	Correctly documented the procedure.				
	Student's Total Points				
	Points Possible				
	Final Score (Student's Total Points/ Possible Points)				

Name _____ **Date** _____ **Score** _____

WORK DOCUMENTATION

_____

Instructor's/Evaluator's Comments and Suggestions:

_____

_____

_____

_____

_____

CHECK #1

Evaluator's Signature: _____ Date: _____

CHECK #2

Evaluator's Signature: _____ Date: _____

CHECK #3

Evaluator's Signature: _____ Date: _____

ABHES Competency: VI.A.1.a.4.h Prepare patient for and assist physician with routine and specialty examinations and treatments and minor office surgeries

CAAHEP Curriculum: I.P.10 Assisting physician with patient care

Name _____   Date _____   Score _____

COMPETENCY ASSESSMENT

Procedure 30-9 Performing Eye Irrigation

Task: To irrigate the patient's eye to remove foreign debris, cleanse discharge, remove chemicals, or apply antiseptic.

Conditions: Sterile irrigation solution as ordered by provider, sterile bulb syringe (rubber), kidney-shaped basin to catch irrigation solution, sterile cotton balls, sterile gloves, biohazard waste container, towel, pillow

Standards: Perform the Task within 15 minutes with a minimum score of _____ points.

**Work
Documentation:** Patient chart entry

No.	Step	Points	Check #1	Check #2	Check #3
1	Organized supplies and room. Selected and prepared the irrigation solution carefully including the amount or dose and expiration date.				
2	Identified and greeted patient appropriately; washed hands.				
3	Prepared the patient for the procedure: • Explained the procedure. • Positioned patient in supine position with towel on shoulder and basin beside affected eye. • Tilted the patient's head toward the affected eye and instructed the patient to stare at a fixed spot during the irrigation.				
4	Checked the solution/medication order carefully again, including the order, amount or dose, and the expiration date.				
5	Performed the irrigation: • Applied sterile gloves. • Correctly cleansed the eyelids and eyelashes of affected eye with cotton balls moistened with irrigation solution, from inner to outer canthus. • Exposed the lower conjunctiva by separating the eyelid with index finger and thumb. • Irrigated the affected eye with sterile solution by resting the bulb on the bridge of the nose. Allowed solution to flow from inner to outer canthus. Did not touch the eye or surrounding area with the tip of the bulb. • After irrigation, dried the eyelid and eyelashes with sterile cotton balls.				

No.	Step	Points	Check #1	Check #2	Check #3
6	Discarded supplies according to OSHA standards; removed gloves and washed hands.				
7	Demonstrated professional behavior in manner, organization, and attire, including communicating clearly and comfortably with patient.				
8	Correctly documented the procedure.				
Student's Total Points					
Points Possible					
Final Score (Student's Total Points/ Possible Points)					

Name _____ **Date** _____ **Score** _____

WORK DOCUMENTATION

_____

Instructor's/Evaluator's Comments and Suggestions:

_____

_____

_____

_____

_____

CHECK #1
Evaluator's Signature: Date:

CHECK #2
Evaluator's Signature: Date:

CHECK #3
Evaluator's Signature: Date:

ABHES Competency: VI.A.1.a.4.h Prepare patient for and assist physician with routine and specialty examinations and treatments and minor office surgeries

CAAHEP Curriculum: I.P.10 Assisting physician with patient care

Name _____ Date _____ Score _____

COMPETENCY ASSESSMENT

Procedure 30-10 Assisting with Audiometry

Task: To assist in testing a patient for hearing loss.

Conditions: Audiometer with headphones, quiet room

Standards: Perform the Task within 20 minutes with a minimum score of _____ points.

Work Documentation: Patient chart entry

No.	Step	Points	Check #1	Check #2	Check #3
1	Organized supplies and area for testing.				
2	Identified and greeted patient appropriately; washed hands.				
3	Prepared the patient for the procedure: • Explained the procedure. • Positioned patient in sitting position. • Instructed patient to put on headphones.				
4	Performed the audiometry test: • Checked one ear first, then the other. • Plotted the graph as the patient indicated a sound was heard.				
5	Gave the results to the provider.				
6	Cleaned and stored equipment properly; washed hands.				
7	Demonstrated professional behavior in manner, organization, and attire, including communicating clearly and comfortably with patient.				
8	Correctly documented the procedure.				
	Student's Total Points				
	Points Possible				
	Final Score (Student's Total Points/ Possible Points)				

Name _____   **Date** _____   **Score** _____

WORK DOCUMENTATION

Instructor's/Evaluator's Comments and Suggestions:

_____

_____

_____

_____

_____

CHECK #1

Evaluator's Signature: _____   Date:

CHECK #2

Evaluator's Signature: _____   Date:

CHECK #3

Evaluator's Signature: _____   Date:

ABHES Competency: VI.A.1.a.4.h Prepare patient for and assist physician with routine and specialty examinations and treatments and minor office surgeries

CAAHEP Curriculum: I.P.10 Assisting physician with patient care

Name _____   **Date** _____   **Score** _____

COMPETENCY ASSESSMENT

Procedure 30-11   Performing Ear Irrigation

Task: To remove impacted cerumen, discharge, or foreign materials from the patient's ear canal as directed by the provider.

Conditions: Irrigation solution as ordered by the provider warmed to 98.6°F to 103°F, ear syringe or bulb or ear irrigation equipment, kidney-shaped basin or ear irrigation basin, larger basin for warmed solution, towel, cotton balls, tissues, otoscope

Standards: Perform the Task within 25 minutes with a minimum score of _____ points.

Work Documentation: Patient chart entry

No.	Step	Points	Check #1	Check #2	Check #3
1	Organized supplies and room. Selected and prepared irrigation solution properly.				
2	Identified and greeted patient appropriately; washed hands.				
3	Prepared the patient for the procedure: • Explained the procedure and that slight discomfort or dizziness may be experienced. • Determined that provider has examined ear. • Positioned patient in sitting position with towel on shoulder and basin against neck. • Cleansed outer ear with moistened cotton ball.				
4	Checked the irrigation solution again for correctness and proper temperature.				
5	Prepared the solution in the syringe.				
6	Performed the irrigation correctly and safely: • Straightened external auditory canal as appropriate for patient's age. • Gently inserted the syringe tip into the ear canal at the appropriate depth. • Directed the flow upward and toward the roof of the canal. • Periodically checked with the patient for discomfort or pain. • Repeated the irrigation until ear canal was clear or solution was finished. • Noted the results by examining the ear with the otoscope. • Dried the outer ear.				

No.	Step	Points	Check #1	Check #2	Check #3
7	Discarded supplies according to OSHA standards; removed gloves and washed hands.				
8	Demonstrated professional behavior in manner, organization, and attire, including communicating clearly and comfortably with patient.				
9	Correctly documented the procedure.				
Student's Total Points					
Points Possible					
Final Score (Student's Total Points/ Possible Points)					

Name _____ Date _____ Score _____

WORK DOCUMENTATION

_____

Instructor's/Evaluator's Comments and Suggestions:

_____

_____

_____

_____

CHECK #1

Evaluator's Signature: Date:

CHECK #2

Evaluator's Signature: Date:

CHECK #3

Evaluator's Signature: Date:

ABHES Competency: VI.A.1.a.4.h Prepare patient for and assist physician with routine and specialty examinations and treatments and minor office surgeries

CAAHEP Curriculum: I.P.10 Assisting physician with patient care

Name _____ Date _____ Score _____

COMPETENCY ASSESSMENT

Procedure 30-12 Performing Ear Instillation

Task: To soften impacted cerumen, treat infection with antibiotics, or relieve pain.

Conditions: Otic medication as prescribed by the provider, sterile ear dropper, cotton balls, gloves

Standards: Perform the Task within 15 minutes with a minimum score of _____ points.

Work Documentation: Patient chart entry

No.	Step	Points	Check #1	Check #2	Check #3
1	Organized supplies and room. Selected medication as ordered and carefully checked dose and expiration date.				
2	Identified and greeted patient appropriately; washed hands.				
3	Prepared the patient for the procedure: • Explained the procedure and that slight discomfort or dizziness may be experienced. • Determined that provider has examined ear. • Positioned patient in sitting position with towel on shoulder and basin against neck.				
4	Checked the medication order again, including the dose and expiration date.				
5	Drew up the prescribed medication.				
6	Performed the irrigation correctly and safely: • Straightened external auditory canal as appropriate for patient's age. • Instilled prescribed dose into the ear. • Instructed patient to maintain position for 5 minutes to retain medication. • When instructed by provider, inserted moistened cotton ball into external canal for 15 minutes.				
7	Discarded supplies according to OSHA standards; removed gloves and washed hands.				

No.	Step	Points	Check #1	Check #2	Check #3
8	Demonstrated professional behavior in manner, organization, and attire, including communicating clearly and comfortably with patient.				
9	Correctly documented the procedure.				
Student's Total Points					
Points Possible					
Final Score (Student's Total Points/ Possible Points)					

Name _____ **Date** _____ **Score** _____

WORK DOCUMENTATION

_____

Instructor's/Evaluator's Comments and Suggestions:

_____

_____

_____

_____

_____

CHECK #1

Evaluator's Signature: _____ Date: _____

CHECK #2

Evaluator's Signature: _____ Date: _____

CHECK #3

Evaluator's Signature: _____ Date: _____

ABHES Competency: VI.A.1.a.4.h Prepare patient for and assist physician with routine and specialty examinations and treatments and minor office surgeries

CAAHEP Curriculum: I.P.10 Assisting physician with patient care

Name _____   Date _____   Score _____

COMPETENCY ASSESSMENT

Procedure 30-13   Assisting with Nasal Examination

Task: To assist the provider with the nasal examination when looking for polyps, engorged superficial blood vessels, and to assist in the possible removal of a foreign object.

Conditions: Nasal speculum, hands-free light source, gloves, kidney basin, bayonet forceps, patient drape

Standards: Perform the Task within 15 minutes with a minimum score of _____ points.

Work Documentation: Patient chart entry

No.	Step	Points	Check #1	Check #2	Check #3
1	Organized supplies and room.				
2	Identified and greeted patient appropriately; washed hands and applied gloves.				
3	Prepared the patient for the procedure: • Explained the procedure. • Positioned patient in a sitting position, slightly reclined (or as directed) with a drape available (in case of bleeding).				
4	Handed provider equipment and supplies as needed.				
5	Discarded supplies according to OSHA standards; removed gloves and washed hands.				
6	Demonstrated professional behavior in manner, organization, and attire, including communicating clearly and comfortably with patient and provider.				
7	Correctly documented the procedure.				
	Student's Total Points				
	Points Possible				
	Final Score (Student's Total Points/ Possible Points)				

Name _____   **Date** _____   **Score** _____

WORK DOCUMENTATION

_____

Instructor's/Evaluator's Comments and Suggestions:

_____

_____

_____

_____

_____

CHECK #1

Evaluator's Signature: _____   Date:

CHECK #2

Evaluator's Signature: _____   Date:

CHECK #3

Evaluator's Signature: _____   Date:

ABHES Competency: VI.A.1.a.4.h Prepare patient for and assist physician with routine and specialty examinations and treatments and minor office surgeries

CAAHEP Curriculum: I.P.10 Assisting physician with patient care

Name _____ **Date** _____ **Score** _____

COMPETENCY ASSESSMENT

Procedure 30-14   Cautery Treatment of Epistaxis

Task: To assist the provider with treatment and control of nose bleeding.

Conditions: Nasal speculum, hands-free light source, gloves, kidney basin, bayonet forceps, silver nitrate applicators, cotton balls, nasal packing material, cotton-tipped applicators, 2 small syringes with large-gauge needles, epinephrine, 2 small medication cups, local anesthetic, antibiotic ointment, other medications as ordered by the provider, patient drape

Standards: Perform the Task within 20 minutes with a minimum score of _____ points.

*Work
Documentation:*   Patient chart entry

No.	Step	Points	Check #1	Check #2	Check #3
1	Organized supplies and room.				
2	Identified and greeted patient appropriately; washed hands and applied gloves.				
3	Prepared the patient for the procedure: • Explained the procedure. • Positioned patient in a sitting position slightly reclined (or as directed) with a drape and basin available.				
4	Prepared the anesthesia as directed by the provider by withdrawing it from the vial and putting it into a medication cup.				
5	Prepared the epinephrine as directed by the provider by withdrawing it from the vial and putting it into a medication cup.				
6	Handed provider equipment and supplies as needed.				
7	Discarded supplies according to OSHA standards; removed gloves and washed hands.				
8	Demonstrated professional behavior in manner, organization, and attire, including communicating clearly and comfortably with patient and provider.				
9	Correctly documented the procedure.				
Student's Total Points					
Points Possible					
Final Score (Student's Total Points/ Possible Points)					

Name _____   Date _____   Score _____

WORK DOCUMENTATION

Instructor's/Evaluator's Comments and Suggestions:

_____

_____

_____

_____

_____

CHECK #1

Evaluator's Signature: _____   Date:

CHECK #2

Evaluator's Signature: _____   Date:

CHECK #3

Evaluator's Signature: _____   Date:

ABHES Competency: VI.A.1.a.4.h Prepare patient for and assist physician with routine and specialty examinations and treatments and minor office surgeries

CAAHEP Curriculum: I.P.10 Assisting physician with patient care

Name _____ **Date** _____ **Score** _____

COMPETENCY ASSESSMENT

Procedure 30-15   Performing Nasal Instillation

Task: To provide medication to the nasal tissues as ordered by the provider.

Conditions: Medication as ordered, sterile medicine dropper, tissues

Standards: Perform the Task within 15 minutes with a minimum score of _____ points.

Work Documentation: Patient chart entry

No.	Step	Points	Check #1	Check #2	Check #3
1	Organized supplies and room. Selected proper medication as ordered and carefully checked dose and expiration date.				
2	Identified and greeted patient appropriately; washed hands and applied gloves.				
3	Prepared the patient for the procedure: • Explained the procedure. • Positioned patient in supine position with head slightly lowered, or sitting with head tilted back. • Helped patient adjust for comfort.				
4	Checked the medication order carefully again including the dose and expiration date.				
5	Instilled the medication properly: • Drew medication into the dropper. • Applied the medication to the affected nostril or both nostrils as directed. • Did not touch the dropper to the nostril. • Handled medication using sterile technique. • Instructed patient to remain in position for 5 minutes. • Handed tissues to patient when head was tilted back or when patient sat up.				
6	Discarded supplies according to OSHA standards; removed gloves and washed hands.				
7	Demonstrated professional behavior in manner, organization, and attire, including communicating clearly and comfortably with patient and provider.				
8	Correctly documented the procedure.				
Student's Total Points					
Points Possible					
Final Score (Student's Total Points/ Possible Points)					

Name _____ **Date** _____ **Score** _____

WORK DOCUMENTATION

_____

Instructor's/Evaluator's Comments and Suggestions:

_____

_____

_____

_____

_____

CHECK #1

Evaluator's Signature: _____   Date: _____

CHECK #2

Evaluator's Signature: _____   Date: _____

CHECK #3

Evaluator's Signature: _____   Date: _____

ABHES Competency: VI.A.1.a.4.h Prepare patient for and assist physician with routine and specialty examinations and treatments and minor office surgeries

CAAHEP Curriculum: I.P.10 Assisting physician with patient care

Name _____   Date _____   Score _____

COMPETENCY ASSESSMENT

Procedure 30-16   Administer Oxygen by Nasal Cannula for Minor Respiratory Distress

Task: To provide a low dose of concentrated oxygen to a patient during periods of respiratory distress.

Conditions: Portable oxygen tank with stand, disposable nasal cannula with connecting tube, flow meter, and pressure regulator

Standards: Perform the Task within 15 minutes with a minimum score of _____ points.

Work Documentation: Patient chart entry

No.	Step	Points	Check #1	Check #2	Check #3
1	Organized supplies and room.				
2	Identified and greeted patient appropriately; washed hands and applied gloves.				
3	Explained procedure to the patient.				
4	Prepared the oxygen equipment properly: • Opened the cylinder one full turn counterclockwise. • Checked the pressure gauge to be sure oxygen was available and flowing. • Attached the nasal cannula to the tubing and then to the flow meter. • Adjusted the flow rate according to the provider's orders. • Placed the tips in the patient's nostrils properly, adjusted around the patient's ears, and secured it under the chin.				
5	Cautioned the patient about safety around oxygen use, answered questions.				
6	Discarded supplies according to OSHA standards; removed gloves and washed hands.				
7	Demonstrated professional behavior in manner, organization, and attire, including communicating clearly and comfortably with patient and provider.				
8	Correctly documented the procedure.				
Student's Total Points					
Points Possible					
Final Score (Student's Total Points/ Possible Points)					

Name _____   **Date** _____   **Score** _____

WORK DOCUMENTATION

_____

Instructor's/Evaluator's Comments and Suggestions:

_____

_____

_____

_____

_____

CHECK #1	
Evaluator's Signature:	Date:

CHECK #2	
Evaluator's Signature:	Date:

CHECK #3	
Evaluator's Signature:	Date:

ABHES Competency: VI.A.1.a.4.h Prepare patient for and assist physician with routine and specialty examinations and treatments and minor office surgeries

CAAHEP Curriculum: I.P.10 Assisting physician with patient care

Name _____ Date _____ Score _____

COMPETENCY ASSESSMENT

Procedure 30-17   Instructing Patient in Use of Metered Dose Inhaler

Task: To instruct the patient in the correct use of a handheld metered dose inhaler.

Conditions: Handheld nebulizer containing medication ordered by the provider

Standards: Perform the Task within 20 minutes with a minimum score of _____ points.

Work Documentation: Patient chart entry

No.	Step	Points	Check #1	Check #2	Check #3
1	Organized supplies and room.				
2	Identified and greeted patient appropriately; washed hands.				
3	Checked medication order three times.				
4	Demonstrated the procedure to the patient, and asked the patient to repeat the demonstration.				
5	Administered the medication: • Instructed patient to sit upright and exhale fully. • Instructed patient to remove cap and shake MDI well. • Helped patient hold nebulizer to mouth, closing the lips and teeth around the mouthpiece. • Instructed patient to tilt head back and take a deep breath while pushing medication container against the mouthpiece. • Instructed patient to continue to inhale deeply until the lungs were full. • Had patient remove the mouthpiece and hold breath for 10 seconds. • Waited one minute and repeated the process (if the provider ordered more than one treatment). • Replaced cap. • If the MDI contained a steroid, instructed patient to rinse mouth well and gargle. • Checked patient for adverse reaction.				

No.	Step	Points	Check #1	Check #2	Check #3
6	Demonstrated professional behavior in manner, organization, and attire, including: • Communicated appropriately and comfortably with the patient				
7	Cleaned/disposed of supplies and equipment appropriately and washed hands.				
8	Documented correctly.				
Student's Total Points					
Points Possible					
Final Score (Student's Total Points/ Possible Points)					

Name _____ **Date** _____ **Score** _____

WORK DOCUMENTATION

_____

Instructor's/Evaluator's Comments and Suggestions:

_____

_____

_____

_____

_____

CHECK #1	
Evaluator's Signature:	Date:

CHECK #2	
Evaluator's Signature:	Date:

CHECK #3	
Evaluator's Signature:	Date:

ABHES Competency: VI.A.1.a.4.h Prepare patient for and assist physician with routine and specialty examinations and treatments and minor office surgeries

CAAHEP Curriculum: I.P.10 Assisting physician with patient care

Name _____ **Date** _____ **Score** _____

COMPETENCY ASSESSMENT

Procedure 30-18   Spirometry

Task: To test a patient's respiratory function.

Conditions: Spirometer, disposable mouthpiece

Standards: Perform the Task within 20 minutes with a minimum score of _____ points.

Work
Documentation: Patient chart entry

No.	Step	Points	Check #1	Check #2	Check #3
1	Organized supplies and area for testing.				
2	Identified and greeted patient appropriately; washed hands.				
3	Prepared the patient and performed the test: • Explained the procedure. • Placed the patient in a comfortable position with instruction to loosen collar if appropriate. • Instructed the patient to not lean forward when blowing into the machine. • Reinforced the inhalation process. • Instructed the patient to continue blowing into the mouthpiece until instructed to stop or patient could not blow any longer. • Was supportive and encouraging throughout the test.				
4	Showed the results to the provider.				
5	Demonstrated professional behavior in manner, organization, and attire, including: • Communicated appropriately and comfortably with the patient.				
6	Cleaned/disposed of supplies and equipment appropriately and washed hands.				
7	Documented correctly.				
Student's Total Points					
Points Possible					
Final Score (Student's Total Points/ Possible Points)					

Name _____   **Date** _____   **Score** _____

WORK DOCUMENTATION

_____

Instructor's/Evaluator's Comments and Suggestions:

_____

_____

_____

_____

_____

CHECK #1 Evaluator's Signature: Date:

CHECK #2 Evaluator's Signature: Date:

CHECK #3 Evaluator's Signature: Date:

ABHES Competency: VI.A.1.a.4.ee Perform respiratory testing

CAAHEP Curriculum: I.P.10 Assisting physician with patient care

Name _____ Date _____ Score _____

COMPETENCY ASSESSMENT

Procedure 30-19   Pulse Oximetry

Task: To measure arterial oxyhemoglobin saturation within seconds by using an external sensor.

Conditions: Pulse oximeter, sensor, soap and water, alcohol wipes, nail polish remover (as needed)

Standards: Perform the Task within 20 minutes with a minimum score of _____ points.

Work
Documentation: Patient chart entry

No.	Step	Points	Check #1	Check #2	Check #3
1	Organized supplies and area for testing.				
2	Identified and greeted patient appropriately; washed hands.				
3	Prepared the patient for the test: • Explained the procedure to the patient. • Selected a site for the sensor, cleaned the site with alcohol (removed nail polish if needed).				
4	Performed the test: • Applied sensor, connected sensor to oximeter. • Turned sensor on and adjusted volume. • Set alarm for abnormal readings. • Checked pulse manually and compared with oximeter, noting results for quality control. • Notified provider of any abnormal results.				
5	Demonstrated professional behavior in manner, organization, and attire, including: • Communicated appropriately and comfortably with the patient.				
6	Cleaned/disposed of supplies and equipment appropriately and washed hands.				
7	Documented correctly.				
	Student's Total Points				
	Points Possible				
	Final Score (Student's Total Points/ Possible Points)				

Name _____ **Date** _____ **Score** _____

WORK DOCUMENTATION

Instructor's/Evaluator's Comments and Suggestions:

_____

_____

_____

_____

_____

CHECK #1

Evaluator's Signature: _____ **Date:**

CHECK #2

Evaluator's Signature: _____ **Date:**

CHECK #3

Evaluator's Signature: _____ **Date:**

ABHES Competency: VI.A.1.a.4.h Prepare patient for and assist physician with routine and specialty examinations and treatments and minor office surgeries

CAAHEP Curriculum: I.P.10 Assisting physician with patient care; I.P.11 Perform quality control measures

Name _____ Date _____ Score _____

COMPETENCY ASSESSMENT

Procedure 30-20   Assisting with Plaster Cast Application

Task: To assist with cast application.

Conditions: Plaster bandage rolls or synthetic cast rolls (for small arm cast, use two to three 2- or 3-inch rolls. For short leg cast, use two to three 3- to 4-inch rolls. For long leg cast, use three to four 4- to 6-inch rolls), container of warm water that is lined with plastic or cloth to catch loose plaster, stockinette (3-inch width for arms, 4- to 6-inch width for legs, etc.), Webril padding rolls, bandage scissors, gloves, walking heel if needed, lotion if using synthetic casting

Standards: Perform the Task within 25 minutes with a minimum score of _____ points.

Work Documentation: Patient chart entry

No.	Step	Points	Check #1	Check #2	Check #3
1	Organized supplies and room.				
2	Identified and greeted patient appropriately; washed hands.				
3	Correctly prepared the patient: • Explained the procedure to the patient. • Properly positioned patient for cast being applied. • Carefully cleaned and dried area to be casted. • Noted open wounds and reported these to the provider.				
4	Correctly assisted the provider: • Prepared stockinette appropriate for the area being casted. • Prepared Webril appropriate for the area being casted. • Assisted provider and patient during the procedure.				
5	After cast application, cleaned patient's skin and provided oral and written instructions to the patient.				
6	Demonstrated professional behavior in manner, organization, and attire, including: • Communicated appropriately and comfortably with the patient and provider.				

No.	Step	Points	Check #1	Check #2	Check #3
7	Cleaned/disposed of supplies and equipment appropriately and washed hands.				
8	Documented correctly.				
Student's Total Points					
Points Possible					
Final Score (Student's Total Points/ Possible Points)					

Name _____   **Date** _____   **Score** _____

WORK DOCUMENTATION

_____

Instructor's/Evaluator's Comments and Suggestions:

_____

_____

_____

_____

_____

CHECK #1

Evaluator's Signature: _____   Date:

CHECK #2

Evaluator's Signature: _____   Date:

CHECK #3

Evaluator's Signature: _____   Date:

ABHES Competency: VI.A.1.a.4.h Prepare patient for and assist physician with routine and specialty examinations and treatments and minor office surgeries

CAAHEP Curriculum: I.P.10 Assisting physician with patient care

Name _____ Date _____ Score _____

COMPETENCY ASSESSMENT

Procedure 30-21   Assisting with Cast Removal

Task: To assist with cast removal.

Conditions: Cast removal saw, cast spreader, cast scissors, patient drape

Standards: Perform the Task within 20 minutes with a minimum score of _____ points.

*Work
Documentation:* Patient chart entry

No.	Step	Points	Check #1	Check #2	Check #3
1	Organized supplies and area.				
2	Identified and greeted patient appropriately; washed hands.				
3	Correctly prepared the patient: • Explained the procedure to the patient. • Reassured the patient. • Properly positioned patient for cast being removed.				
4	Removed the cast properly or assisted the provider as needed. Handed provider equipment as requested.				
5	After cast removal, helped clean patient's skin and provided oral and written instructions to the patient.				
6	Demonstrated professional behavior in manner, organization, and attire, including: • Communicated appropriately and comfortably with the patient and provider.				
7	Cleaned/disposed of supplies and equipment appropriately and washed hands.				
8	Documented correctly.				
Student's Total Points					
Points Possible					
Final Score (Student's Total Points/ Possible Points)					

Name _____   **Date** _____   **Score** _____

WORK DOCUMENTATION

_____

Instructor's/Evaluator's Comments and Suggestions:

_____

_____

_____

_____

_____

CHECK #1	
Evaluator's Signature:	Date:

CHECK #2	
Evaluator's Signature:	Date:

CHECK #3	
Evaluator's Signature:	Date:

ABHES Competency: VI.A.1.a.4.h Prepare patient for and assist physician with routine and specialty examinations and treatments and minor office surgeries

CAAHEP Curriculum: I.P.10 Assisting physician with patient care

Name _____   Date _____   Score _____

COMPETENCY ASSESSMENT

Procedure 30-22   Assisting the Physician during a Lumbar Puncture or Cerebrospinal Fluid Aspiration

Task: To position the patient and assist with removal of cerebrospinal fluid (CSF).

Conditions: Patient drape; Xylocaine 1–2%; syringe and needle for anesthetic; sterile gloves; disposable sterile lumbar puncture tray to include: skin antiseptic with applicator, adhesive bandage, spinal puncture needle, three to four test tubes with secure tops, laboratory requisition, specimen transport bag, patient gown and drape, manometer, laboratory requisition, examination light, gauze sponges

Standards: Perform the Task within 30 minutes with a minimum score of _____ points.

Work Documentation: Patient chart entry, laboratory requisition

No.	Step	Points	Check #1	Check #2	Check #3
1	Organized supplies and area for procedure.				
2	Identified and greeted patient appropriately; washed hands.				
3	Correctly prepared the patient: • Explained the procedure to the patient. • Instructed patient to empty bladder, bowel. • Verified that the patient signed a consent form. • Instructed patient to undress and gown; covered patient with additional drape. • Positioned patient on edge of table. • Applied gloves and cleansed puncture site. • Positioned patient in fetal position.				
4	Assisted the provider and patient during the procedure as needed: • Assisted the provider to aspirate anesthetic. • Helped the patient maintain position until needle was inserted into spinal canal. • Reminded patient to breathe evenly. • At the provider's direction, instructed patient to straighten the legs. • Assisted the physician in collecting CSF as needed. • When the puncture was completed, assisted the provider in applying dressing to the puncture site.				

No.	Step	Points	Check #1	Check #2	Check #3
5	Repositioned the patient into prone position for 2–3 hours, and had the patient drink fluids as directed.				
6	Applied gloves and labeled the specimens, put into transfer bag, and completed lab requisition.				
7	Demonstrated professional behavior in manner, organization, and attire, including: • Communicated appropriately and comfortably with the patient and provider.				
8	Cleaned/disposed of supplies and equipment appropriately and washed hands.				
9	Documented correctly.				
Student's Total Points					
Points Possible					
Final Score (Student's Total Points/ Possible Points)					

Name _____ **Date** _____ **Score** _____

WORK DOCUMENTATION

_____

Instructor's/Evaluator's Comments and Suggestions:

_____

_____

_____

_____

_____

CHECK #1   Evaluator's Signature: Date:

CHECK #2   Evaluator's Signature: Date:

CHECK #3   Evaluator's Signature: Date:

ABHES Competency: VI.A.1.a.4.h Prepare patient for and assist physician with routine and specialty examinations and treatments and minor office surgeries

CAAHEP Curriculum: I.P.10 Assisting physician with patient care

Name _____   **Date** _____   **Score** _____

COMPETENCY ASSESSMENT

Procedure 30-23   Assisting the Provider with a Neurologic Screening Examination

Task: To determine a patient's neurologic status.

Conditions: Percussion hammer, safety pin or sensory wheel, material for odor identification, cotton ball, tuning fork, flashlight, tongue blade, ophthalmoscope

Standards: Perform the Task within 20 minutes with a minimum score of _____ points.

Work Documentation: Patient chart entry

No.	Step	Points	Check #1	Check #2	Check #3
1	Organized supplies and area for procedure.				
2	Identified and greeted patient appropriately; washed hands.				
3	While taking patient's medical history, observed level of awareness, memory, cognition, and mood.				
4	Assisted the provider as needed during examination.				
5	Demonstrated professional behavior in manner, organization, and attire, including: • Communicated appropriately and comfortably with the patient and provider.				
6	Cleaned/disposed of supplies and equipment appropriately and washed hands.				
7	Documented correctly.				
Student's Total Points					
Points Possible					
Final Score (Student's Total Points/ Possible Points)					

Name _____   **Date** _____   **Score** _____

WORK DOCUMENTATION

_____

Instructor's/Evaluator's Comments and Suggestions:

_____

_____

_____

_____

_____

CHECK #1

Evaluator's Signature: _____   Date:

CHECK #2

Evaluator's Signature: _____   Date:

CHECK #3

Evaluator's Signature: _____   Date:

ABHES Competency: VI.A.1.a.4.h Prepare patient for and assist physician with routine and specialty examinations and treatments and minor office surgeries

CAAHEP Curriculum: I.P.10 Assisting physician with patient care

Name _____   **Date** _____   **Score** _____

COMPETENCY ASSESSMENT

Procedure 31-1   Applying Sterile Gloves

Task: Applying sterile gloves.

Conditions: Packaged pair of sterile gloves of appropriate size and a flat, clean, dry surface

Standards: Perform the Task within 10 minutes with a minimum score of _____ points.

No.	Step	Points	Check #1	Check #2	Check #3
1	Removed ring(s) and watch and washed hands.				
2	Selected proper glove size and type, inspected package, and placed on a clean, dry, flat surface above waist level.				
3	Opened package properly: • Peeled open outer package. • Positioned inner package properly. • Opened inner package with care not to contaminate. • Determined that gloves were in position or adjusted.				
4	Applied both gloves properly without contamination.				
Student's Total Points					
Points Possible					
Final Score (Student's Total Points/ Possible Points)					

Name _____ **Date** _____ **Score** _____

Instructor's/Evaluator's Comments and Suggestions:

_____

_____

_____

_____

_____

CHECK #1

Evaluator's Signature: Date:

CHECK #2

Evaluator's Signature: Date:

CHECK #3

Evaluator's Signature: Date:

ABHES Competency: VI.A.1.a.4.c Apply principles of aseptic techniques and infection control

CAAHEP Curriculum: III.P.3 Select appropriate barrier/personal protective equipment (PPE) for potentially infectious situations

Name _____ Date _____ Score _____

COMPETENCY ASSESSMENT

Procedure 31-2   Chemical "Cold" Sterilization of Endoscopes

Task:　　　　To sterilize heat-sensitive items such as fiber-optic endoscopes, using chemical solution.

Conditions:　Chemical solution, timer, sterile water, airtight container, heavy-duty gloves, sterile towels, poly-lined sterile drapes

Standards:　Perform the Task within 30 minutes with a minimum score of _____ points.

No.	Step	Points	Check #1	Check #2	Check #3
1	Sanitized and dried instrument/scope following manufacturer's instructions.				
2	Read manufacturer's instructions regarding use of sterilizing chemicals.				
3	Applied PPE.				
4	Prepared solution according to instructions. Recorded the solution and ratio. Poured solution into container with a tight-fitting lid.				
5	Placed scope into the solution, closed lid, timed properly.				
6	When time was up, prepared sterile field, applied PPE and sterile gloves, removed endoscope from solution, rinsed and applied to sterile tray without contaminating.				
Student's Total Points					
Points Possible					
Final Score (Student's Total Points/ Possible Points)					

Name _____ **Date** _____ **Score** _____

Instructor's/Evaluator's Comments and Suggestions:

_____

_____

_____

_____

_____

CHECK #1

Evaluator's Signature: _____ Date:

CHECK #2

Evaluator's Signature: _____ Date:

CHECK #3

Evaluator's Signature: _____ Date:

ABHES Competency: VI.A.1.a.4.p Perform sterilization techniques

CAAHEP Curriculum: III.P.3 Select appropriate barrier/personal protective equipment (PPE) for potentially infectious situations; III.P.6 Perform sterilization procedures

Name _____ **Date** _____ **Score** _____

COMPETENCY ASSESSMENT

Procedure 31-3 Preparing Instruments for Sterilization in Autoclave

Task: To properly wrap sanitized instruments for sterilization in an autoclave.

Conditions: Sanitized instruments, wrapping materials (muslin, disposable wrapping paper), sterilization indicators, 2 × 2 gauze (if instrument has hinges), autoclave wrapping tape, tip protectors as indicated, marking pen for labeling

Standards: Perform the Task within 10 minutes with a minimum score of _____ points.

No.	Step	Points	Check #1	Check #2	Check #3
1	Washed hands. Prepared a clean, dry, flat surface of adequate size to lay the wrapping material on.				
2	Selected appropriate size and type of wrap.				
3	Wrapped first layer properly so it was snug and neat. Included sterilization indicator, tip protectors, and gauze as appropriate.				
4	Wrapped second layer properly so it was snug and neat.				
5	Taped package closed and labeled properly.				
Student's Total Points					
Points Possible					
Final Score (Student's Total Points/ Possible Points)					

Name _____ **Date** _____ **Score** _____

Instructor's/Evaluator's Comments and Suggestions:

_____

_____

_____

_____

_____

CHECK #1

Evaluator's Signature: _____ Date:

CHECK #2

Evaluator's Signature: _____ Date:

CHECK #3

Evaluator's Signature: _____ Date:

ABHES Competency: VI.A.1.a.4.o Wrap items for autoclaving

CAAHEP Curriculum: III.P.5 Prepare items for autoclaving

Name _____   **Date** _____   **Score** _____

COMPETENCY ASSESSMENT

Procedure 31-4   Sterilization of Instruments (Autoclave)

Task: To rid instruments of all forms of microbial (microorganism) life for use in invasive procedures.

Conditions: Steam sterilizer (autoclave), autoclave manufacturer procedure manual, wrapped sanitized instrument package(s) with sterilization indicators placed inside the package (or unwrapped item, if removed with sterile transfer forceps)

Standards: Perform the Task within 45 minutes with a minimum score of _____ points.

No.	Step	Points	Check #1	Check #2	Check #3
1	Washed hands. Checked water level in autoclave, and added distilled water, if necessary.				
2	Loaded packages into autoclave properly.				
3	Sealed door, turned on autoclave, and set proper time.				
4	When cycle completed, turned off autoclave and allowed instruments to cool before removing.				
5	When cooled, removed wrapped contents with dry, clean hands and stored in clean, dry, closed storage area.				
6	Removed unwrapped contents with sterile transfer forceps.				
Student's Total Points					
Points Possible					
Final Score (Student's Total Points/ Possible Points)					

Name _____   **Date** _____   **Score** _____

Instructor's/Evaluator's Comments and Suggestions:

_____

_____

_____

_____

_____

CHECK #1	
Evaluator's Signature:	Date:

CHECK #2	
Evaluator's Signature:	Date:

CHECK #3	
Evaluator's Signature:	Date:

ABHES Competency: VI.A.1.a.4.p Perform sterilization techniques

CAAHEP Curriculum: III.P.6 Perform sterilization procedures

Name _____ **Date** _____ **Score** _____

COMPETENCY ASSESSMENT

Procedure 31-5   Setting Up and Covering a Sterile Field

Task: To lay a sterile field onto a Mayo tray suitable for surgery or a sterile procedure, and to cover the sterile tray with another sterile drape.

Conditions: Disposable sterile poly-lined field drapes or sterile towels (two), Mayo instrument tray/stand positioned above the waist with stem to the right, at right angle to the counter

Standards: Perform the Task within 15 minutes with a minimum score of _____ points.

No.	Step	Points	Check #1	Check #2	Check #3
1	Washed hands.				
2	Sanitized and disinfected a Mayo instrument tray. Positioned tray above waist level with the stem to the right.				
3	Set up sterile field onto tray without contaminating it.				
4	Applied instruments and supplies properly without contamination, was able to problem-solve as needed.				
5	Covered tray using proper sterile technique.				
Student's Total Points					
Points Possible					
Final Score (Student's Total Points/ Possible Points)					

Name _____   **Date** _____   **Score** _____

Instructor's/Evaluator's Comments and Suggestions:

_____

_____

_____

_____

_____

CHECK #1

Evaluator's Signature: _____   Date:

CHECK #2

Evaluator's Signature: _____   Date:

CHECK #3

Evaluator's Signature: _____   Date:

ABHES Competency: VI.A.1.a.4.g Prepare and maintain examination and treatment area

Name _____ Date _____ Score _____

COMPETENCY ASSESSMENT

Procedure 31-6   Opening Sterile Packages of Instruments and Supplies and Applying Them to a Sterile Field

Task: To open sterile packages of surgical instruments and supplies and place them onto a sterile field using sterile technique.

Conditions: Mayo instrument tray draped with a sterile field, sterile gloves, wrapped-twice sterile surgical instruments, prepackaged sterile surgical supplies

Standards: Perform the Task within 20 minutes with a minimum score of _____ points.

No.	Step	Points	Check #1	Check #2	Check #3
1	Washed hands and assembled supplies.				
2	Set up sterile tray correctly.				
3	Properly opened packages without contaminating contents.				
4	Transferred sterile instruments and supplies to sterile tray using sterile technique.				
5	Applied sterile gloves and arranged instruments and supplies on the tray in an organized and logical manner according to the provider's preference.				
6	Applied the sterile cover (as described in Procedure 31-5).				
Student's Total Points					
Points Possible					
Final Score (Student's Total Points/ Possible Points)					

Name _____ **Date** _____ **Score** _____

Instructor's/Evaluator's Comments and Suggestions:

_____

_____

_____

_____

_____

CHECK #1

Evaluator's Signature: _____ Date:

CHECK #2

Evaluator's Signature: _____ Date:

CHECK #3

Evaluator's Signature: _____ Date:

ABHES Competency: VI.A.1.a.4.g Prepare and maintain examination and treatment area

Name _____   Date _____   Score _____

COMPETENCY ASSESSMENT

Procedure 31-7   Pouring a Sterile Solution into a Cup on a Sterile Field

Task: To pour a sterile solution into a cup on a sterile tray in a sterile manner.

Conditions: Covered sterile surgical tray with a sterile cup in upper right corner, container of sterile scrub solution (as ordered)

Standards: Perform the Task within 5 minutes with a minimum score of _____ points.

No.	Step	Points	Check #1	Check #2	Check #3
1	Washed hands.				
2	Selected the appropriate solution, read the label of the solution container two times, and checked expiration date.				
3	Transported the covered surgical tray to the surgical area before pouring solution.				
4	Read the label again just before pouring to ensure accuracy. Palmed the label and handled the cap properly.				
5	Exposed the cup and poured the solution without splashing or contaminating the sterile field.				
Student's Total Points					
Points Possible					
Final Score (Student's Total Points/ Possible Points)					

Name _____ **Date** _____ **Score** _____

Instructor's/Evaluator's Comments and Suggestions:

_____

_____

_____

_____

_____

CHECK #1

Evaluator's Signature: _____ Date:

CHECK #2

Evaluator's Signature: _____ Date:

CHECK #3

Evaluator's Signature: _____ Date:

ABHES Competency: VI.A.1.a.4.g Prepare and maintain examination and treatment area

Name _____   Date _____   Score _____

COMPETENCY ASSESSMENT

Procedure 31-8   Assisting with Office/Ambulatory Surgery

Task: To maintain sterility while assisting with office surgery.

Conditions: *On Mayo stand:* sterile field and cover drapes (two), gauze sponges, scalpel (handle and blade), operating scissors, thumb forceps, hemostats (curved and straight), dressing forceps, suture pack, needle holder, skin retractor, transfer forceps. *May be on sterile field or on the side (provider preference):* fenestrated drape, needles and syringe for anesthesia, prep bowl/cup, Betadine® solution. *On counter or side table:* sterile gloves in package, labeled biopsy containers with formalin, laboratory requisition, anesthesia vial, alcohol wipes, dressings, tape, bandages, biohazard container, extra gauze in sterile package

Standards: Perform the Task within 30 minutes with a minimum score of _____ points.

Work
Documentation: Laboratory requisition (if appropriate)

No.	Step	Points	Check #1	Check #2	Check #3
1	Checked room for equipment, readiness, cleanliness, and washed hands.				
2	Set up side table or counter for nonsterile items.				
3	Performed surgical asepsis hand washing and applied appropriate PPE.				
4	Set up sterile surgical tray.				
5	Prepared the patient: • Greeted and identified patient, introduced self, and explained the procedure. • Checked for signed informed consent form. • Identified health concerns, allergies, tetanus status, possible complications, and current medications. • Positioned and prepped the patient.				
6	Assisted the physician and patient as needed.				
7	Prepared lab specimens and requisitions as needed.				
8	Demonstrated professional behavior in manner, organization, and attire, including: • Communicatied appropriately and comfortably with the patient and provider.				

No.	Step	Points	Check #1	Check #2	Check #3
9	Cleaned/disposed of supplies and equipment appropriately and washed hands.				
	Student's Total Points				
	Points Possible				
	Final Score (Student's Total Points/ Possible Points)				

Name _____   **Date** _____   **Score** _____

WORK DOCUMENTATION

*Also attach lab requisition.

Instructor's/Evaluator's Comments and Suggestions:

_____

_____

_____

_____

_____

CHECK #1	
Evaluator's Signature:	Date:

CHECK #2	
Evaluator's Signature:	Date:

CHECK #3	
Evaluator's Signature:	Date:

ABHES Competency: VI.A.1.a.4.g Prepare and maintain examination and treatment area; VI.A.1.a.4.h Prepare patient for and assist physician with routine and specialty examinations and treatments and minor office surgeries

CAAHEP Curriculum: I.P.10 Assist physician with patient care; III.P.4 Select appropriate barrier/personal protective equipment (PPE) for potentially infectious situations

Name _____ **Date** _____ **Score** _____

COMPETENCY ASSESSMENT

Procedure 31-9   Dressing Change

Task: To remove a wound dressing, clean the wound, and apply a dry, sterile dressing.

Conditions: *On the sterile field:* several sterile gauze sponges and other dressing material as needed, sterile bowl/cup with Betadine® solution or prepared sterile Betadine swab sticks, sterile dressing forceps, sterile sponge forceps. *On counter side area:* nonsterile gloves, sterile gloves in package, container of sterile water, sterile cotton-tipped applicators in package, sterile adhesive strips, antibacterial ointment/cream as ordered, tape, sponge forceps, bandage scissors, waterproof waste bag, biohazard waste container

Standards: Perform the Task within 20 minutes with a minimum score of _____ points.

**Work
Documentation:** Patient chart entry

No.	Step	Points	Check #1	Check #2	Check #3
1	Checked provider's orders and washed hands.				
2	Prepared the supplies and room: • Prepared sterile field, added supplies using sterile technique. • Positioned a waterproof bag and biohazard container away from the sterile area. • Prepared Betadine® solution into sterile bowl or used swab sticks.				
3	Greeted and identified the patient, introduced self, and explained the procedure.				
4	Correctly removed old bandage and cleaned the wound: • Applied gloves. • Removed dressing and/or bandage, placing into biohazard container. • Assessed wound and noted any drainage or signs of infection. • Cleaned the wound with antiseptic solution as ordered. • Applied topical medication as ordered.				
5	Correctly applied sterile dressing: • Removed gloves, washed hands, applied sterile gloves. • Applied sterile dressing and bandaging as appropriate. • Disposed of contaminated supplies properly, washed hands.				

No.	Step	Points	Check #1	Check #2	Check #3
6	Demonstrated professional behavior in manner, organization, and attire, including: • Communicated appropriately and comfortably with the patient.				
7	Cleaned/disposed of supplies and equipment appropriately and washed hands.				
8	Correctly documented the procedure.				
Student's Total Points					
Points Possible					
Final Score (Student's Total Points/ Possible Points)					

Name _____ **Date** _____ **Score** _____

WORK DOCUMENTATION

_____

Instructor's/Evaluator's Comments and Suggestions:

_____
_____
_____
_____

CHECK #1	
Evaluator's Signature:	Date:

CHECK #2	
Evaluator's Signature:	Date:

CHECK #3	
Evaluator's Signature:	Date:

ABHES Competency: VI.A.1.a.4.h Prepare patient for and assist physician with routine and specialty examinations and treatments and minor office surgeries

CAAHEP Curriculum: I.P.10 Assist physician with patient care; III.P.4 Select appropriate barrier/personal protective equipment (PPE) for potentially infectious situations

Name _____ **Date** _____ **Score** _____

COMPETENCY ASSESSMENT

Procedure 31-10   Wound Irrigation

Task: To irrigate a wound to remove the accumulation of excessive exudates, which impair and delay healing.

Conditions: Sterile gloves, sterile irrigation kit, sterile dressing material, waterproof pad, sterile solution (according to doctor's orders), nonsterile gloves, waterproof waste bag

Standards: Perform the Task within 20 minutes with a minimum score of _____ points.

Work
Documentation: Patient chart entry

No.	Step	Points	Check #1	Check #2	Check #3
1	Checked provider's order. Selected the appropriate solution, verifying expiration date.				
2	Greeted and identified the patient, introduced self. Explained the procedure.				
3	Washed hands.				
4	Removed old dressing properly: • Applied nonsterile gloves, removed the dressing, and disposed of it into waterproof waste bag. • Noted the wound's appearance, color, amount of discharge, and odor of discharge. • Removed and discarded gloves into biohazard container and washed hands, applied sterile gloves.				
5	Irrigated the wound properly: • Checked the irrigation solution order again, verifying amount and expiration date. • Maintained sterile technique. • Prepared the irrigation supplies. • Irrigated the wound. • Dried with sterile gauze. • Applied sterile dressing and bandage as appropriate.				
6	Demonstrated professional behavior in manner, organization, and attire, including: • Communicated appropriately and comfortably with the patient.				
7	Cleaned/disposed of supplies and equipment appropriately and washed hands.				
8	Correctly documented the procedure.				
Student's Total Points					
Points Possible					
Final Score (Student's Total Points/ Possible Points)					

Name _____   **Date** _____   **Score** _____

WORK DOCUMENTATION

_____

Instructor's/Evaluator's Comments and Suggestions:

_____

_____

_____

_____

_____

CHECK #1

Evaluator's Signature: _____   Date:

CHECK #2

Evaluator's Signature: _____   Date:

CHECK #3

Evaluator's Signature: _____   Date:

ABHES Competency: VI.A.1.a.4.h Prepare patient for and assist physician with routine and specialty examinations and treatments and minor office surgeries

CAAHEP Curriculum: I.P.10 Assist physician with patient care; III.P.4 Select appropriate barrier/personal protective equipment (PPE) for potentially infectious situations

Name _____   Date _____   Score _____

COMPETENCY ASSESSMENT

Procedure 31-11   Preparation of Patient's Skin before Surgery

Task: To remove as many microorganisms as possible from the patient's skin before surgery.

Conditions: Absorbent pad, sterile drapes (two), one fenestrated drape if doctor prefers, disposable skin prep kit (includes antiseptic soap, several sponges, razor, and a container for water), sterile water, antiseptic solution (as ordered), sterile bowl, sterile gloves (two pair)

Standards: Perform the Task within 20 minutes with a minimum score of _____ points.

No.	Step	Points	Check #1	Check #2	Check #3
1	Assembled supplies and washed hands.				
2	Greeted and identified the patient, introduced self, explained the procedure, and checked for signed informed consent.				
3	Positioned patient for comfort and access to site. Laid protective absorbent pad under site. Provided good lighting.				
4	Washed hands and applied sterile gloves.				
5	Applied antiseptic soap with gauze sponges, beginning in center of operative site and moving in concentric circles outward. Shaved hair as indicated, washed skin again, rinsed and dried area using sterile technique.				
6	Removed and discarded absorbent pad, gauze sponges, disposable prep kit, and gloves. Washed hands again.				
7	Using sterile technique, placed sterile towel/drape under operative site. Covered site with another sterile drape. Instructed the patient not to touch the area. Explained rationale.				
8	Poured antiseptic solution into bowl for provider to apply with sterile gauze. Used fenestrated drape according to provider's preference.				
9	Demonstrated professional behavior in manner, organization, and attire, including: • Communicated appropriately and comfortably with the patient.				
Student's Total Points					
Points Possible					
Final Score (Student's Total Points/ Possible Points)					

Name _____ **Date** _____ **Score** _____

Instructor's/Evaluator's Comments and Suggestions:

_____

_____

_____

_____

_____

CHECK #1

Evaluator's Signature: _____ Date:

CHECK #2

Evaluator's Signature: _____ Date:

CHECK #3

Evaluator's Signature: _____ Date:

ABHES Competency: VI.A.1.a.4.h Prepare patient for and assist physician with routine and specialty examinations and treatments and minor office surgeries

CAAHEP Curriculum: I.P.10 Assist physician with patient care

Name _____ **Date** _____ **Score** _____

COMPETENCY ASSESSMENT

Procedure 31-12   Suturing of Laceration or Incision Repair

Task: To set up and assist with the procedure of suturing a wound.

Conditions: *On the sterile tray:* syringe and needle for anesthetic, hemostats (curved), Adson with teeth or thumb tissue forceps, needle holder with cutting edge or plain needle holder and curved iris scissors, suture pack (suture material and needle, sized and typed according to provider's preference), gauze sponges. *On the counter:* anesthetic as ordered by the physician, dressings, bandages, tape, splint/brace/sling (optional), sterile gloves in package

Standards: Perform the Task within 30 minutes with a minimum score of _____ points.

*Work
Documentation:*   Patient chart entry

No.	Step	Points	Check #1	Check #2	Check #3
1	Assembled the supplies and washed hands.				
2	Greeted and identified the patient, introduced self, explained the procedure, checked for signed informed consent form.				
3	Prepared the patient for the procedure: • Identified known allergies, tetanus status, health concerns. • Positioned patient for comfort and safety and accessed the site. • Reassured the patient as needed. • Assessed the cause of wound and severity. • Soaked or irrigated wound in antiseptic solution as ordered. • Cleaned and dried wound.				
4	Assisted the provider and patient as needed.				
5	Provided post-op care: • Applied sterile gloves. • Cleaned area around the wound and dried the wound. • Dressed/bandaged/splinted the area, following provider's orders. • Removed gloves and washed hands. • Checked patient's color and blood pressure. • Gave wound care instructions, both orally and written, symptoms of infection, after-hours phone numbers. • Assisted the patient with concerns and questions. • Arranged for follow-up care, medications, and scheduled return appointment.				

No.	Step	Points	Check #1	Check #2	Check #3
6	Demonstrated professional behavior in manner, organization, and attire, including: • Communicated appropriately and comfortably with the patient.				
7	Cleaned/disposed of supplies and equipment appropriately and washed hands.				
8	Correctly documented the procedure.				
Student's Total Points					
Points Possible					
Final Score (Student's Total Points/ Possible Points)					

Name _____ **Date** _____ **Score** _____

WORK DOCUMENTATION

_____

Instructor's/Evaluator's Comments and Suggestions:

_____

_____

_____

_____

_____

CHECK #1
Evaluator's Signature: Date:

CHECK #2
Evaluator's Signature: Date:

CHECK #3
Evaluator's Signature: Date:

ABHES Competency: VI.A.1.a.4.h Prepare patient for and assist physician with routine and specialty examinations and treatments and minor office surgeries

CAAHEP Curriculum: I.P.10 Assist physician with patient care

Name _____ **Date** _____ **Score** _____

COMPETENCY ASSESSMENT

Procedure 31-13   Sebaceous Cyst Excision

Task: To remove an inflamed or infected sebaceous cyst or to remove a sebaceous cyst that is not inflamed or infected but is located on an area of the body where the cyst is unsightly or where it may become irritated from rubbing.

Conditions: *On the sterile field:* syringe and needle for anesthesia, iris scissors (curved), mosquito hemostat (curved), scalpel blade and handle, tissue forceps (two), suture material with needle, needle holder, Mayo scissors (curved). *On the counter:* skin prep supplies, extra sterile gauze (in package), fenestrated drape in package, antiseptic solution as ordered, gloves (sterile in package and nonsterile), personal protective equipment, anesthesia as directed, sterile dressing in package, bandages, tape, biohazard waste container, alcohol pledgets, sterile culture tube, requisition and transport bag (optional), wicking material (optional)

Standards: Perform the Task within 30 minutes with a minimum score of _____ points.

Work Documentation: Patient chart entry, lab requisition

No.	Step	Points	Check #1	Check #2	Check #3
1	Washed hands, assembled the supplies, and set up the sterile tray.				
2	Greeted and identified the patient, introduced self, explained the procedure, and checked for signed informed consent form.				
3	Prepared the patient for the procedure: • Identified known allergies, tetanus status, health concerns. • Positioned patient for comfort and safety and accessed the site. • Applied PPE and prepared the patient's skin as directed.				
4	Assisted the provider during the procedure: • Assisted with drawing up anesthesia as needed. • Blotted surgical site as needed. • Handed and received supplies and equipment as directed. • Supported the patient during surgery. • Prepared lab specimen and requisition as directed.				

No.	Step	Points	Check #1	Check #2	Check #3
5	Provided post-op care: • Applied sterile gloves. • Cleaned area around the wound and dried the wound. • Dressed and bandaged the wound. • Removed gloves and washed hands. • Checked patient's color and blood pressure. • Gave wound care instructions, both orally and written, symptoms of infection, after-hours phone numbers. • Assisted the patient with concerns and questions. • Arranged for follow-up care, medications, and scheduled return appointment.				
6	Demonstrated professional behavior in manner, organization, and attire, including: • Communicated appropriately and comfortably with the patient.				
7	Cleaned/disposed of supplies and equipment appropriately and washed hands.				
8	Correctly documented the procedure.				
Student's Total Points					
Points Possible					
Final Score (Student's Total Points/ Possible Points)					

Name _____ Date _____ Score _____

WORK DOCUMENTATION

*Also attach lab requisition.

_____

Instructor's/Evaluator's Comments and Suggestions:

_____

_____

_____

_____

_____

CHECK #1	
Evaluator's Signature:	Date:

CHECK #2	
Evaluator's Signature:	Date:

CHECK #3	
Evaluator's Signature:	Date:

ABHES Competency: VI.A.1.a.4.h Prepare patient for and assist physician with routine and specialty examinations and treatments and minor office surgeries

CAAHEP Curriculum: I.P.10 Assist physician with patient care

Name _____ Date _____ Score _____

COMPETENCY ASSESSMENT

Procedure 31-14   Incision and Drainage of Localized Infection

Task: To assist with the incision and drainage of an abscess (localized infection).

Conditions: *On sterile tray:* syringe/needle for anesthesia; instruments as determined by physician: scalpel blade and handle, tissue forceps (two), thumb dressing forceps, Mayo scissors (curved), iris scissors (curved), mosquito hemostat (curved), gauze sponges (many), fenestrated drape, antiseptic solution in sterile cup. *On side area:* skin prep supplies, gloves (sterile unopened and nonsterile), personal protective equipment (PPE), anesthesia as directed, sterile dressing unopened, bandages, tape, culture container, requisition
and transport bag (optional), biohazard waste container, extra gauze sponges unopened, io-doform gauze wicking, alcohol pledgets, antiseptic solution

Standards: Perform the Task within 30 minutes with a minimum score of _____ points.

Work
Documentation: Patient chart entry, lab requisition

No.	Step	Points	Check #1	Check #2	Check #3
1	Washed hands, assembled the supplies, and set up the sterile tray.				
2	Greeted and identified the patient, introduced self, explained the procedure, and checked for signed informed consent form.				
3	Prepared the patient for the procedure: • Identified known allergies, tetanus status, health concerns. • Positioned patient for comfort and safety and accessed the site. • Applied PPE and prepared the patient's skin as directed.				
4	Assisted the provider during the procedure: • Assisted with drawing up anesthesia as needed. • Blotted surgical site as needed. • Handed and received supplies and equipment as directed. • Supported the patient during surgery. • Prepared lab specimen and requisition as directed.				

No.	Step	Points	Check #1	Check #2	Check #3
5	Provided post-op care: • Applied sterile gloves. • Cleaned area around the wound and dried the wound. • Dressed and bandaged the wound. • Removed gloves and washed hands. • Checked patient's color and blood pressure. • Gave wound care instructions, both orally and written, symptoms of infection, after-hours phone numbers. • Assisted the patient with concerns and questions. • Arranged for follow-up care, medications, and scheduled return appointment.				
6	Demonstrated professional behavior in manner, organization, and attire, including: • Communicated appropriately and comfortably with the patient.				
7	Cleaned/disposed of supplies and equipment appropriately and washed hands.				
8	Correctly documented the procedure.				
Student's Total Points					
Points Possible					
Final Score (Student's Total Points/ Possible Points)					

Name _____   **Date** _____   **Score** _____

WORK DOCUMENTATION

*Also attach lab requisition.

_____

Instructor's/Evaluator's Comments and Suggestions:

_____

_____

_____

_____

_____

CHECK #1	
Evaluator's Signature:	Date:

CHECK #2	
Evaluator's Signature:	Date:

CHECK #3	
Evaluator's Signature:	Date:

ABHES Competency: VI.A.1.a.4.h Prepare patient for and assist physician with routine and specialty examinations and treatments and minor office surgeries

CAAHEP Curriculum: I.P.10 Assist physician with patient care

Name _____   Date _____   Score _____

COMPETENCY ASSESSMENT

Procedure 31-15   Aspiration of Joint Fluid

Task: To remove excess synovial fluid from a joint after injury.

Conditions: *On surgical field:* syringe/needle for anesthesia (size and gauge as directed), syringe/needle for drainage (size and gauge as directed), sturdy hemostat or needle driver (to remove needle from syringe), gauze sponges (many, sterile), sterile basin for aspirated fluid, fenestrated drape (optional). *On side counter:* skin prep supplies, gloves (sterile, in package and nonsterile), personal protective equipment (PPE), anesthesia as directed, cortisone medication as directed, culture tube, specimen container, pathology requisition, biohazard specimen transfer bag, alcohol swabs, dressings, bandages, tape, biohazard waste container

Standards: Perform the Task within 30 minutes with a minimum score of _____ points.

**Work
Documentation:**   Patient chart entry, lab requisition

No.	Step	Points	Check #1	Check #2	Check #3
1	Washed hands, assembled the supplies, and set up the sterile tray.				
2	Greeted and identified the patient, introduced self, explained the procedure, and checked for signed informed consent form.				
3	Prepared the patient for the procedure: • Identified known allergies, tetanus status, health concerns. • Positioned patient for comfort and safety and accessed the site. • Applied PPE and prepared the patient's skin as directed.				
4	Assisted the provider during the procedure: • Assisted with drawing up anesthesia as needed. • Blotted surgical site as needed. • Handed and received supplies and equipment as directed. • Supported the patient during surgery. • Prepared lab specimen and requisition as directed.				

No.	Step	Points	Check #1	Check #2	Check #3
5	Provided post-op care: • Applied sterile gloves. • Cleaned area around the wound and dried the wound. • Dressed and bandaged the wound. • Removed gloves and washed hands. • Checked patient's color and blood pressure. • Gave wound care instructions, both orally and written, symptoms of infection, after-hours phone numbers. • Assisted the patient with concerns and questions. • Arranged for follow-up care, medications, and scheduled return appointment.				
6	Demonstrated professional behavior in manner, organization, and attire, including: • Communicated appropriately and comfortably with the patient.				
7	Cleaned/disposed of supplies and equipment appropriately and washed hands.				
8	Correctly documented the procedure.				
Student's Total Points					
Points Possible					
Final Score (Student's Total Points/ Possible Points)					

Name _____ **Date** _____ **Score** _____

WORK DOCUMENTATION
*Also attach lab requisition.

_____

Instructor's/Evaluator's Comments and Suggestions:

_____
_____
_____
_____
_____

| **CHECK #1** |
| Evaluator's Signature: Date: |

| **CHECK #2** |
| Evaluator's Signature: Date: |

| **CHECK #3** |
| Evaluator's Signature: Date: |

ABHES Competency: VI.A.1.a.4.h Prepare patient for and assist physician with routine and specialty examinations and treatments and minor office surgeries

CAAHEP Curriculum: I.P.10 Assist physician with patient care

Name _____ **Date** _____ **Score** _____

COMPETENCY ASSESSMENT

Procedure 31-16   Hemorrhoid Thrombectomy

Task: To incise inflamed hemorrhoids and remove thrombus. To remove hemorrhoids with laser, electrosurgery, cryosurgery, or banding.

Conditions: *On surgical field:* syringe/needle for anesthesia, mosquito hemostat (curved), sterile basin, gauze sponges, rubber bands (optional), fenestrated drape. *On side counter:* skin prep supplies, gloves (sterile in package and nonsterile), personal protective equipment (PPE), anesthesia as directed, biohazard waste container, extra gauze sponges, soft absorbent pad (similar to sanitary napkin), T-bandage (to hold pad in place)

Standards: Perform the Task within 30 minutes with a minimum score of _____ points.

Work
Documentation: Patient chart entry

No.	Step	Points	Check #1	Check #2	Check #3
1	Washed hands, assembled the supplies, and set up the sterile tray.				
2	Greeted and identified the patient, introduced self, explained the procedure, and checked for signed informed consent form.				
3	Prepared the patient for the procedure: • Identified known allergies, tetanus status, health concerns. • Positioned the patient for comfort, safety, and access to the site. • Applied PPE and prepared the surgical site as directed.				
4	Assisted the provider during the procedure: • Assisted with drawing up anesthesia as needed. • Blotted surgical site as needed. • Handed and received supplies and equipment as directed. • Supported the patient during surgery. • Prepared lab specimen and requisition as directed.				

No.	Step	Points	Check #1	Check #2	Check #3
5	Provided post-op care: • Applied sterile gloves. • Cleaned area around the wound and dried the wound. • Applied absorbent pad as necessary. • Removed gloves and washed hands. • Checked patient's color and blood pressure. • Gave wound care instructions, both orally and written, symptoms of infection, after-hours phone numbers. • Assisted the patient with concerns and questions. • Arranged for follow-up care, medications, and scheduled return appointment.				
6	Demonstrated professional behavior in manner, organization, and attire, including: • Communicated appropriately and comfortably with the patient.				
7	Cleaned/disposed of supplies and equipment appropriately and washed hands.				
8	Correctly documented the procedure.				
Student's Total Points					
Points Possible					
Final Score (Student's Total Points/ Possible Points)					

Name _____ **Date** _____ **Score** _____

WORK DOCUMENTATION

―――――――――――――――――――――――――――――――――――

Instructor's/Evaluator's Comments and Suggestions:

_____

_____

_____

_____

_____

CHECK #1	
Evaluator's Signature:	Date:

CHECK #2	
Evaluator's Signature:	Date:

CHECK #3	
Evaluator's Signature:	Date:

ABHES Competency: VI.A.1.a.4.h Prepare patient for and assist physician with routine and specialty examinations and treatments and minor office surgeries

CAAHEP Curriculum: I.P.10 Assist physician with patient care

Name _____   Date _____   Score _____

COMPETENCY ASSESSMENT

Procedure 31-17   Suture/Staple Removal

Task:　　　　　　To remove sutures or staples from a healed surgical wound.

Conditions:　　　*To remove bandage:* bandage scissors, gloves. *To remove sutures/staples:* sterile gloves, suture/staple removal kit (suture scissors and thumb dressing forceps, or staple remover, and 4×4 pads) *To redress:* antibiotic cream if ordered, cotton-tipped applicators, gauze sponges, and tape or adhesive strip. *Clean up:* sharps container for staples, biohazard waste container

Standards:　　　Perform the Task within 15 minutes with a minimum score of _____ points.

*Work
Documentation:*　Patient chart entry

No.	Step	Points	Check #1	Check #2	Check #3
1	Checked provider's orders, washed hands, assembled the supplies, set up the sterile field.				
2	Greeted and identified the patient, introduced self, explained the procedure, and positioned patient properly for comfort and safety.				
3	Performed the removal of all sutures and staples using proper technique.				
4	Cleaned and bandaged the wound, explained follow-up care as directed.				
5	Demonstrated professional behavior in manner, organization, and attire, including: • Communicated appropriately and comfortably with the patient.				
6	Cleaned/disposed of supplies and equipment appropriately and washed hands.				
7	Correctly documented the procedure.				
Student's Total Points					
Points Possible					
Final Score (Student's Total Points/ Possible Points)					

Name _____   **Date** _____   **Score** _____

WORK DOCUMENTATION

Instructor's/Evaluator's Comments and Suggestions:

_____

_____

_____

_____

_____

CHECK #1

Evaluator's Signature: _____   Date: _____

CHECK #2

Evaluator's Signature: _____   Date: _____

CHECK #3

Evaluator's Signature: _____   Date: _____

ABHES Competency: VI.A.1.a.4.h Prepare patient for and assist physician with routine and specialty examinations and treatments and minor office surgeries

CAAHEP Curriculum: I.P.10 Assist physician with patient care

Name _____ Date _____ Score _____

COMPETENCY ASSESSMENT

Procedure 31-18   Application of Sterile Adhesive Skin Closure Strips

Task: To approximate the edges of a wound after the removal of sutures. Sometimes used in lieu of sutures or to give additional support together with sutures.

Conditions: *On sterile field:* suture removal instruments and supplies (as indicated), sterile adhesive skin closure strips, iris scissors (straight), Adson dressing forceps, tincture of benzoin (optional), sterile cotton-tipped applicators (for tincture of benzoin). *On side area:* sterile gloves in package, dressings, bandages, tape

Standards: Perform the Task within 15 minutes with a minimum score of _____ points.

Work Documentation: Patient chart entry

No.	Step	Points	Check #1	Check #2	Check #3
1	Checked provider's orders, washed hands, assembled the supplies, set up the sterile field.				
2	Greeted and identified the patient, introduced self, explained the procedure, and positioned patient properly for comfort and safety.				
3	Applied sterile adhesive skin closure strips using proper technique.				
4	Cleaned and bandaged the wound, explained follow-up care as directed.				
5	Demonstrated professional behavior in manner, organization, and attire, including: • Communicated appropriately and comfortably with the patient.				
6	Cleaned/disposed of supplies and equipment appropriately and washed hands.				
7	Correctly documented the procedure.				
Student's Total Points					
Points Possible					
Final Score (Student's Total Points/ Possible Points)					

Name _____   **Date** _____   **Score** _____

WORK DOCUMENTATION

Instructor's/Evaluator's Comments and Suggestions:

_____

_____

_____

_____

_____

CHECK #1

Evaluator's Signature: _____   Date:

CHECK #2

Evaluator's Signature: _____   Date:

CHECK #3

Evaluator's Signature: _____   Date:

ABHES Competency: VI.A.1.a.4.h Prepare patient for and assist physician with routine and specialty examinations and treatments and minor office surgeries

CAAHEP Curriculum: I.P.10 Assist physician with patient care

Name _____ Date _____ Score _____

COMPETENCY ASSESSMENT

Procedure 33-1   Transferring Patient from Wheelchair to Examination Table

Task: To safely transfer a patient from a wheelchair to an examination table using a one-person transfer technique, and then using a two-person transfer technique.

Conditions: Wheelchair, examination table, gait belt, step stool with rubber tips and a handle for gripping

Standards: Perform the Task within 15 minutes with a minimum score of _____ points.

No.	Step	Points	Check #1	Check #2	Check #3
1	Checked provider's orders, checked room for cleanliness, equipment, and readiness, and washed hands.				
2	Greeted and identified the patient, introduced self, and explained the procedure.				
3	Transferred the patient correctly and safely by self.				
4	Transferred the patient correctly and safely with the assistance of another person.				
5	Demonstrated professional behavior in manner, organization, and attire, including: • Communicated appropriately and comfortably with the patient.				
Student's Total Points					
Points Possible					
Final Score (Student's Total Points/ Possible Points)					

Name _____   **Date** _____   **Score** _____

Instructor's/Evaluator's Comments and Suggestions:

_____

_____

_____

_____

_____

CHECK #1

Evaluator's Signature: Date:

CHECK #2

Evaluator's Signature: Date:

CHECK #3

Evaluator's Signature: Date:

ABHES Competency: VI.A.1.a.4.h Prepare patient for and assist physician with routine and specialty examinations and treatments and minor office surgeries

CAAHEP Curriculum: XI.P.11 Use proper body mechanics

Name _____ **Date** _____ **Score** _____

COMPETENCY ASSESSMENT

Procedure 33-2   Transferring Patient from Examination Table to Wheelchair

Task: To safely transfer a patient from the examination table to a wheelchair.

Conditions: Wheelchair, examination table, gait belt, step stool with rubber tips and a handle for gripping

Standards: Perform the Task within 15 minutes with a minimum score of _____ points.

No.	Step	Points	Check #1	Check #2	Check #3
1	Checked provider's orders, checked room for cleanliness, equipment, and readiness, and washed hands.				
2	Greeted and identified the patient, introduced self, and explained the procedure.				
3	Transferred the patient correctly and safely by self.				
4	Transferred the patient correctly and safely with the assistance of another person.				
5	Demonstrated professional behavior in manner, organization, and attire, including: • Communicated appropriately and comfortably with the patient.				
	Student's Total Points				
	Points Possible				
	Final Score (Student's Total Points/ Possible Points)				

Name _____   **Date** _____   **Score** _____

Instructor's/Evaluator's Comments and Suggestions:

_____

_____

_____

_____

_____

CHECK #1

Evaluator's Signature: _____   Date:

CHECK #2

Evaluator's Signature: _____   Date:

CHECK #3

Evaluator's Signature: _____   Date:

ABHES Competency: VI.A.1.a.4.h Prepare patient for and assist physician with routine and specialty examinations and treatments and minor office surgeries

CAAHEP Curriculum: XI.P.11 Use proper body mechanics

Name _____   **Date** _____   **Score** _____

COMPETENCY ASSESSMENT

Procedure 33-3 Assisting the Patient to Stand and Walk

Task: To help a patient ambulate safely.

Conditions: Gait belt, chair, or wheelchair

Standards: Perform the Task within 20 minutes with a minimum score of _____ points.

Work Documentation: Patient chart entry

No.	Step	Points	Check #1	Check #2	Check #3
1	Checked provider's orders, checked room for cleanliness, equipment, and readiness, and washed hands.				
2	Greeted and identified the patient, introduced self, and explained the procedure.				
3	Assisted the patient to stand and walk correctly and safely.				
4	Demonstrated professional behavior in manner, organization, and attire, including: • Communicated appropriately and comfortably with the patient.				
5	Documented the procedure correctly.				
Student's Total Points					
Points Possible					
Final Score (Student's Total Points/ Possible Points)					

Name _____   **Date** _____   **Score** _____

WORK DOCUMENTATION

_____

Instructor's/Evaluator's Comments and Suggestions:

_____
_____
_____
_____
_____

CHECK #1

Evaluator's Signature: _____   Date:

CHECK #2

Evaluator's Signature: _____   Date:

CHECK #3

Evaluator's Signature: _____   Date:

ABHES Competency: VI.A.1.a.4.h Prepare patient for and assist physician with routine and specialty examinations and treatments and minor office surgeries

CAAHEP Curriculum: XI.P.11 Use proper body mechanics

Name _____ Date _____ Score _____

COMPETENCY ASSESSMENT

Procedure 33-4   Care of the Falling Patient

Task: To help a patient fall safely to avoid injury.

Conditions: Gait belt may already be on the patient.

Standards: Perform the Task within 5 minutes with a minimum score of _____ points.

***Work
Documentation:***   Patient chart entry, incident report

No.	Step	Points	Check #1	Check #2	Check #3
1	Assisted the patient to fall gently, safely, and without harm to either the patient or self.				
2	Alerted the provider for patient examination before further moving the fallen patient.				
3	Demonstrated professional behavior in manner, organization, and attire, including: • Communicated appropriately and comfortably with the patient.				
4	Documented correctly and completed an accident report per clinic policy.				
Student's Total Points					
Points Possible					
Final Score (Student's Total Points/ Possible Points)					

Name _____ **Date** _____ **Score** _____

WORK DOCUMENTATION
*Also attach incident report.

_____

Instructor's/Evaluator's Comments and Suggestions:

_____

_____

_____

_____

_____

CHECK #1

Evaluator's Signature: Date:

CHECK #2

Evaluator's Signature: Date:

CHECK #3

Evaluator's Signature: Date:

ABHES Competency: VI.A.1.a.4.e Recognize emergencies; VI.A.1.a.5.a Determine needs for documentation and reporting; VI.A.1.a.5.h Perform risk management procedures

CAAHEP Curriculum: IX.P.6 Complete an incident report; XI.P.11 Use proper body mechanics

Name _____   Date _____   Score _____

COMPETENCY ASSESSMENT

Procedure 33-5   Assisting a Patient to Ambulate with a Walker

Task: To help a patient to ambulate safely and independently with a walker.

Conditions: Gait belt, walker

Standards: Perform the Task within 20 minutes with a minimum score of _____ points.

Work
Documentation: Patient chart entry

No.	Step	Points	Check #1	Check #2	Check #3
1	Checked provider's orders, checked area for cleanliness, equipment, and readiness, and washed hands.				
2	Greeted and identified the patient, introduced self, and explained the procedure.				
3	Assisted the patient to stand and walk correctly and safely using a walker. Demonstrated proper technique, then assisted the patient to follow the instructions. Provided the patient with written instructions.				
4	Demonstrated professional behavior in manner, organization, and attire, including: • Communicated appropriately and comfortably with the patient.				
5	Documented the procedure correctly.				
Student's Total Points					
Points Possible					
Final Score (Student's Total Points/ Possible Points)					

Name _____ **Date** _____ **Score** _____

WORK DOCUMENTATION

_____

Instructor's/Evaluator's Comments and Suggestions:

_____

_____

_____

_____

_____

CHECK #1

Evaluator's Signature: _____   Date:

CHECK #2

Evaluator's Signature: _____   Date:

CHECK #3

Evaluator's Signature: _____   Date:

ABHES Competency: VI.A.1.a.7.b Instruct patients with special needs

CAAHEP Curriculum: IV.P.5 Instruct patients according to their needs to promote health maintenance and disease prevention

Name _____   **Date** _____   **Score** _____

COMPETENCY ASSESSMENT

Procedure 33-6   Teaching the Patient to Ambulate with Crutches

Task: To help a patient to ambulate safely using crutches.

Conditions: Gait belt, crutches

Standards: Perform the Task within 20 minutes with a minimum score of _____ points.

Work Documentation: Patient chart entry

No.	Step	Points	Check #1	Check #2	Check #3
1	Checked provider's orders, checked area for cleanliness, equipment, and readiness, and washed hands.				
2	Greeted and identified the patient, introduced self, and explained the procedure.				
3	Assisted the patient to stand and walk correctly and safely using crutches. Demonstrated proper technique, then assisted the patient to follow the instructions. Provided the patient with written instructions.				
4	Demonstrated professional behavior in manner, organization, and attire, including: • Communicated appropriately and comfortably with the patient.				
5	Documented the procedure correctly.				
Student's Total Points					
Points Possible					
Final Score (Student's Total Points/ Possible Points)					

Name _____   **Date** _____   **Score** _____

WORK DOCUMENTATION

Instructor's/Evaluator's Comments and Suggestions:

_____

_____

_____

_____

_____

CHECK #1

Evaluator's Signature: _____   Date: _____

CHECK #2

Evaluator's Signature: _____   Date: _____

CHECK #3

Evaluator's Signature: _____   Date: _____

ABHES Competency: VI.A.1.a.7.b Instruct patients with special needs

CAAHEP Curriculum: IV.P.5 Instruct patients according to their needs to promote health maintenance and disease prevention

Name _____   **Date** _____   **Score** _____

COMPETENCY ASSESSMENT

Procedure 33-7   Assisting a Patient to Ambulate with a Cane

Task: To help a patient to ambulate safely with a cane.

Conditions: Gait belt, appropriate cane for patient

Standards: Perform the Task within 20 minutes with a minimum score of _____ points.

Work
Documentation: Patient chart entry

No.	Step	Points	Check #1	Check #2	Check #3
1	Checked provider's orders, checked area for cleanliness, equipment, and readiness, and washed hands.				
2	Greeted and identified the patient, introduced self, and explained the procedure.				
3	Assisted the patient to stand and walk correctly and safely using crutches. Demonstrated proper technique, then assisted the patient to follow the instructions. Provided the patient with written instructions.				
4	Demonstrated professional behavior in manner, organization, and attire, including: • Communicated appropriately and comfortably with the patient.				
5	Documented the procedure correctly.				
Student's Total Points					
Points Possible					
Final Score (Student's Total Points/ Possible Points)					

Name _____   **Date** _____   **Score** _____

WORK DOCUMENTATION

Instructor's/Evaluator's Comments and Suggestions:

_____

_____

_____

_____

_____

CHECK #1

Evaluator's Signature: _____   Date: _____

CHECK #2

Evaluator's Signature: _____   Date: _____

CHECK #3

Evaluator's Signature: _____   Date: _____

ABHES Competency: VI.A.1.a.7.b Instruct patients with special needs

CAAHEP Curriculum: IV.P.5 Instruct patients according to their needs to promote health maintenance and disease prevention

Name _____ **Date** _____ **Score** _____

COMPETENCY ASSESSMENT

Procedure 34-1 Provide Instruction for Health Maintenance and Disease Prevention

Task: To instruct patients about how to exercise more responsibly and control their health in order to extend their lives and enjoy healthy years.

Conditions: Discussion, DVDs, videos, print material, authentic Web-based interactive information, community resources directories

Standards: Perform the Task within 20 minutes with a minimum score of _____ points.

Work Documentation: Patient chart entry

No.	Step	Points	Check #1	Check #2	Check #3
1	Checked provider's orders, gathered materials and supplies for education, and arranged for a quiet area.				
2	Greeted and identified the patient and introduced self.				
3	Discussed the patient education topic per the provider's orders.				
4	Reinforced discussion by giving patient written materials and resources.				
5	Demonstrated professional behavior in manner, organization, and attire, including: • Communicated appropriately and comfortably with the patient.				
6	Documented patient education session on the patient's chart.				
Student's Total Points					
Points Possible					
Final Score (Student's Total Points/ Possible Points)					

Name _____   **Date** _____   **Score** _____

WORK DOCUMENTATION

_____

Instructor's/Evaluator's Comments and Suggestions:

_____

_____

_____

_____

_____

CHECK #1

Evaluator's Signature: _____   Date:

CHECK #2

Evaluator's Signature: _____   Date:

CHECK #3

Evaluator's Signature: _____   Date:

ABHES Competency: VI.A.1.a.7.c Teach patients methods of health promotion and disease prevention

CAAHEP Curriculum: IV.P.5 Instruct patients according to their needs to promote health maintenance and disease prevention

Name _____   **Date** _____   **Score** _____

COMPETENCY ASSESSMENT

Procedure 35-1   Proper Disposal of Drugs

Task: To properly dispose of drugs that have reached their expiration dates.

Conditions: Drugs (oral and parenteral) that have reached their expiration dates

Standards: Perform the Task within 10 minutes with a minimum score of _____ points.

Work Documentation: Medication disposal log

No.	Step	Points	Check #1	Check #2	Check #3
1	Gathered all expired drugs.				
2	Properly disposed of the drugs per agency policy and state law.				
3	Documented instructions in the office log that the drugs with expired use-by dates were disposed of either by returning them to the pharmacy or by having the contracted agency incinerate them. Saved all receipts associated with disposal.				
Student's Total Points					
Points Possible					
Final Score (Student's Total Points/ Possible Points)					

Name _____ **Date** _____ **Score** _____

WORK DOCUMENTATION
*Attach medication disposal log.

_____

Instructor's/Evaluator's Comments and Suggestions:

_____

_____

_____

_____

CHECK #1
Evaluator's Signature: Date:

CHECK #2
Evaluator's Signature: Date:

CHECK #3
Evaluator's Signature: Date:

ABHES Competency: VI.A.1.a.5.e Dispose of controlled substances in compliance with government regulations

CAAHEP Curriculum: IX.P.8 Apply local, state and federal health care legislation and regulation appropriate to the medical assisting practice setting

Name _____   **Date** _____   **Score** _____

COMPETENCY ASSESSMENT

Procedure 36-1   Administration of Oral Medications

Task: To correctly administer an oral medication after receiving a physician's order.

Conditions: Patient chart, medication order from provider, medication, medicine tray, medicine cup, water

Standards: Perform the Task within 10 minutes with a minimum score of _____ points.

Work
Documentation: Patient chart entry

No.	Step	Points	Check #1	Check #2	Check #3
1	Checked provider's orders; organized equipment and supplies; checked room for cleanliness, equipment, and readiness; washed hands.				
2	Correctly prepared the medication: • Selected the proper medication, checked the expiration date. • Calculated the proper dosage according to the provider's order. • Prepared the medication tray for transport to the exam room.				
3	Correctly prepared the patient: • Greeted and identified patient and introduced self. • Identified health concerns, allergies, tetanus status, possible complications, and current medications. • Positioned the patient appropriately and comfortably.				
4	Administered the medication correctly and safely: • Followed the six rights of medication administration. • Checked the medication order, dosage calculation, and expiration date again. • Gave the patient adequate water to swallow the medication.				
5	Demonstrated professional behavior in manner, organization, and attire, including: • Communicated appropriately and comfortably with the patient.				
6	Documented correctly and returned medication bottle to storage.				
Student's Total Points					
Points Possible					
Final Score (Student's Total Points/ Possible Points)					

Name _____   **Date** _____   **Score** _____

WORK DOCUMENTATION

_____

Instructor's/Evaluator's Comments and Suggestions:

_____

_____

_____

_____

_____

CHECK #1

Evaluator's Signature: _____   Date:

CHECK #2

Evaluator's Signature: _____   Date:

CHECK #3

Evaluator's Signature: _____   Date:

ABHES Competency: VI.A.1.a.4.m Prepare and administer oral and parenteral medications as directed by physician

CAAHEP Curriculum: I.P.8 Administer oral medications; II.P.1 Prepare proper dosages of medication for administration

Name _____ Date _____ Score _____

COMPETENCY ASSESSMENT

Procedure 36-2   Withdrawing Medication from a Vial

Task: To correctly withdraw medication from a vial with 100% accuracy.

Conditions: Medication order by provider, vial of medication, medication note, appropriately sized safety syringe and needle, alcohol wipes, gloves, sharps container

Standards: Perform the Task within 5 minutes with a minimum score of _____ points.

No.	Step	Points	Check #1	Check #2	Check #3
1	Checked provider's orders; organized equipment and supplies; washed hands.				
2	Correctly prepared and withdrew the medication: • Selected the proper medication and checked the expiration date. • Calculated the proper dosage according to the provider's order. • Prepared the syringe and needle using sterile technique. • Prepped the vial properly. • Withdrew the appropriate amount of medication, releasing any bubbles, and recapped safely. • Changed needles according to office protocol.				
3	Performed the six rights of medication administration as appropriate.				
4	Demonstrated professional behavior in manner, organization, and attire.				
5	Documented correctly.				
Student's Total Points					
Points Possible					
Final Score (Student's Total Points/ Possible Points)					

Name _____   **Date** _____   **Score** _____

Instructor's/Evaluator's Comments and Suggestions:

_____

_____

_____

_____

_____

CHECK #1

Evaluator's Signature: _____   Date: _____

CHECK #2

Evaluator's Signature: _____   Date: _____

CHECK #3

Evaluator's Signature: _____   Date: _____

ABHES Competency: VI.A.1.a.4.m Prepare and administer oral and parenteral medications as directed by physician

CAAHEP Curriculum: II.P.1 Prepare proper dosages of medication for administration

Name _____ **Date** _____ **Score** _____

COMPETENCY ASSESSMENT

Procedure 36-3 Withdrawing Medication from an Ampule

Task:　　　　To properly withdraw medication from an ampule with 100% accuracy.

Conditions:　Medicine tray, medication order by physician, ampule of medication, medication note, appropriately sized safety syringe and filter needle and regular needle, antiseptic wipes (alcohol), sharps container

Standards:　Perform the Task within 5 minutes with a minimum score of _____ points.

No.	Step	Points	Check #1	Check #2	Check #3
1	Checked provider's orders; organized equipment and supplies; washed hands.				
2	Correctly prepared and withdrew the medication: • Selected the proper medication and checked the expiration date. • Calculated the proper dosage according to the provider's order. • Prepared the syringe and needle using sterile technique. • Prepped the ampule properly. • Withdrew the appropriate amount of medication, releasing any bubbles and recapped safely. • Changed filter needle to a regular needle.				
3	Performed the six rights of medication administration as appropriate.				
4	Demonstrated professional behavior in manner, organization, and attire.				
5	Documented correctly.				
Student's Total Points					
Points Possible					
Final Score (Student's Total Points/ Possible Points)					

Name _____ **Date** _____ **Score** _____

Instructor's/Evaluator's Comments and Suggestions:

_____

_____

_____

_____

_____

CHECK #1

Evaluator's Signature: _____ Date: _____

CHECK #2

Evaluator's Signature: _____ Date: _____

CHECK #3

Evaluator's Signature: _____ Date: _____

ABHES Competency: VI.A.1.a.4.m Prepare and administer oral and parenteral medications as directed by physician

CAAHEP Curriculum: II.P.1 Prepare proper dosages of medication for administration

Name _____ Date _____ Score _____

COMPETENCY ASSESSMENT

Procedure 36-4   Administration of Subcutaneous, Intramuscular, and Intradermal Injections

Task: To correctly administer subcutaneous, intramuscular, and intradermal injections with 100% accuracy.

Conditions: Medication order by provider, medication vial or ampule, medication note, appropriately sized safety needle-syringe unit, antiseptic (alcohol) wipes, gloves, cotton balls, adhesive strip, sharps container

Standards: Perform the Task within 10 minutes with a minimum score of _____ points.

Work Documentation: Patient chart entry

No.	Step	Points	Check #1	Check #2	Check #3
1	Checked provider's orders; organized equipment and supplies; checked room for cleanliness, equipment, and readiness; washed hands.				
2	Properly and accurately selected and withdrew the medication using all safety precautions.				
3	Correctly prepared the patient: • Greeted and identified patient and introduced self; explained procedure and checked for signed informed consent form. • Identified health concerns, allergies, tetanus status, possible complications, and current medications. • Positioned patient appropriately and comfortably. • Exposed, calculated, and prepped the appropriate site. • Reassured the patient as needed.				
4	Administered medication properly and safely: • Followed the six rights of medication administration. • Correctly administered medication. • Activated safety mechanism immediately and disposed of syringe/needle unit properly.				

No.	Step	Points	Check #1	Check #2	Check #3
5	Checked patient for adverse reactions, applied adhesive strip as needed, and instructed the patient about precautions to watch for as appropriate.				
6	Demonstrated professional behavior in manner, organization, and attire, including: • Communicated appropriately and comfortably with the patient.				
7	Documented correctly.				
Student's Total Points					
Points Possible					
Final Score (Student's Total Points/ Possible Points)					

Name _____ Date _____ Score _____

WORK DOCUMENTATION

_____

Instructor's/Evaluator's Comments and Suggestions:

_____
_____
_____
_____
_____

CHECK #1

Evaluator's Signature: _____   Date:

CHECK #2

Evaluator's Signature: _____   Date:

CHECK #3

Evaluator's Signature: _____   Date:

ABHES Competency: VI.A.1.a.4.m Prepare and administer oral and parenteral medications as directed by physician

CAAHEP Curriculum: I.P.9 Administer parenteral (excluding IV) medications; II.P.1 Prepare proper dosages of medication for administration

Name _____   Date _____   Score _____

COMPETENCY ASSESSMENT

Procedure 36-5   Administering a Subcutaneous Injection

Task: To correctly administer a subcutaneous injection with 100% accuracy.

Conditions: Medication order by provider, medication vial or ampule, medication note, appropriately sized safety needle-syringe unit, antiseptic (alcohol) wipes, gloves, cotton balls, adhesive strip, sharps container

Standards: Perform the Task within 10 minutes with a minimum score of _____ points.

Work Documentation: Patient chart entry

No.	Step	Points	Check #1	Check #2	Check #3
1	Checked provider's orders; organized equipment and supplies; checked room for cleanliness, equipment, and readiness; washed hands.				
2	Properly and accurately selected and withdrew the medication using all safety precautions.				
3	Correctly prepared the patient: • Greeted and identified patient and introduced self; explained procedure and checked for signed informed consent form. • Identified health concerns, allergies, tetanus status, possible complications, and current medications. • Positioned patient appropriately and comfortably. • Exposed, calculated, and prepped the appropriate site. • Reassured the patient as needed.				
4	Administered medication properly and safely: • Followed the six rights of medication administration. • Correctly administered medication. • Activated safety mechanism immediately and disposed of syringe/needle unit properly.				
5	Checked patient for adverse reactions, applied adhesive strip as needed, and instructed the patient about precautions to watch for as appropriate.				

No.	Step	Points	Check #1	Check #2	Check #3
6	Demonstrated professional behavior in manner, organization, and attire, including: • Communicated appropriately and comfortably with the patient.				
7	Documented correctly.				
Student's Total Points					
Points Possible					
Final Score (Student's Total Points/ Possible Points)					

Name _____ **Date** _____ **Score** _____

WORK DOCUMENTATION

_____

Instructor's/Evaluator's Comments and Suggestions:

_____
_____
_____
_____
_____

CHECK #1	
Evaluator's Signature:	Date:

CHECK #2	
Evaluator's Signature:	Date:

CHECK #3	
Evaluator's Signature:	Date:

ABHES Competency: VI.A.1.a.4.m Prepare and administer oral and parenteral medications as directed by physician

CAAHEP Curriculum: I.P.9 Administer parenteral (excluding IV) medications; II.P.1 Prepare proper dosages of medication for administration

Name _____ Date _____ Score _____

COMPETENCY ASSESSMENT

Procedure 36-6   Administering an Intramuscular Injection

Task:　　　　　To correctly administer an intramuscular injection with 100% accuracy.

Conditions:　　Medication order by provider, medication vial or ampule, medication note, appropriately sized safety needle-syringe unit, antiseptic (alcohol) wipes, gloves, cotton balls, adhesive strip, sharps container

Standards:　　Perform the Task within 10 minutes with a minimum score of _____ points.

Work Documentation:　　Patient chart entry

No.	Step	Points	Check #1	Check #2	Check #3
1	Checked provider's orders; organized equipment and supplies; checked room for cleanliness, equipment, and readiness; washed hands.				
2	Properly and accurately selected and withdrew the medication using all safety precautions.				
3	Correctly prepared the patient: • Greeted and identified patient and introduced self; explained procedure and checked for signed informed consent form. • Identified health concerns, allergies, tetanus status, possible complications, and current medications. • Positioned patient appropriately and comfortably. • Exposed, calculated, and prepped the appropriate site. • Reassured the patient as needed.				
4	Administered medication properly and safely: • Followed the six rights of medication administration. • Correctly administered medication. • Activated safety mechanism immediately and disposed of syringe/needle unit properly.				
5	Checked patient for adverse reactions, applied adhesive strip as needed, and instructed the patient about precautions to watch for as appropriate.				

No.	Step	Points	Check #1	Check #2	Check #3
6	Demonstrated professional behavior in manner, organization, and attire, including: • Communicated appropriately and comfortably with the patient.				
7	Documented correctly.				
Student's Total Points					
Points Possible					
Final Score (Student's Total Points/ Possible Points)					

Name _____ **Date** _____ **Score** _____

WORK DOCUMENTATION

_____

Instructor's/Evaluator's Comments and Suggestions:

_____

_____

_____

_____

_____

CHECK #1

Evaluator's Signature: Date:

CHECK #2

Evaluator's Signature: Date:

CHECK #3

Evaluator's Signature: Date:

ABHES Competency: VI.A.1.a.4.m Prepare and administer oral and parenteral medications as directed by physician

CAAHEP Curriculum: I.P.9 Administer parenteral (excluding IV) medications; II.P.1 Prepare proper dosages of medication for administration

Name _____ Date _____ Score _____

COMPETENCY ASSESSMENT

Procedure 36-7 Administering an Intradermal Injection of Purified Protein Derivative (PPD)

Task: To correctly administer an intradermal injection of PPD with 100% accuracy.

Conditions: Medication order by provider, medication vial, medication note, appropriately sized safety needle-syringe unit, antiseptic (alcohol) wipes, gloves, cotton balls, adhesive strip, sharps container, disclosure form

Standards: Perform the Task within 15 minutes with a minimum score of _____ points.

Work Documentation: Patient chart entry

No.	Step	Points	Check #1	Check #2	Check #3
1	Checked provider's orders; organized equipment and supplies; checked room for cleanliness, equipment, and readiness; washed hands.				
2	Properly and accurately selected and withdrew the medication using all safety precautions.				
3	Correctly prepared the patient: • Greeted and identified patient and introduced self, explained procedure. • Determined if patient could return for the TB reading in 48 hours; checked for signed disclosure form. • Identified health concerns, allergies, tetanus status, possible complications, and current medications. • Positioned patient appropriately and comfortably. • Exposed, calculated, and prepped the appropriate site. • Reassured the patient as needed.				
4	Administered medication properly and safely: • Followed the six rights of medication administration. • Correctly administered medication. • Activated safety mechanism immediately and disposed of syringe/needle unit properly.				

No.	Step	Points	Check #1	Check #2	Check #3
5	Checked patient for adverse reactions, applied adhesive strip as needed, and instructed the patient about precautions to watch for as appropriate.				
6	Scheduled follow-up appointment for reading the TB test.				
7	Demonstrated professional behavior in manner, organization, and attire, including: • Communicated appropriately and comfortably with the patient.				
8	Documented correctly.				
Student's Total Points					
Points Possible					
Final Score (Student's Total Points/ Possible Points)					

Name _____ **Date** _____ **Score** _____

WORK DOCUMENTATION

_____

Instructor's/Evaluator's Comments and Suggestions:

_____

_____

_____

_____

_____

CHECK #1	
Evaluator's Signature:	Date:

CHECK #2	
Evaluator's Signature:	Date:

CHECK #3	
Evaluator's Signature:	Date:

ABHES Competency: VI.A.1.a.4.m Prepare and administer oral and parenteral medications as directed by physician

CAAHEP Curriculum: I.P.9 Administer parenteral (excluding IV) medications; II.P.1 Prepare proper dosages of medication for administration

Name _____ Date _____ Score _____

COMPETENCY ASSESSMENT

Procedure 36-8 Reconstituting a Powder Medication for Administration

Task: To correctly reconstitute a powder medication and calculate correct dosage with 100% accuracy.

Conditions: Medication order by provider, vial of medication, vial of diluent, medication note, two appropriately sized safety syringes and needles, alcohol wipes, gloves, sharps container

Standards: Perform the Task within 10 minutes with a minimum score of _____ points.

No.	Step	Points	Check #1	Check #2	Check #3
1	Checked provider's orders; organized equipment and supplies; washed hands.				
2	Correctly prepared the medication: • Selected proper medication and diluent, checked the expiration dates. • Calculated proper strength and dosage according to the provider's order. • Prepared syringe and needle using sterile technique. • Prepped the vials properly. • Withdrew appropriate amount of diluent and injected it properly into the powdered medication. • Mixed well. • Drew up correct dosage of mixed medication, releasing any bubbles, and recapped safely. • Changed needles according to office protocol.				
3	Performed the six rights of medication administration as appropriate.				
4	Demonstrated professional behavior in manner, organization, and attire.				
5	Documented correctly.				
Student's Total Points					
Points Possible					
Final Score (Student's Total Points/ Possible Points)					

Name _____ **Date** _____ **Score** _____

Instructor's/Evaluator's Comments and Suggestions:

_____

_____

_____

_____

_____

CHECK #1

Evaluator's Signature: _____ Date: _____

CHECK #2

Evaluator's Signature: _____ Date: _____

CHECK #3

Evaluator's Signature: _____ Date: _____

ABHES Competency: VI.A.1.a.4.m Prepare and administer oral and parenteral medications as directed by physician

CAAHEP Curriculum: II.P.1 Prepare proper dosages of medication for administration

Name _____ Date _____ Score _____

COMPETENCY ASSESSMENT

Procedure 36-9   Z-Track Intramuscular Injection Technique

Task: To correctly administer a Z-track intramuscular injection with 100% accuracy.

Conditions: Medication order by provider, medication note, medication vial, appropriately sized safety needle-syringe unit, antiseptic (alcohol) wipes, gloves, cotton balls, adhesive strip, sharps container

Standards: Perform the Task within 10 minutes with a minimum score of ___ points.

Work Documentation: Patient chart entry

No.	Step	Points	Check #1	Check #2	Check #3
1	Checked provider's orders; organized equipment and supplies; checked room for cleanliness, equipment, and readiness; washed hands.				
2	Properly and accurately selected and withdrew the medication using all safety precautions.				
3	Correctly prepared the patient: • Greeted and identified patient and introduced self; explained procedure and checked for signed informed consent form. • Identified health concerns, allergies, tetanus status, possible complications, and current medications. • Positioned patient appropriately and comfortably. • Exposed, calculated, and prepped the appropriate site. • Reassured the patient as needed.				
4	Administered medication properly and safely: • Followed the six rights of medication administration. • Correctly administered medication. • Activated safety mechanism immediately and disposed of syringe/needle unit properly.				

No.	Step	Points	Check #1	Check #2	Check #3
5	Checked patient for adverse reactions, applied adhesive strip as needed, and instructed the patient about precautions to watch for as appropriate.				
6	Demonstrated professional behavior in manner, organization, and attire, including: • Communicated appropriately and comfortably with the patient.				
7	Documented correctly.				
Student's Total Points					
Points Possible					
Final Score (Student's Total Points/ Possible Points)					

Name _____ **Date** _____ **Score** _____

WORK DOCUMENTATION

_____

Instructor's/Evaluator's Comments and Suggestions:

_____
_____
_____
_____
_____

CHECK #1

Evaluator's Signature: _____ Date: _____

CHECK #2

Evaluator's Signature: _____ Date: _____

CHECK #3

Evaluator's Signature: _____ Date: _____

ABHES Competency: VI.A.1.a.4.m Prepare and administer oral and parenteral medications as directed by physician

CAAHEP Curriculum: I.P.9 Administer parenteral (excluding IV) medications; II.P.1 Prepare proper dosages of medication for administration

Name _____   Date _____   Score _____

COMPETENCY ASSESSMENT

Procedure 37-1   Perform Single-Channel or Multichannel Electrocardiogram

Task: To perform a standard 12-lead electrocardiogram (ECG).

Conditions: Electrocardiograph machine, lead wires with end clips, tabbed adhesive electrodes, tracing paper, patient gown, small pillow, blanket/sheet, alcohol, razor (optional), mounting card/paper

Standards: Perform the Task within 20 minutes with a minimum score of _____ points.

Work Documentation: Patient chart entry, output from ECG machine

No.	Step	Points	Check #1	Check #2	Check #3
1	Checked provider's orders; organized equipment and supplies, ensuring ECG machine is ready; checked room for cleanliness, equipment, and readiness; washed hands.				
2	Correctly prepared the patient: • Greeted and identified patient and introduced self; explained procedure and checked for signed informed consent form. • Identified health concerns, allergies, tetanus status, possible complications, and current medications; obtained blood pressure. • Positioned patient appropriately and comfortably. • Exposed chest, arms, and legs, shaving hair if needed. • Reassured the patient as needed.				
3	Performed the ECG properly, mounting it if needed.				
4	Alerted provider immediately if any abnormalities were shown; otherwise, showed ECG to provider before removing the electrodes, following clinic protocol.				
5	Demonstrated professional behavior in manner, organization, and attire, including: • Communicated appropriately and comfortably with the patient.				
6	Documented correctly.				
	Student's Total Points				
	Points Possible				
	Final Score (Student's Total Points/ Possible Points)				

Name _____ **Date** _____ **Score** _____

WORK DOCUMENTATION

*Also attach ECG output.

_____

Instructor's/Evaluator's Comments and Suggestions:

_____

_____

_____

_____

_____

CHECK #1
Evaluator's Signature: _____ Date: _____

CHECK #2
Evaluator's Signature: _____ Date: _____

CHECK #3
Evaluator's Signature: _____ Date: _____

ABHES Competency: VI.A.1.a.4.l Screen and follow up patient test results; VI.A.1.a.4.dd Perform electrocardiograms

CAAHEP Curriculum: I.P.5 Perform electrocardiography; I.P.16 Screen test results

Name _____ **Date** _____ **Score** _____

COMPETENCY ASSESSMENT

Procedure 37-2 Holter Monitor Application (Cassette and Digital)

Task: To apply a Holter or cardiac event monitor and teach the patient how to wear the monitor, record the incidents, keep the activity log/diary, and when to return.

Conditions: Holter or cardiac event monitor, patient activity diary/log, blank magnetic tape cassette, disposable electrodes, alcohol, razor, gauze, carrying case, belt or shoulder strap

Standards: Perform the Task within 20 minutes with a minimum score of _____ points.

Work Documentation: Patient chart entry

No.	Step	Points	Check #1	Check #2	Check #3
1	Checked provider's orders; organized equipment and supplies, ensuring monitor is in working order; checked room for cleanliness, equipment, and readiness; washed hands.				
2	Correctly prepared the patient: • Greeted and identified patient and introduced self; explained procedure and checked for signed informed consent form. • Identified health concerns, allergies, tetanus status, possible complications, and current medications; obtained blood pressure. • Positioned patient appropriately and comfortably. • Exposed chest, shaving hair if needed. • Reassured the patient as needed.				
3	Performed the procedure properly: • Applied monitor properly. • Instructed patient clearly in the proper use of the monitor and provided written instruction. • Instructed patient clearly in the use of activity log. • Answered patient questions as needed, discussed solutions to any problems that could arise. • Provided patient with 24-hour numbers to call if needed. • Arranged for follow-up appointment.				
4	Demonstrated professional behavior in manner, organization, and attire, including: • Communicated appropriately and comfortably with the patient.				
5	Documented correctly.				
Student's Total Points					
Points Possible					
Final Score (Student's Total Points/ Possible Points)					

Name _____ **Date** _____ **Score** _____

WORK DOCUMENTATION

_____

Instructor's/Evaluator's Comments and Suggestions:

_____

_____

_____

_____

_____

CHECK #1

Evaluator's Signature: _____ Date:

CHECK #2

Evaluator's Signature: _____ Date:

CHECK #3

Evaluator's Signature: _____ Date:

ABHES Competency: VI.A.1.a.4.dd Perform electrocardiograms

CAAHEP Curriculum: I.P.5 Perform electrocardiography

Name _____ **Date** _____ **Score** _____

COMPETENCY ASSESSMENT

Procedure 39-1   Using the Microscope

Task: To properly use a microscope to view organisms using the coarse and fine adjustments, as well as the low- and high-power and oil-immersion objectives.

Conditions: Microscope, lens paper, lens cleaner, prepared slides, immersion oil, disinfectant

Standards: Perform the Task within 15 minutes with a minimum score of _____ points.

No.	Step	Points	Check #1	Check #2	Check #3
1	Washed hands.				
2	Set up the microscope, cleaned lens, turned on light, adjusted as needed.				
3	Placed slide properly, adjusted vision.				
4	Handled objectives properly, moved away from the field while using coarse adjustments.				
5	Examined the slide, turned off the light, notified the provider that the slide was ready.				
6	When provider completed the PPMP, cleaned microscope properly and disposed of slide(s) and other samples according to OSHA standards.				
7	Demonstrated professional behavior in manner, organization, and attire, including: • Communicated appropriately and comfortably with the physician.				
Student's Total Points					
Points Possible					
Final Score (Student's Total Points/ Possible Points)					

Name _____   **Date** _____   **Score** _____

Instructor's/Evaluator's Comments and Suggestions:

_____

_____

_____

_____

_____

CHECK #1

Evaluator's Signature: _____   Date:

CHECK #2

Evaluator's Signature: _____   Date:

CHECK #3

Evaluator's Signature: _____   Date:

ABHES Competency: VI.A.1.a.4.g Prepare and maintain examination and treatment area

Name _____   **Date** _____   **Score** _____

COMPETENCY ASSESSMENT

Procedure 40-1   Palpating a Vein and Preparing a Patient for Venipuncture

Task: To palpate for an appropriate vein for venipuncture using a tourniquet.

Conditions: Gloves, alcohol swab, tourniquet

Standards: Perform the Task within 5 minutes with a minimum score of _____ points.

No.	Step	Points	Check #1	Check #2	Check #3
1	Organized equipment and supplies; checked room for cleanliness, equipment, and readiness; washed hands.				
2	Greeted and identified patient and introduced self.				
3	Performed the procedure correctly and safely: • Positioned patient correctly for proper body mechanics. • Exposed arm appropriately. • Applied tourniquet correctly. • Palpated veins to determine depth, direction, characteristics. • Ruled out a pulse that would indicate an artery rather than a vein. • Released tourniquet. • Repeated procedure on other arm if needed.				
4	Demonstrated professional behavior in manner, organization, and attire, including: • Communicated appropriately and comfortably with the patient.				
5	Washed hands.				
Student's Total Points					
Points Possible					
Final Score (Student's Total Points/ Possible Points)					

Name _____ **Date** _____ **Score** _____

Instructor's/Evaluator's Comments and Suggestions:

_____

_____

_____

_____

_____

CHECK #1

Evaluator's Signature: _____ Date: _____

CHECK #2

Evaluator's Signature: _____ Date: _____

CHECK #3

Evaluator's Signature: _____ Date: _____

ABHES Competency: VI.A.1.a.4.b Prepare patients for procedures

Name _____ **Date** _____ **Score** _____

COMPETENCY ASSESSMENT

Procedure 40-2   Venipuncture by Syringe

Task: Using a syringe to obtain venous blood acceptable for laboratory testing as requisitioned by a physician.

Conditions: Gloves, goggles, and mask, 10-mL syringe, 21-gauge safety needle, vacuum tube(s) or special collection tube(s), vacuum tube safety holder, tourniquet, 70% isopropyl alcohol swab, cotton balls, gauze, adhesive bandage or tape, sharps container, test tube rack

Standards: Perform the Task within 15 minutes with a minimum score of _____ points.

*Work
Documentation:*   Patient chart entry, lab requisition

No.	Step	Points	Check #1	Check #2	Check #3
1	Checked provider's orders; organized equipment and supplies; checked room for cleanliness, equipment, and readiness; washed hands.				
2	Correctly prepared the patient: • Greeted and identified patient and introduced self, explained procedure, washed hands. • Identified health concerns, allergies, tetanus status, possible complications, and current medications. • Positioned patient appropriately and comfortably. • Reassured the patient as needed.				
3	Applied appropriate PPE.				
4	Performed the procedure correctly and safely: • Applied tourniquet correctly. • Palpated veins correctly, ruled out artery, planned approach. • Prepped skin. • Performed puncture correctly and safely with minimum of discomfort to patient, did not unduly move the needle during the procedure. • Released tourniquet. • Removed needle safely and comfortably while applying pressure on site. • Selected correct tubes in order and filled them correctly using a rack. • Implemented safety mechanism on syringe/needle unit and disposed of properly. • Applied appropriate dressing.				

No.	Step	Points	Check #1	Check #2	Check #3
5	Disposed of contaminated supplies following OSHA regulations and washed hands.				
6	Demonstrated professional behavior in manner, organization, and attire, including: • Communicated appropriately and comfortably with the patient.				
7	Labeled tubes properly, completed requisition correctly and completely, packaged specimens for transport correctly.				
8	Documented correctly.				
Student's Total Points					
Points Possible					
Final Score (Student's Total Points/ Possible Points)					

Name _____ **Date** _____ **Score** _____

WORK DOCUMENTATION
*Also attach lab requisition.

_____

Instructor's/Evaluator's Comments and Suggestions:

_____

_____

_____

_____

_____

CHECK #1

Evaluator's Signature: Date:

CHECK #2

Evaluator's Signature: Date:

CHECK #3

Evaluator's Signature: Date:

ABHES Competency: VI.A.1.a.4.s Perform venipuncture

CAAHEP Curriculum: I.P.2 Perform venipuncture; III.P.3 Select appropriate barrier/personal protective equipment (PPE) for potentially infectious situations

Name _____ Date _____ Score _____

COMPETENCY ASSESSMENT

Procedure 40-3   Venipuncture by Vacuum Tube System

Task: Using a vacuum tube system to obtain venous blood acceptable for laboratory testing as requisitioned by a physician.

Conditions: Gloves, goggles, and mask, vacuum tube adapter/holder, 21-gauge multidraw needle, vacuum tube(s) or special collection tube(s), tourniquet, 70% isopropyl alcohol swab, cotton balls, adhesive bandage or tape, sharps container

Standards: Perform the Task within 15 minutes with a minimum score of _____ points.

Work Documentation: Patient chart entry, lab requisition

No.	Step	Points	Check #1	Check #2	Check #3
1	Checked provider's orders; organized equipment and supplies; checked room for cleanliness, equipment, and readiness; washed hands.				
2	Correctly prepared the patient: • Greeted and identified patient and introduced self, explained procedure, washed hands. • Identified health concerns, allergies, tetanus status, possible complications, and current medications. • Positioned patient appropriately and comfortably. • Reassured the patient as needed.				
3	Applied appropriate PPE.				
4	Performed the procedure correctly and safely: • Applied tourniquet correctly. • Palpated veins correctly, ruled out artery, planned approach. • Prepped skin. • Performed puncture correctly and safely with minimum of discomfort to the patient, did not move needle during tube changes. • Selected correct tubes in order and filled them correctly. • Released tourniquet. • Removed needle safely and comfortably while applying pressure on site. • Implemented safety mechanism and disposed of properly. • Applied appropriate dressing.				

No.	Step	Points	Check #1	Check #2	Check #3
5	Disposed of contaminated supplies following OSHA regulations; washed hands.				
6	Demonstrated professional behavior in manner, organization, and attire, including: • Communicated appropriately and comfortably with the patient.				
7	Labeled tubes properly, completed requisition correctly and completely, packaged specimens for transport correctly.				
8	Documented correctly.				
Student's Total Points					
Points Possible					
Final Score (Student's Total Points/ Possible Points)					

Name _____ **Date** _____ **Score** _____

WORK DOCUMENTATION

*Also attach lab requisition.

_____

Instructor's/Evaluator's Comments and Suggestions:

_____

_____

_____

_____

_____

CHECK #1

Evaluator's Signature: _____ Date:

CHECK #2

Evaluator's Signature: _____ Date:

CHECK #3

Evaluator's Signature: _____ Date:

ABHES Competency: VI.A.1.a.4.s Perform venipuncture

CAAHEP Curriculum: I.P.2 Perform venipuncture; III.P.3 Select appropriate barrier/personal protective equipment (PPE) for potentially infectious situations

Name _____   Date _____   Score _____

COMPETENCY ASSESSMENT

Procedure 40-4   Venipuncture by Butterfly Needle System

Task: Using a butterfly needle system to obtain venous blood acceptable for laboratory testing as requisitioned by a provider.

Conditions: Gloves, goggles, and mask, vacuum tube adapter/holder (if using a vacuum tube connection), a 10- to 15-mL syringe (if using a syringe connection), butterfly needle system with 21-gauge needle (use a multi-sample needle system with a luer adapter for attaching to the vacuum tube and a hypodermic needle for syringe attachment), vacuum tube rack (syringe collection), vacuum tubes, tourniquet, 70% isopropyl alcohol swab, gauze or cotton balls, adhesive bandage or tape, sharps container

Standards: Perform the Task within 15 minutes with a minimum score of _____ points.

Work Documentation: Patient chart entry, lab requisition

No.	Step	Points	Check #1	Check #2	Check #3
1	Checked provider's orders; organized equipment and supplies; checked room for cleanliness, equipment, and readiness; washed hands.				
2	Correctly prepared the patient: • Greeted and identified patient and introduced self, explained procedure, washed hands. • Identified health concerns, allergies, tetanus status, possible complications, and current medications. • Positioned patient appropriately and comfortably. • Reassured the patient as needed.				
3	Applied appropriate PPE.				
4	Performed the procedure correctly and safely: • Applied tourniquet correctly. • Palpated veins correctly, ruled out artery, planned approach. • Prepped skin. • Performed puncture correctly and safely with minimum of discomfort to the patient, did not move needle during procedure. • If using vacuum system: Selected correct tubes in order and filled them correctly. • Released tourniquet.				

No.	Step	Points	Check #1	Check #2	Check #3
	• Removed needle safely and comfortably while applying pressure on site. • If transferring blood to tubes from syringe: Selected correct tubes in order and filled them correctly using a rack. • Implemented safety mechanism on butterfly unit and disposed of properly. • Applied appropriate dressing.				
5	Disposed of contaminated supplies following OSHA regulations; washed hands.				
6	Demonstrated professional behavior in manner, organization, and attire, including: • Communicated appropriately and comfortably with the patient.				
7	Labeled tubes properly, completed requisition correctly and completely, packaged specimens for transport correctly.				
8	Documented correctly.				
Student's Total Points					
Points Possible					
Final Score (Student's Total Points/ Possible Points)					

Name _____ **Date** _____ **Score** _____

WORK DOCUMENTATION

*Also attach lab requisition.

Instructor's/Evaluator's Comments and Suggestions:

_____

_____

_____

_____

CHECK #1

Evaluator's Signature: Date:

CHECK #2

Evaluator's Signature: Date:

CHECK #3

Evaluator's Signature: Date:

ABHES Competency: VI.A.1.a.4.s Perform venipuncture

CAAHEP Curriculum: I.P.2 Perform venipuncture; III.P.3 Select appropriate barrier/personal protective equipment (PPE) for potentially infectious situations

Name _____ **Date** _____ **Score** _____

COMPETENCY ASSESSMENT

Procedure 40-5   Capillary Puncture

Task: To obtain capillary blood acceptable for laboratory testing as required by a provider.

Conditions: Gloves, goggles, and mask (optional), alcohol swab, microcollection tubes, capillary tubes or specific test kit, safety lancet, gauze, cotton balls, adhesive bandage or tape, sharps container

Standards: Perform the Task within 20 minutes with a minimum score of _____ points.

Work Documentation: Patient chart entry, lab requisition

No.	Step	Points	Check #1	Check #2	Check #3
1	Checked provider's orders; organized equipment and supplies; checked room for cleanliness, equipment, and readiness; washed hands.				
2	Correctly prepared the patient: • Greeted and identified patient and introduced self, explained procedure, washed hands. • Identified health concerns, allergies, tetanus status, possible complications, and current medications. • Positioned patient appropriately and comfortably.				
3	Applied appropriate PPE.				
4	Performed the procedure correctly and safely: • Encouraged good blood flow: Had patient wash hands in warm water. If needed, applied warming pack to fingers. • Encouraged patient to relax and provided a comfortable, relaxing atmosphere. • Selected an appropriate puncture site. • Cleansed the site with alcohol. • Held the finger securely and comfortably. • Performed the puncture correctly and safely with minimum of discomfort to the patient. • Disposed of puncture lancet safely and properly. • Disposed of first drop. • Acquired specimen as needed for test(s). • Applied appropriate dressing to puncture site and held pressure as needed.				

No.	Step	Points	Check #1	Check #2	Check #3
5	Demonstrated professional behavior in manner, organization, and attire, including: • Communicated appropriately and comfortably with the patient.				
6	Disposed of contaminated supplies following OSHA regulations; washed hands.				
7	Processed specimens as requisitioned or labeled containers properly, completed requisition correctly and completely, packaged specimens for transport correctly.				
8	Documented correctly.				
Student's Total Points					
Points Possible					
Final Score (Student's Total Points/ Possible Points)					

Name _____ **Date** _____ **Score** _____

WORK DOCUMENTATION

*Also attach lab requisition.

Instructor's/Evaluator's Comments and Suggestions:

_____

_____

_____

_____

_____

CHECK #1	
Evaluator's Signature:	Date:

CHECK #2	
Evaluator's Signature:	Date:

CHECK #3	
Evaluator's Signature:	Date:

ABHES Competency: VI.A.1.a.4.t Perform capillary puncture

CAAHEP Curriculum: I.P.3 Perform capillary puncture; III.P.3 Select appropriate barrier/personal protective equipment (PPE) for potentially infectious situations

Name _____ Date _____ Score _____

COMPETENCY ASSESSMENT

Procedure 40-6   Obtaining a Capillary Specimen for Transport Using a Microtainer Transport Unit

Task: To obtain a specimen of capillary blood for transport to a laboratory for testing, using a Microtainer transport unit.

Standards: Capillary puncture supplies (gloves, alcohol pad, safety lancet, cotton ball, adhesive bandage), Microtainer transport unit, laboratory requisition, small sturdy container with a tightly fitting lid (such as a urine specimen cup), pen, biohazard specimen transport bag

Standards: Perform the Task within 20 minutes with a minimum score of _____ points.

Work Documentation: Patient chart entry

No.	Step	Points	Check #1	Check #2	Check #3
1	Checked provider's orders; organized equipment and supplies; checked room for cleanliness, equipment, and readiness; washed hands.				
2	Correctly prepared the patient: • Greeted and identified patient and introduced self, explained procedure, washed hands. • Identified health concerns, allergies, tetanus status, possible complications, and current medications. • Positioned patient appropriately and comfortably.				
3	Applied appropriate PPE.				
4	Performed the procedure correctly and safely: • Encouraged good blood flow: Had patient wash hands in warm water. If needed, applied warming pack to the fingers. • Encouraged the patient to relax and provided a comfortable, relaxing atmosphere. • Selected an appropriate puncture site. • Cleansed the site with alcohol. • Held the finger securely and comfortably. • Performed puncture correctly and safely with minimum of discomfort to patient.				

No.	Step	Points	Check #1	Check #2	Check #3
	• Disposed of puncture lancet safely and properly. • Disposed of first drop. • Scooped the blood drops into Microtainer tube properly, agitating tube after each drop to mix well. Filled Microtainer tube as needed for tests. • Removed scoop and capped tube. • Applied appropriate dressing to puncture site and held pressure as needed.				
5	Disposed of contaminated supplies following OSHA regulations.				
6	Placed tube into capped transport container and washed hands.				
7	Demonstrated professional behavior in manner, organization, and attire, including: • Communicated appropriately and comfortably with the patient.				
8	Labeled containers properly, completed requisition correctly and completely, packaged specimens for transport correctly.				
9	Documented correctly.				
Student's Total Points					
Points Possible					
Final Score (Student's Total Points/ Possible Points)					

Name _____ **Date** _____ **Score** _____

WORK DOCUMENTATION

_____

Instructor's/Evaluator's Comments and Suggestions:

_____

_____

_____

_____

_____

CHECK #1

Evaluator's Signature: Date:

CHECK #2

Evaluator's Signature: Date:

CHECK #3

Evaluator's Signature: Date:

ABHES Competency: VI.A.1.a.4.t Perform capillary puncture

CAAHEP Curriculum: I.P.3 Perform capillary puncture; III.P.3 Select appropriate barrier/personal protective equipment (PPE) for potentially infectious situations

Name _____ **Date** _____ **Score** _____

COMPETENCY ASSESSMENT

Procedure 40-7   Obtaining Blood for Blood Culture

Task: While performing venipuncture from two separate sites, prepare two culture bottles of blood from each site for culture (four total).

Conditions: Nonsterile gloves for use with povidone-iodine solution; sterile gloves; laboratory requisition; blood cultures, anaerobic and aerobic (usually four: two bottles each for two sets of cultures); 70% isopropyl alcohol; povidone-iodine solution swabs or towelettes; venipuncture supplies (according to method used) for two separate sites; biohazard red bag; biohazard sharps container; labeling pen

Standards: Perform the Task within 20 minutes with a minimum score of _____ points.

*Work
Documentation:* Patient chart entry, lab requisition, bottle labels

No.	Step	Points	Check #1	Check #2	Check #3
1	Checked provider's orders; organized equipment and supplies; checked room for cleanliness, equipment, and readiness; washed hands.				
2	Correctly prepared the patient: • Greeted and identified patient and introduced self, explained procedure, washed hands. • Identified health concerns, allergies, tetanus status, possible complications, and current medications. • Determined that the patient has not already started antibiotic therapy. • Positioned patient appropriately and comfortably.				
3	Applied appropriate PPE.				
4	Performed the procedures correctly and safely: • Prepped the skin with iodine surgical prep, allowing the prep to air dry for 1 full minute. • Did not touch the prepped area. • Cleansed the culture bottle tops with surgical prep solution. • Applied sterile gloves. • Performed venipuncture properly and safely. • Mixed the specimens into the culture media by inverting 8–10 times. • Repeated procedure at a second site within 30 minutes.				

No.	Step	Points	Check #1	Check #2	Check #3
5	Disposed of contaminated supplies following OSHA regulations, disinfected surfaces, and washed hands.				
6	Demonstrated professional behavior in manner, organization, and attire, including: • Communicated appropriately and comfortably with the patient.				
7	Labeled bottles correctly and completed the requisitions correctly according to the laboratory manual instructions. Provided all the information required and held pressure as needed.				
8	Documented correctly.				
	Student's Total Points				
	Points Possible				
	Final Score (Student's Total Points/ Possible Points)				

Name _____   **Date** _____   **Score** _____

WORK DOCUMENTATION

*Also attach lab requisition.

_____

Instructor's/Evaluator's Comments and Suggestions:

_____

_____

_____

_____

_____

CHECK #1

Evaluator's Signature: _____   Date:

CHECK #2

Evaluator's Signature: _____   Date:

CHECK #3

Evaluator's Signature: _____   Date:

ABHES Competency: VI.A.1.a.4.s Perform venipuncture

CAAHEP Curriculum: I.P.2 Perform venipuncture; III.P.3 Select appropriate barrier/personal protective equipment (PPE) for potentially infectious situations

Name _____ Date _____ Score _____

COMPETENCY ASSESSMENT

Procedure 41-1   Hemoglobin Determination Using a CLIA Waived Hemoglobin Analyzer

Task: To properly and safely perform an automated hemoglobin determination to evaluate the oxygen capacity of the blood.

Conditions: Gloves, disinfectant, capillary puncture equipment or blood samples collected in EDTA, HemoCue® system or other hemoglobin analyzer with supplies appropriate for the analyzer, biohazard red bag, biohazard sharps container

Standards: Perform the Task within 20 minutes with a minimum score of _____ points.

Work Documentation: Patient chart entry, lab report

No.	Step	Points	Check #1	Check #2	Check #3
1	Checked provider's orders; organized equipment and supplies, turned on instrument; checked room for cleanliness, equipment, and readiness.				
2	Correctly prepared the patient: • Greeted and identified patient and introduced self, explained procedure, washed hands. • Identified health concerns, allergies, tetanus status, possible complications, and current medications. • Positioned patient appropriately and comfortably.				
3	Applied appropriate PPE.				
4	Performed the procedure correctly and safely: • Performed capillary puncture correctly and safely. • Obtained specimen properly. • Inserted specimen into machine following manufacturer's instructions. • Performed test according to instructions. • Recorded the results.				
5	Disposed of contaminated supplies following OSHA regulations; cleaned and stored machine, disinfected surfaces, washed hands.				

No.	Step	Points	Check #1	Check #2	Check #3
6	Demonstrated professional behavior in manner, organization, and attire, including: • Communicated appropriately and comfortably with the patient.				
7	Documented correctly.				
Student's Total Points					
Points Possible					
Final Score (Student's Total Points/ Possible Points)					

Name _____ **Date** _____ **Score** _____

WORK DOCUMENTATION
*Also attach lab report.

_____

Instructor's/Evaluator's Comments and Suggestions:

_____

_____

_____

_____

_____

CHECK #1 Evaluator's Signature: Date:

CHECK #2 Evaluator's Signature: Date:

CHECK #3 Evaluator's Signature: Date:

ABHES Competency: VI.A.1.a.4.j Collect and process specimens; VI.A.1.a.4.t Perform capillary puncture; VI.A.1.a.4.z Perform hematology

CAAHEP Curriculum: I.P.3 Perform capillary puncture; I.P.12 Perform hematology testing

Name _____ Date _____ Score _____

COMPETENCY ASSESSMENT

Procedure 41-2   Microhematocrit Determination

Task: To properly and safely perform the microhematocrit procedure using a few microliters of blood in a capillary tube to separate the cellular elements of the blood from the plasma by centrifugation.

Conditions: Gloves, capillary tubes (heparinized), sealing clay, microhematocrit centrifuge and reader, alcohol swabs, gauze and cotton balls, safety lancets, adhesive strip, disinfectant, biohazard red bag, sharps container. OPTIONAL: If obtaining blood from a vacuum tube: vacuum tube of anticoagulated blood, safety shield for cap removal, face shield

Standards: Perform the Task within 15 minutes with a minimum score of _____ points.

Work Documentation: Patient chart entry, lab report

No.	Step	Points	Check #1	Check #2	Check #3
1	Checked provider's orders; organized equipment and supplies, turned on instrument; checked room for cleanliness, equipment, and readiness.				
2	Correctly prepared the patient: • Greeted and identified patient and introduced self, explained procedure, washed hands. • Identified health concerns, allergies, tetanus status, possible complications, and current medications. • Positioned patient appropriately and comfortably.				
3	Applied appropriate PPE.				
4	Performed the procedure correctly and safely: • Performed capillary puncture correctly and safely. • Filled two tubes using proper technique. • Loaded tubes into machine correctly. • Centrifuged correctly. • Read and recorded the averaged results.				
5	Disposed of contaminated supplies following OSHA regulations; cleaned and stored machine, disinfected surfaces, washed hands.				
6	Demonstrated professional behavior in manner, organization, and attire, including: • Communicated appropriately and comfortably with the patient.				
7	Documented correctly.				
	Student's Total Points				
	Points Possible				
	Final Score (Student's Total Points/ Possible Points)				

Name _____   **Date** _____   **Score** _____

WORK DOCUMENTATION
*Also attach lab report.

_____

Instructor's/Evaluator's Comments and Suggestions:

_____

_____

_____

_____

_____

CHECK #1

Evaluator's Signature: _____   Date: _____

CHECK #2

Evaluator's Signature: _____   Date: _____

CHECK #3

Evaluator's Signature: _____   Date: _____

ABHES Competency: VI.A.1.a.4.j Collect and process specimens; VI.A.1.a.4.t Perform capillary puncture; VI.A.1.a.4.z Perform hematology

CAAHEP Curriculum: I.P.3 Perform capillary puncture; I.P.12 Perform hematology testing

Name _____   Date _____   Score _____

COMPETENCY ASSESSMENT

Procedure 41-3   Erythrocyte Sedimentation Rate

Task: To properly and safely perform an erythrocyte sedimentation rate (ESR).

Conditions: Gloves, sample of venous blood collected in EDTA, Sediplast® or other ESR kit (sedivial and sedirack, Sediplast® autozeroing pipette, pipette capable of delivering up to 1.0 mL), Wintrobe method (Wintrobe sedimentation tube, Wintrobe sedimentation rack, long-stem Pasteur-type pipette with rubber bulb), timer, 10% chlorine bleach solution/disinfectant, face shield or goggles and mask, biohazard red bag for waste, sharps container

Standards: Perform the Task within 75 minutes with a minimum score of _____ points.

Work Documentation: Patient chart entry, lab report

No.	Step	Points	Check #1	Check #2	Check #3
1	Checked provider's orders; organized equipment and supplies, turned on instrument; checked room for cleanliness, equipment, and readiness.				
2	Correctly prepared the patient: • Greeted and identified patient and introduced self, explained procedure, washed hands. • Identified health concerns, allergies, tetanus status, possible complications, and current medications. • Positioned patient appropriately and comfortably.				
3	Applied appropriate PPE.				
4	Performed the procedure correctly and safely: • Performed venipuncture correctly and safely. • Performed either the Sediplast ESR or Wintrobe method correctly, following manufacturer's and lab manual instructions. • After 1 hour of undisturbed sedimentation, observed and recorded the ESR results.				
5	Disposed of contaminated supplies following OSHA regulations; cleaned and stored equipment, disinfected surfaces, washed hands.				
6	Demonstrated professional behavior in manner, organization, and attire, including: • Communicated appropriately and comfortably with the patient.				
7	Documented correctly.				
Student's Total Points					
Points Possible					
Final Score (Student's Total Points/ Possible Points)					

Name _____ **Date** _____ **Score** _____

WORK DOCUMENTATION
*Also attach lab report.

_____

Instructor's/Evaluator's Comments and Suggestions:

_____
_____
_____
_____
_____

CHECK #1

Evaluator's Signature: Date:

CHECK #2

Evaluator's Signature: Date:

CHECK #3

Evaluator's Signature: Date:

ABHES Competency: VI.A.1.a.4.j Collect and process specimens; VI.A.1.a.4.s Perform venipuncture; VI.A.1.a.4.z Perform hematology

CAAHEP Curriculum: I.P.2 Perform venipuncture; I.P.12 Perform hematology testing

Name _____   Date _____   Score _____

COMPETENCY ASSESSMENT

Procedure 41-4   Prothrombin Time (Using CLIA Waived ProTime Analyzer)

Task: Properly and safely perform an automated prothrombin time determination to evaluate the clotting time of a drop of blood.

Condition: Gloves, biohazard container, sharps container, capillary puncture equipment, alcohol wipes, safety lancet, cotton ball, gauze 2 × 2, adhesive bandage, CLIA Waived ProTime Analyzer with accessories

Standards: Perform the Task within 15 minutes with a minimum score of _____ points.

Work Documentation: Patient chart entry, lab report

No.	Step	Points	Check #1	Check #2	Check #3
1	Checked provider's orders; checked room for cleanliness, equipment, and readiness; organized equipment and supplies, turned on and prepared instrument.				
2	Correctly prepared the patient: • Greeted and identified patient and introduced self, explained procedure, washed hands. • Identified health concerns, allergies, tetanus status, possible complications, and current medications. • Positioned patient appropriately and comfortably.				
3	Applied appropriate PPE.				
4	Performed the procedure correctly and safely: • Performed capillary puncture correctly and safely. • Filled Tenderlett lancet cup to fill line and placed onto the cuvette; pressed start. • Applied cotton ball to patient's arm and held pressure for 3–5 minutes. • When prompted by machine, removed device and discarded into sharps container. • Read and recorded clotting time and INR.				
	Alerted provider immediately if results fell into critical range.				

No.	Step	Points	Check #1	Check #2	Check #3
5	Disposed of contaminated supplies following OSHA regulations; cleaned and stored equipment, disinfected surfaces, washed hands.				
6	Demonstrated professional behavior in manner, organization, and attire, including: • Communicated appropriately and comfortably with the patient.				
7	Documented correctly.				
Student's Total Points					
Points Possible					
Final Score (Student's Total Points/ Possible Points)					

Name _____   **Date** _____   **Score** _____

WORK DOCUMENTATION
*Also attach lab report.

Instructor's/Evaluator's Comments and Suggestions:

_____

_____

_____

_____

_____

| **CHECK #1** | |
| Evaluator's Signature: | Date: |

| **CHECK #2** | |
| Evaluator's Signature: | Date: |

| **CHECK #3** | |
| Evaluator's Signature: | Date: |

ABHES Competency: VI.A.1.a.4.j Collect and process specimens; VI.A.1.a.4.t Perform capillary puncture; VI.A.1.a.4.z Perform hematology

CAAHEP Curriculum: I.P.3 Perform capillary puncture; I.P.12 Perform hematology testing

Name _____ Date _____ Score _____

COMPETENCY ASSESSMENT

Procedure 42-1 Assessing Urine Volume, Color, and Clarity

Task: Determine and document the volume, color, and clarity of a urine sample.

Conditions: Gloves, urine specimen in labeled, clear urine cup with secure lid, biohazard container, disinfectant cleaner, laboratory report form

Standards: Perform the Task within 5 minutes with a minimum score of _____ points.

Work Documentation: Patient chart entry, lab report

No.	Step	Points	Check #1	Check #2	Check #3
1	Washed hands, organized supplies and equipment, and applied appropriate PPE.				
2	Examined specimen for proper labeling. With lid tightly sealed, mixed urine well.				
3	Noted the amount of urine in the cup (in milliliters).				
4	Assessed and noted the urine color against a white background with good lighting.				
5	Assessed the clarity of the urine using the white background. Recorded any cloudiness as appropriate.				
6	Disposed of contaminated supplies following OSHA regulations; disinfected surfaces; washed hands.				
7	Demonstrated professional behavior in manner, organization, and attire.				
8	Documented correctly.				
Student's Total Points					
Points Possible					
Final Score (Student's Total Points/ Possible Points)					

Name _____ **Date** _____ **Score** _____

WORK DOCUMENTATION
*Also attach lab report.

_____

Instructor's/Evaluator's Comments and Suggestions:

_____

_____

_____

_____

_____

CHECK #1	
Evaluator's Signature:	Date:

CHECK #2	
Evaluator's Signature:	Date:

CHECK #3	
Evaluator's Signature:	Date:

ABHES Competency: VI.A.1.a.4.j Collect and process specimens; VI.A.1.a.4.y Perform urinalysis

CAAHEP Curriculum: I.P.14 Perform urinalysis

Name _____   **Date** _____   **Score** _____

COMPETENCY ASSESSMENT

Procedure 42-2   Using the Refractometer to Measure Specific Gravity

Task: Measure and record the specific gravity of a urine specimen.

Conditions: Refractometer, gloves, urine sample, pipettes, distilled water, lint-free (lens) tissues, bio-hazard container, disinfectant, laboratory report form

Standards: Perform the Task within 5 minutes with a minimum score of _____ points.

Work Documentation: Patient chart entry

No.	Step	Points	Check #1	Check #2	Check #3
1	Washed hands, organized supplies and equipment, and applied appropriate PPE.				
2	Performed quality control on the refractometer by checking it using distilled water. Calibrated as needed.				
3	Examined specimen for proper labeling. With lid tightly sealed, mixed urine well.				
4	Applied urine to the refractometer according to manufacturer's instructions. Read and noted the specific gravity.				
5	Disposed of contaminated supplies following OSHA regulations; cleaned and stored equipment; disinfected surfaces; washed hands.				
6	Demonstrated professional behavior in manner, organization, and attire.				
7	Documented correctly.				
Student's Total Points					
Points Possible					
Final Score (Student's Total Points/ Possible Points)					

Name _____   **Date** _____   **Score** _____

WORK DOCUMENTATION

Instructor's/Evaluator's Comments and Suggestions:

_____

_____

_____

_____

_____

CHECK #1 Evaluator's Signature: Date:

CHECK #2 Evaluator's Signature: Date:

CHECK #3 Evaluator's Signature: Date:

ABHES Competency: VI.A.1.a.4.i Use quality control; VI.A.1.a.4.j Collect and process specimens; VI.A.1.a.4.y Perform urinalysis

CAAHEP Curriculum: I.P.11 Perform quality control measures; I.P.14 Perform urinalysis

Name _____ **Date** _____ **Score** _____

COMPETENCY ASSESSMENT

Procedure 42-3   Performing a Urinalysis Chemical Examination

Task: Detect any abnormal chemical constituents of a urine specimen.

Conditions: Gloves, urine test strips, urine specimen, paper towel, biohazard container, disinfectant cleaner, laboratory report form

Standards: Perform the Task within 15 minutes with a minimum score of _____ points.

Work Documentation: Patient chart entry, lab report

No.	Step	Points	Check #1	Check #2	Check #3
1	Washed hands, organized supplies and equipment, checked expiration date on bottle of test strips, applied appropriate PPE.				
2	Examined specimen for proper labeling. With lid tightly sealed, mixed urine well.				
3	Performed the procedure correctly and safely: • Opened container of test strips, set lid down properly. Selected one test strip properly without contaminating other strips. Secured lid back onto container. • Dipped the strip into the urine completely, tapped edge onto paper towel. • Held strip close to color chart but did not touch it. Timed each test properly while comparing strip with chart, noting results.				
4	Disposed of contaminated supplies following OSHA regulations; disinfected surfaces; washed hands.				
5	Demonstrated professional behavior in manner, organization, and attire.				
6	Documented correctly.				
Student's Total Points					
Points Possible					
Final Score (Student's Total Points/ Possible Points)					

Name _____   **Date** _____   **Score** _____

WORK DOCUMENTATION
*Also attach lab report.

_____

Instructor's/Evaluator's Comments and Suggestions:

_____

_____

_____

_____

_____

CHECK #1
Evaluator's Signature: Date:

CHECK #2
Evaluator's Signature: Date:

CHECK #3
Evaluator's Signature: Date:

ABHES Competency: VI.A.1.a.4.j Collect and process specimens; VI.A.1.a.4.y Perform urinalysis

CAAHEP Curriculum: I.P.14 Perform urinalysis

Name _____   **Date** _____   **Score** _____

COMPETENCY ASSESSMENT

Procedure 42-4   Preparing Slide for Microscopic Examination of Urine Sediment

Task: Prepare a slide for a microscopic examination of urine sediment.

Conditions: Gloves, microscope, centrifuge, microscope slides, cover slips, disposable pipette, centrifuge tubes and holder, urine specimen, urine atlas guide, disinfectant cleaner, biohazard container, sharps container, Sedi-Stain® (optional)

Standards: Perform the Task within 15 minutes with a minimum score of _____ points.

Work Documentation: Patient chart entry, lab report

No.	Step	Points	Check #1	Check #2	Check #3
1	Washed hands, organized supplies and equipment, set up microscope, applied appropriate PPE.				
2	Examined specimen for proper labeling. With lid tightly sealed, mixed urine well.				
3	Correctly processed specimen in centrifuge: • Labeled centrifuge tube. • Poured 12–15 mL of urine into tube. • Placed tube into centrifuge, balancing as needed. • Secured lid on centrifuge. • Centrifuged specimen at 1500 rpm for 5 minutes.				
4	Poured off supernatant.				
5	Correctly prepared slide: • Mixed sediment to dislodge and evenly disperse. Applied 2 drops of Sedi-Stain® to sediment if desired. Mixed well. • Used pipette to apply one drop of sediment to center of microscope slide. Applied cover slip smoothly, without air bubbles. • Placed slide onto microscope stage, adjusting for provider viewing. Turned light off until provider was ready. If medical assistant viewed slide for educational purposes, prepared fresh slide for provider.				

No.	Step	Points	Check #1	Check #2	Check #3
6	Removed PPE, washed hands, and prepared lab report for provider to complete.				
7	Disposed of contaminated supplies following OSHA regulations; disinfected surfaces; washed hands.				
8	Demonstrated professional behavior in manner, organization, and attire.				
9	Documented correctly.				
Student's Total Points					
Points Possible					
Final Score (Student's Total Points/ Possible Points)					

Name _____ **Date** _____ **Score** _____

WORK DOCUMENTATION
*Also attach lab report.

_____

Instructor's/Evaluator's Comments and Suggestions:

_____

_____

_____

_____

_____

CHECK #1 Evaluator's Signature: Date:

CHECK #2 Evaluator's Signature: Date:

CHECK #3 Evaluator's Signature: Date:

ABHES Competency: VI.A.1.a.4.j Collect and process specimens; VI.A.1.a.4.y Perform urinalysis

CAAHEP Curriculum: I.P.14 Perform urinalysis

Name _____ **Date** _____ **Score** _____

COMPETENCY ASSESSMENT

Procedure 42-5   Performing a Complete Urinalysis

Task:　　　　　Perform a complete urinalysis, including the physical and chemical examinations, and prepare for the microscopic examination test within 30 minutes of obtaining the specimen.

Conditions:　　Gloves, patient preparation supplies and information, urine specimen, pipettes, centrifuge tube, centrifuge, microscope, microscope slides, cover slip, permanent marker, urine test strips, urine atlas, refractometer, distilled water, lint-free tissues, biohazard container, sharps container, disinfectant cleaner, laboratory report form, Sedi-Stain® (optional)

Standards:　　Perform the Task within 15 minutes with a minimum score of _____ points.

Work Documentation:　　Patient chart entry, lab report

No.	Step	Points	Check #1	Check #2	Check #3
1	Washed hands, organized supplies and equipment, set up microscope, applied appropriate PPE.				
2	Examined specimen for proper labeling. With lid tightly sealed, mixed urine well.				
3	Properly performed centrifugation of 12–15 mL of urine.				
4	While specimen was spinning, properly performed physical and chemical examination of urine, documenting results correctly and completely.				
5	After specimen was spun, prepared microscope slide for provider. Turned light off to preserve specimen. If desired, prepared another slide for self to view for educational purposes.				
6	Disposed of contaminated supplies following OSHA regulations; disinfected surfaces; removed PPE; washed hands.				
7	Demonstrated professional behavior in manner, organization, and attire.				
8	Documented correctly.				
Student's Total Points					
Points Possible					
Final Score (Student's Total Points/ Possible Points)					

Name _____   **Date** _____   **Score** _____

WORK DOCUMENTATION
*Also attach lab report.

_____

Instructor's/Evaluator's Comments and Suggestions:

_____

_____

_____

_____

_____

CHECK #1
Evaluator's Signature: Date:

CHECK #2
Evaluator's Signature: Date:

CHECK #3
Evaluator's Signature: Date:

ABHES Competency: VI.A.1.a.4.i Use quality control; VI.A.1.a.4.j Collect and process specimens; VI.A.1.a.4.y Perform urinalysis

CAAHEP Curriculum: I.P.11 Perform quality control measures; I.P.14 Perform urinalysis

Name _____   Date _____   Score _____

COMPETENCY ASSESSMENT

Procedure 42-6   Utilizing a Urine Transport System for C&S

Task: Perform a complete urinalysis, including the physical and chemical examinations, and prepare for the microscopic examination test within 30 minutes of obtaining the specimen.

Conditions: Gloves, patient preparation supplies and information, urine specimen, pipettes, centrifuge tube, centrifuge, microscope, microscope slides, cover slip, permanent marker, urine test strips, urine atlas, refractometer, distilled water, lint-free tissues, biohazard container, sharps container, disinfectant cleaner, laboratory report form, Sedi-Stain® (optional)

Standards: Perform the Task within 15 minutes with a minimum score of _____ points.

Work Documentation: Patient chart entry, lab requisition, practice label

No.	Step	Points	Check #1	Check #2	Check #3
1	Washed hands, organized supplies and equipment, set up microscope, applied appropriate PPE.				
2	Examined specimen for proper labeling. With lid tightly sealed, mixed urine well.				
3	Correctly performed the procedure: • Checked the urine culture and sensitivity transport kit expiration date. • Followed the manufacturer's instructions exactly, which will vary, depending on the system being used. • Secured and labeled the transport container and placed it into biohazard transport bag.				
4	Completed requisition correctly and placed it into biohazard transport bag.				
5	Disposed of contaminated supplies following OSHA regulations; disinfected surfaces; removed PPE; washed hands.				
6	Demonstrated professional behavior in manner, organization, and attire.				
7	Documented correctly.				
Student's Total Points					
Points Possible					
Final Score (Student's Total Points/ Possible Points)					

Name _____ Date _____ Score _____

WORK DOCUMENTATION
*Also attach lab requisition.

_____

Instructor's/Evaluator's Comments and Suggestions:

_____
_____
_____
_____
_____

CHECK #1

Evaluator's Signature: _____ Date:

CHECK #2

Evaluator's Signature: _____ Date:

CHECK #3

Evaluator's Signature: _____ Date:

ABHES Competency: VI.A.1.a.4.j Collect and process specimens; VI.A.1.a.4.y Perform urinalysis

CAAHEP Curriculum: I.P.14 Perform urinalysis

Name _____   Date _____   Score _____

COMPETENCY ASSESSMENT

Procedure 42-7   Instructing a Patient in the Collection of a Clean-Catch, Midstream Urine Specimen

Task: To instruct a patient in the proper technique of collecting a urine specimen suitable for urinalysis testing.

Conditions: Gloves, urine cup with a secure lid, cleansing towelettes, marking pen, written instructions posted appropriately in the bathroom

Standards: Perform the Task within 15 minutes with a minimum score of _____ points.

No.	Step	Points	Check #1	Check #2	Check #3
1	Checked room for cleanliness, equipment, and readiness; organized supplies and equipment; washed hands.				
2	Greeted and identified the patient and introduced self. Explained the procedure. Provided patient with written instructions so she could read along as medical assistant instructs.				
3	Provided patient with cleansing wipes, gloves, and labeled urine container with lid.				
4	Escorted patient to restroom and pointed out the written instructions on the wall beside the toilet. Instructed her where to place specimen when finished and how to get back to the examination room if not available to escort her. If possible, escorted patient back to examination room.				
5	Demonstrated professional behavior in manner, organization, and attire, including: • Communicated appropriately and comfortably with the patient.				
Student's Total Points					
Points Possible					
Final Score (Student's Total Points/ Possible Points)					

Name _____   **Date** _____   **Score** _____

Instructor's/Evaluator's Comments and Suggestions:

_____

_____

_____

_____

_____

CHECK #1

Evaluator's Signature: _____   Date:

CHECK #2

Evaluator's Signature: _____   Date:

CHECK #3

Evaluator's Signature: _____   Date:

ABHES Competency: VI.A.1.a.4.w Instruct patients in the collection of a clean-catch mid-stream urine specimen

CAAHEP Curriculum: IV.P.2 Report relevant information to others succinctly and accurately; IV.P.6 Prepare a patient for procedures and/or treatments

Name _____   Date _____   Score _____

COMPETENCY ASSESSMENT

Procedure 43-1   Procedure for Obtaining a Throat Specimen for Culture

Task: To obtain secretions from the nasopharnyx and tonsillar area as a means of identifying pathogenic microorganisms.

Conditions: Tongue depressor, culture tube with applicator stick or commercially prepared culture collection system (culturette), label and requisition form, gloves and face shield, good light source, emesis basin and tissues

Standards: Perform the Task within 15 minutes with a minimum score of _____ points.

Work Documentation: Patient chart entry, lab report

No.	Step	Points	Check #1	Check #2	Check #3
1	Washed hands; checked room for cleanliness, equipment, and readiness; organized supplies and equipment.				
2	Greeted and identified the patient and introduced self. Explained the procedure and washed hands.				
3	Provided the patient with emesis basin and tissues and positioned the patient appropriately. Applied appropriate PPE.				
4	Obtained the specimen properly.				
5	Handled and labeled the specimen properly.				
6	Disposed of contaminated supplies following OSHA regulations; disinfected surfaces; washed hands.				
7	Demonstrated professional behavior in manner, organization, and attire, including: • Communicated appropriately and comfortably with the patient.				
8	Documented correctly.				
Student's Total Points					
Points Possible					
Final Score (Student's Total Points/ Possible Points)					

Name _____ **Date** _____ **Score** _____

WORK DOCUMENTATION
*Also attach lab report.

_____

Instructor's/Evaluator's Comments and Suggestions:

_____

_____

_____

_____

_____

CHECK #1

Evaluator's Signature: Date:

CHECK #2

Evaluator's Signature: Date:

CHECK #3

Evaluator's Signature: Date:

ABHES Competency: VI.A.1.a.4.u Obtain throat specimen for microbiological testing

CAAHEP Curriculum: III.P.7 Obtain specimens for microbiological testing

Name _____ **Date** _____ **Score** _____

COMPETENCY ASSESSMENT

Procedure 43-2   Wet Mount and Hanging Drop Slide Preparations

Task: To prepare a slide for viewing live microorganisms for motility and identifying characteristics.

Conditions: Gloves, glass slide and cover slip, special slide with a well, petroleum jelly, dropper

Standards: Perform the Task within 15 minutes with a minimum score of _____ points.

No.	Step	Points	Check #1	Check #2	Check #3
1	Washed hands; organized supplies and equipment; applied appropriate PPE.				
2	Prepared the wet mount appropriately.				
3	Prepared the hanging drop slide appropriately.				
4	Obtained the specimen properly.				
5	Disposed of contaminated supplies following OSHA regulations; disinfected surfaces; washed hands.				
6	Demonstrated professional behavior in manner, organization, and attire.				
Student's Total Points					
Points Possible					
Final Score (Student's Total Points/ Possible Points)					

Name _____ **Date** _____ **Score** _____

Instructor's/Evaluator's Comments and Suggestions:

_____

_____

_____

_____

_____

CHECK #1

Evaluator's Signature: _____ Date:

CHECK #2

Evaluator's Signature: _____ Date:

CHECK #3

Evaluator's Signature: _____ Date:

ABHES Competency: VI.A.1.a.4.j Collect and process specimens

Name _____   Date _____   Score _____

COMPETENCY ASSESSMENT

Procedure 43-3   Performing Strep Throat Testing

Task: To test for streptococcus infection of the throat for diagnostic purposes. The following steps are intentionally general, so a variety of kits can be used.

Conditions: Gloves, commercial strep throat testing kit including controls and standards, disinfectant, tongue blade, adjustable light source, biohazard container

Standards: Perform the Task within 15 minutes with a minimum score of _____ points.

Work Documentation: Patient chart entry, lab report

No.	Step	Points	Check #1	Check #2	Check #3
1	Washed hands; checked room for cleanliness, equipment, and readiness; organized supplies and equipment.				
2	Greeted and identified the patient and introduced self. Explained the procedure and washed hands.				
3	Provided the patient with emesis basin and tissues and positioned the patient appropriately. Applied appropriate PPE.				
4	Obtained the specimen properly.				
5	Handled and labeled the specimen properly.				
6	Tested the specimen according to the test kit's manufacturer's instructions, following instructions exactly.				
7	Disposed of contaminated supplies following OSHA regulations; disinfected surfaces; washed hands.				
8	Demonstrated professional behavior in manner, organization, and attire, including: • Communicated appropriately and comfortably with the patient.				
9	Documented correctly.				
Student's Total Points					
Points Possible					
Final Score (Student's Total Points/ Possible Points)					

Name _____   **Date** _____   **Score** _____

WORK DOCUMENTATION

*Also attach lab report.

_____

Instructor's/Evaluator's Comments and Suggestions:

_____

_____

_____

_____

_____

CHECK #1

Evaluator's Signature: Date:

CHECK #2

Evaluator's Signature: Date:

CHECK #3

Evaluator's Signature: Date:

ABHES Competency: VI.A.1.a.4.u Obtain throat specimen for microbiological testing; VI.A.1.a.4.cc Perform microbiology testing

CAAHEP Curriculum: III.P.7 Obtain specimens for microbiological testing; III.P.8 Perform CLIA waived microbiology testing

Name _____ **Date** _____ **Score** _____

COMPETENCY ASSESSMENT

Procedure 43-4 Instructing a Patient on Obtaining a Fecal Specimen

Task: To instruct a patient in the correct collection of a fecal sample.

Condition: Gloves, biohazard container, sturdy and opaque waterproof specimen container with a securely fitting lid, special laboratory manual instructions if needed

Standards: Perform the Task within 15 minutes with a minimum score of _____ points.

Work Documentation: Patient chart entry

No.	Step	Points	Check #1	Check #2	Check #3
1	Checked room for cleanliness, equipment, and readiness; organized supplies and equipment; washed hands.				
2	Greeted and identified the patient and introduced self. Explained the procedure and provided patient with written instructions as well.				
3	Handed patient the labeled specimen container and instructed patient to deposit a sample of stool into the cup, then securely set the lid. Cautioned patient not to contaminate specimen with urine.				
4	Gave the patient a biohazard transport bag and instructions on which pocket to put the specimen into and how to secure the bag.				
5	Instructed patient to transport the specimen as soon as possible to the lab, keeping the specimen at or just below body temperature.				
6	Demonstrated professional behavior in manner, organization, and attire, including: • Communicated appropriately and comfortably with the patient.				
7	Documented correctly.				
	Student's Total Points				
	Points Possible				
	Final Score (Student's Total Points/ Possible Points)				

Name _____ **Date** _____ **Score** _____

WORK DOCUMENTATION

_____

Instructor's/Evaluator's Comments and Suggestions:

_____

_____

_____

_____

_____

| **CHECK #1** | |
| Evaluator's Signature: | Date: |

| **CHECK #2** | |
| Evaluator's Signature: | Date: |

| **CHECK #3** | |
| Evaluator's Signature: | Date: |

ABHES Competency: VI.A.1.a.4.x Instruct patient in the collection of fecal specimen

CAAHEP Curriculum: IV.P.2 Report relevant information to others succinctly and accurately

Name _____   **Date** _____   **Score** _____

COMPETENCY ASSESSMENT

Procedure 44-1   Pregnancy Test

Task: To perform the enzyme immunoassay or agglutination inhibition test to detect human chorionic gonadotropin (hCG) in urine to determine positive or negative pregnancy results.

Conditions: Gloves, urine specimen, timer, surface disinfectant, biohazard container, hCG negative and positive urine control, pregnancy test kit

Standards: Perform the Task within 15 minutes with a minimum score of _____ points.

Work Documentation: Patient chart entry, lab report

No.	Step	Points	Check #1	Check #2	Check #3
1	Washed hands; organized supplies and equipment; applied appropriate PPE.				
2	Performed urine pregnancy test properly.				
3	Disposed of contaminated supplies following OSHA regulations; disinfected surfaces; washed hands.				
4	Demonstrated professional behavior in manner, organization, and attire.				
5	Documented correctly.				
Student's Total Points					
Points Possible					
Final Score (Student's Total Points/ Possible Points)					

Name _____ **Date** _____ **Score** _____

WORK DOCUMENTATION
*Also attach lab report.

_____

Instructor's/Evaluator's Comments and Suggestions:

_____

_____

_____

_____

_____

CHECK #1

Evaluator's Signature: _____   Date:

CHECK #2

Evaluator's Signature: _____   Date:

CHECK #3

Evaluator's Signature: _____   Date:

ABHES Competency: VI.A.1.a.4.k Perform selected CLIA-waived tests (i.e. kit tests such as pregnancy, quick strep, dip sticks) that assist with diagnosis and treatment

Name _____ Date _____ Score _____

COMPETENCY ASSESSMENT

Procedure 44-2   Performing Infectious Mononucleosis Test

Task: To perform an accurate test of serum or plasma to detect the presence or absence of antibodies of mononucleosis.

Conditions: Gloves, goggles (optional), safety lancet, alcohol swabs, cotton balls, gauze, adhesive strip, glucose analyzer, control solutions for glucose analyzer, test strips for glucose analyzer, laboratory tissue

Standards: Perform the Task within 15 minutes with a minimum score of _____ points.

Work Documentation: Patient chart entry, lab report

No.	Step	Points	Check #1	Check #2	Check #3
1	Washed hands; organized supplies and equipment; applied appropriate PPE.				
2	Performed infectious mononucleosis test properly.				
3	Disposed of contaminated supplies following OSHA regulations; disinfected surfaces; washed hands.				
4	Demonstrated professional behavior in manner, organization, and attire.				
5	Documented correctly.				
Student's Total Points					
Points Possible					
Final Score (Student's Total Points/ Possible Points)					

Name _____   **Date** _____   **Score** _____

WORK DOCUMENTATION
*Also attach lab report.

_____

Instructor's/Evaluator's Comments and Suggestions:

_____

_____

_____

_____

_____

CHECK #1

Evaluator's Signature: _____   Date:

CHECK #2

Evaluator's Signature: _____   Date:

CHECK #3

Evaluator's Signature: _____   Date:

ABHES Competency: VI.A.1.a.4.bb Perform immunology testing

CAAHEP Curriculum: I.P.15 Perform immunology testing

Name _____ Date _____ Score _____

COMPETENCY ASSESSMENT

Procedure 44-3   Obtaining Blood Specimen for Phenylketonuria (PKU) Test

Task: To obtain a blood specimen using a PKU test card or "filter paper" to determine phenylalanine levels in newborns who are at least 3 days old.

Conditions: Gloves, PKU filter paper test card and mailing envelope, alcohol swabs, cotton balls or gauze pad, sterile pediatric-sized lancet, biohazard waste container

Standards: Perform the Task within 20 minutes with a minimum score of _____ points.

Work Documentation: Patient chart entry, PKU card

No.	Step	Points	Check #1	Check #2	Check #3
1	Washed hands; checked room for cleanliness, equipment, and readiness; organized supplies and equipment.				
2	Greeted and identified the patient and parents, and introduced self.				
3	Explained the procedure, gave parents information documents, obtained written informed consent, obtained patient information as required for PKU forms.				
4	Washed hands; positioned the patient properly for comfort and safety; applied PPE.				
5	Obtained the blood specimens properly and safely, filling the appropriate areas on the card as required for proper testing. Comforted the patient and assisted the parents as needed.				
6	Completed the forms properly, packaged the specimen for mailing, following manufacturer's instructions exactly.				
7	Disposed of contaminated supplies following OSHA regulations; disinfected surfaces; washed hands.				
8	Demonstrated professional behavior in manner, organization, and attire, including: • Communicated appropriately and comfortably with the patient.				
9	Documented correctly.				
	Student's Total Points				
	Points Possible				
	Final Score (Student's Total Points/ Possible Points)				

Name _____   **Date** _____   **Score** _____

WORK DOCUMENTATION
*Also attach PKU card.

Instructor's/Evaluator's Comments and Suggestions:

_____

_____

_____

_____

_____

CHECK #1

Evaluator's Signature: Date:

CHECK #2

Evaluator's Signature: Date:

CHECK #3

Evaluator's Signature: Date:

ABHES Competency: VI.A.1.a.4.aa Perform chemistry testing

CAAHEP Curriculum: I.P.13 Perform chemistry testing

Name _____ **Date** _____ **Score** _____

COMPETENCY ASSESSMENT

Procedure 44-4   Screening Test for PKU

Task:	Test a urine specimen using the diaper test or the Phenistik test to determine phenylalanine levels in infants who are at least 6 weeks old. This is a quick screening test only and *does not* take the place of the blood test.
Conditions:	Gloves, 10% ferric chloride for the diaper test or Phenistik Method Test, biohazard waste container
Standards:	Perform the Task within 5 minutes with a minimum score of _____ points.
Work Documentation:	Patient chart entry

No.	Step	Points	Check #1	Check #2	Check #3
1	Washed hands; checked room for cleanliness, equipment, and readiness; organized supplies and equipment.				
2	Greeted and identified the patient and parents, and introduced self.				
3	Explained the procedure and that this does not take the place of the PKU blood test. Determined that the patient was at least 6 weeks of age. Applied PPE.				
4	Removed diaper from the infant, replaced with clean diaper. Performed the test on urine in the diaper safely and away from patient and parent(s).				
5	If the test was positive, alerted the physician and followed up with the PKU test.				
6	Disposed of contaminated supplies following OSHA regulations; disinfected surfaces; washed hands.				
7	Demonstrated professional behavior in manner, organization, and attire, including: • Communicated appropriately and comfortably with the patient.				
8	Documented correctly.				
	Student's Total Points				
	Points Possible				
	Final Score (Student's Total Points/ Possible Points)				

Name _____   Date _____   Score _____

WORK DOCUMENTATION

_____

Instructor's/Evaluator's Comments and Suggestions:

_____

_____

_____

_____

_____

CHECK #1

Evaluator's Signature: Date:

CHECK #2

Evaluator's Signature: Date:

CHECK #3

Evaluator's Signature: Date:

ABHES Competency: VI.A.1.a.4.1 Screen and follow up patient test results; VI.A.1.a.4.aa Perform chemistry testing

CAAHEP Curriculum: I.P.13 Perform chemistry testing; I.P.16 Screen test results

Name _____ Date _____ Score _____

COMPETENCY ASSESSMENT

Procedure 44-5   Measurement of Blood Glucose Using an Automated Analyzer

Task: To measure blood glucose.

Conditions: Gloves, goggles (optional), safety lancet, alcohol swabs, cotton balls, gauze, adhesive strip, glucose analyzer, control solutions for glucose analyzer, test strips for glucose analyzer, laboratory tissue

Standards: Perform the Task within 15 minutes with a minimum score of _____ points.

Work Documentation: Patient chart entry, lab report

No.	Step	Points	Check #1	Check #2	Check #3
1	Washed hands; organized supplies and equipment; applied appropriate PPE.				
2	Performed instrument calibrations and quality controls.				
3	Obtained blood specimen using proper technique.				
4	Tested specimen following the manufacturer's instructions exactly. Repeated test if indicated.				
5	Disposed of contaminated supplies following OSHA regulations; disinfected surfaces; washed hands.				
6	Demonstrated professional behavior in manner, organization, and attire.				
7	Documented correctly.				
Student's Total Points					
Points Possible					
Final Score (Student's Total Points/ Possible Points)					

Name _____ **Date** _____ **Score** _____

WORK DOCUMENTATION
*Also attach lab report.

_____

Instructor's/Evaluator's Comments and Suggestions:

_____

_____

_____

_____

_____

CHECK #1

Evaluator's Signature: _____   Date:

CHECK #2

Evaluator's Signature: _____   Date:

CHECK #3

Evaluator's Signature: _____   Date:

ABHES Competency: VI.A.1.a.4.k Perform selected CLIA-waived tests (i.e. kit tests such as pregnancy, quick strep, dip sticks) that assist with diagnosis and treatment; VI.A.1.a.4.i Use quality control; VI.A.1.a.4.aa Perform chemistry testing

CAAHEP Curriculum: I.P.11 Perform quality control measures; I.P.13 Perform chemistry testing

Name _____ Date _____ Score _____

COMPETENCY ASSESSMENT

Procedure 44-6 Cholesterol Testing

Task: To test for cholesterol, high-density lipoprotein, or triglyceride level for monitoring purposes. The following steps are intentionally general, so a variety of kits can be used.

Conditions: Gloves, blood collection equipment, pipettes with disposable tips, chlorine bleach, commercial kit for manual determination of cholesterol, controls and standards, marking pen, biohazard container

Standards: Perform the Task within 15 minutes with a minimum score of _____ points.

Work Documentation: Patient chart entry, lab report

No.	Step	Points	Check #1	Check #2	Check #3
1	Washed hands; organized supplies and equipment; applied appropriate PPE.				
2	Performed instrument calibrations and quality controls.				
3	Obtained blood specimen using proper technique.				
4	Tested specimen following the manufacturer's instructions exactly.				
5	Disposed of contaminated supplies following OSHA regulations; disinfected surfaces; washed hands.				
6	Demonstrated professional behavior in manner, organization, and attire.				
7	Documented correctly.				
Student's Total Points					
Points Possible					
Final Score (Student's Total Points/ Possible Points)					

Name _____   **Date** _____   **Score** _____

WORK DOCUMENTATION
*Also attach lab report.

_____

Instructor's/Evaluator's Comments and Suggestions:

_____

_____

_____

_____

_____

CHECK #1 Evaluator's Signature: Date:

CHECK #2 Evaluator's Signature: Date:

CHECK #3 Evaluator's Signature: Date:

ABHES Competency: VI.A.1.a.4.k Perform selected CLIA-waived tests (i.e. kit tests such as pregnancy, quick strep, dip sticks) that assist with diagnosis and treatment; VI.A.1.a.4.i Use quality control; VI.A.1.a.4.aa Perform chemistry testing

CAAHEP Curriculum: I.P.11 Perform quality control measures; I.P.13 Perform chemistry testing

Name _____   **Date** _____   **Score** _____

COMPETENCY ASSESSMENT

Procedure 45-1   Completing a Medical Incident Report

Task: To complete a medical incident report and submit it in a timely manner.

Condition: Appropriate medical incident report form or computer with Incident Report Software

Standards: Perform the Task within 15 minutes with a minimum score of _____ points.

Work Documentation: Completed incident report form

No.	Step	Points	Check #1	Check #2	Check #3
1	Accurately completed the incident report form, filling in each section of the report, including: • Used quotes when referring to un-witnessed statements. • Wrote the names of all witnesses to the incident in the report.				
2	Submitted the completed incident report to the appropriate person.				
Student's Total Points					
Points Possible					
Final Score (Student's Total Points/ Possible Points)					

Name _____ **Date** _____ **Score** _____

WORK DOCUMENTATION

*Attach completed incident report form.

Instructor's/Evaluator's Comments and Suggestions:

_____

_____

_____

_____

_____

CHECK #1

Evaluator's Signature: _____ Date: _____

CHECK #2

Evaluator's Signature: _____ Date: _____

CHECK #3

Evaluator's Signature: _____ Date: _____

ABHES Competency: VI.A.1.a.5.h Perform risk management procedures

CAAHEP Curriculum: IX.P.6 Complete an incident report

Name _____   **Date** _____   **Score** _____

COMPETENCY ASSESSMENT

Procedure 45-2   Preparing a Meeting Agenda

Task: To prepare a meeting agenda with an established list of specific items to be discussed or acted on, or both.

Condition: List of participants, the order of business, names of individuals giving reports, names of any guest speakers, a computer, paper on which to print agendas

Standards: Perform the Task within 20 minutes with a minimum score of _____ points.

Work Documentation: Printed agenda

No.	Step	Points	Check #1	Check #2	Check #3
1	Confirmed the proposed dates and place of meeting.				
2	Prepared and typed agenda: • Collected information from previous meetings' minutes for old agenda items. • Checked with others for report items and determined any new business.				
3	When completed, had agenda approved by the meeting chair.				
4	Sent agenda to participants.				
5	Reserved meeting room and arranged for food items, equipment, and supplies that may be needed.				
Student's Total Points					
Points Possible					
Final Score (Student's Total Points/ Possible Points)					

Name _____ **Date** _____ **Score** _____

WORK DOCUMENTATION

*Attach printed agenda.

Instructor's/Evaluator's Comments and Suggestions:

_____

_____

_____

_____

_____

CHECK #1

Evaluator's Signature: _____ Date: _____

CHECK #2

Evaluator's Signature: _____ Date: _____

CHECK #3

Evaluator's Signature: _____ Date: _____

ABHES Competency: VI.A.1.a.2.j Use correct grammar, spelling and formatting techniques in written works; VI.A.1.a.2.o Fundamental writing skills; VI.A.1.a.3.a Perform basic secretarial skills

CAAHEP Curriculum: IV.P.2 Report relevant information to others succinctly and accurately

Name _____ Date _____ Score _____

COMPETENCY ASSESSMENT

Procedure 45-3 Supervising a Student Practicum

Task: To prepare a training path for a student extern being assigned to the office, make the involved personnel aware of their responsibilities, preplan the jobs the student will perform and in what sequence they will be assigned, and try to make the externship successful by providing as much supervision and assistance as necessary.

Condition: A schedule log, calendar, office procedures manual, any criteria presented by the program director

Standards: Perform the Task within 30 minutes with a minimum score of _____ points.

No.	Step	Points	Check #1	Check #2	Check #3
1	Reviewed the clinical practicum contract between your agency and the educational institution.				
2	Identified student's supervisor, planned tasks that the student will perform, and created a schedule for the student and staff.				
3	Oriented the student to the facility and staff upon arrival.				
4	Maintained an accurate record of hours the student worked, including missed days and late arrivals.				
5	Consulted with providers, staff, and the student for feedback.				
6	Reported student progress to the medical assistants program director and prepared student's evaluation report using input from all who worked with student.				
Student's Total Points					
Points Possible					
Final Score (Student's Total Points/ Possible Points)					

Name _____   **Date** _____   **Score** _____

Instructor's/Evaluator's Comments and Suggestions:

_____

_____

_____

_____

_____

CHECK #1

Evaluator's Signature: _____   Date: _____

CHECK #2

Evaluator's Signature: _____   Date: _____

CHECK #3

Evaluator's Signature: _____   Date: _____

ABHES Competency: VI.A.1.a.2.m Adaptation for individualized needs; VI.A.1.a.7.d orient and train personnel

CAAHEP Curriculum: IV.P.4 Explain general office policies

Name _____ Date _____ Score _____

COMPETENCY ASSESSMENT

Procedure 45-3   Supervising a Student Practicum

Task: To prepare a training path for a student extern being assigned to the office, make the involved personnel aware of their responsibilities, preplan the jobs the student will perform and in what sequence they will be assigned, and try to make the externship successful by providing as much supervision and assistance as necessary.

Condition: A schedule log, calendar, office procedures manual, any criteria presented by the program director

Standards: Perform the Task within 30 minutes with a minimum score of _____ points.

No.	Step	Points	Check #1	Check #2	Check #3
1	Reviewed the clinical practicum contract between your agency and the educational institution.				
2	Identified student's supervisor, planned tasks that the student will perform, and created a schedule for the student and staff.				
3	Oriented the student to the facility and staff upon arrival.				
4	Maintained an accurate record of hours the student worked, including missed days and late arrivals.				
5	Consulted with providers, staff, and the student for feedback.				
6	Reported student progress to the medical assistants program director and prepared student's evaluation report using input from all who worked with student.				
	Student's Total Points				
	Points Possible				
	Final Score (Student's Total Points/ Possible Points)				

Name _____ **Date** _____ **Score** _____

Instructor's/Evaluator's Comments and Suggestions:

_____

_____

_____

_____

_____

CHECK #1

Evaluator's Signature: _____   Date:

CHECK #2

Evaluator's Signature: _____   Date:

CHECK #3

Evaluator's Signature: _____   Date:

ABHES Competency: VI.A.1.a.2.m Adaptation for individualized needs; VI.A.1.a.7.d orient and train personnel

CAAHEP Curriculum: IV.P.4 Explain general office policies

Name _____ **Date** _____ **Score** _____

COMPETENCY ASSESSMENT

Procedure 45-4   Developing and Maintaining a Procedure Manual

Task: To develop and maintain a comprehensive, up-to-date procedures manual covering each medical, technical, and administrative procedure in the office with step-by-step directions and rationale for performing each task.

Condition: A computer, three-ring binder, paper, procedures, and criteria

Standards: Perform the Task within 20 minutes with a minimum score of _____ points.

Work Documentation: Binder with procedure entries

No.	Step	Points	Check #1	Check #2	Check #3
1	Wrote detailed, step-by-step procedures and rationale for each medical, technical, and administrative function. Each procedure was written by experienced employees close to the function and reviewed by a supervisor or the office manager.				
2	Included regular maintenance (cleaning, servicing, and calibrating) instructions and flow sheets for all office equipment, both in the clinical area and in the office/ business areas.				
3	Included step-by-step procedures on how to accomplish each task, both in the clinical area and in the office/business areas.				
4	Included local and out of the area resources for clinical staff, office/business staff, physicians/providers, and patients. Provided a listing in each area with contact information and services available.				
5	Included basic rules and regulations, state and federal, which are related to processes performed in both clinical and office/business areas.				
6	Included the clinic procedures and flow sheets for taking inventory in each of the areas, and instructions on ordering procedures.				
7	Collected the procedures into the office procedures manual.				
Student's Total Points					
Points Possible					
Final Score (Student's Total Points/ Possible Points)					

Name _____ **Date** _____ **Score** _____

WORK DOCUMENTATION
*Attach completed procedure manual entries.

Instructor's/Evaluator's Comments and Suggestions:

_____

_____

_____

_____

_____

CHECK #1

Evaluator's Signature: _____ Date:

CHECK #2

Evaluator's Signature: _____ Date:

CHECK #3

Evaluator's Signature: _____ Date:

ABHES Competency: VI.A.1.a.6.a Maintain physical plant; VI.A.1.a.7.d Orient and train personnel

CAAHEP Curriculum: IX.P.5 Incorporate the Patient's Bill of Rights into personal practice and medical office policies and procedures; IX.P.8 Apply local, state and federal health care legislation and regulation appropriate to the medical assisting practice setting

Name _____   **Date** _____   **Score** _____

COMPETENCY ASSESSMENT

Procedure 45-8   Perform an Inventory of Equipment and Supplies

Task: To develop an inventory of expendable administrative and clinical supplies in a medical office.

Condition: Printout of most recent inventory spreadsheet, clipboard, pad of reorder forms, pen or pencil

Standards: Perform the Task within 15 minutes with a minimum score of _____ points.

Work Documentation: Completed inventory list

No.	Step	Points	Check #1	Check #2	Check #3
1	Assembled equipment and supplies to be inventoried.				
2	Accurately counted and recorded the quantity of each item and completed an inventory form.				
3	If a supply or equipment was below the minimum amount, indicated that reordering was necessary.				
4	Signed form and gave to person responsible for ordering supplies. Or filled out an order form for the additional supplies.				
Student's Total Points					
Points Possible					
Final Score (Student's Total Points/ Possible Points)					

Name _____   **Date** _____   **Score** _____

WORK DOCUMENTATION

*Attach completed inventory list.

_____

Instructor's/Evaluator's Comments and Suggestions:

_____

_____

_____

_____

_____

CHECK #1

Evaluator's Signature: _____   Date:

CHECK #2

Evaluator's Signature: _____   Date:

CHECK #3

Evaluator's Signature: _____   Date:

ABHES Competency: VI.A.1.a.6.c Inventory equipment and supplies; VI.A.1.a.6.d Evaluate and recommend equipment and supplies for practice

CAAHEP Curriculum: V.P.10 Perform an office inventory

Name _____ **Date** _____ **Score** _____

COMPETENCY ASSESSMENT

Procedure 45-9   Perform Routine Maintenance or Calibration of Administrative and Clinical Equipment

Task: To ensure the operability and calibration of administrative and clinical equipment.

Condition: Equipment list with maintenance or calibration requirements; clipboard, pen, maintenance record sheets, and deficiency tags; access to operation and service manuals of equipment to be serviced; access to any necessary maintenance tools and supplies

Standards: Perform the Task within 30 minutes with a minimum score of _____ points.

Work Documentation: Maintenance record form

No.	Step	Points	Check #1	Check #2	Check #3
1	Inspected appropriate administrative and clinical equipment. Inspected for cleanliness, safety, and operability. Noted and recorded equipment that required repairs.				
2	Properly completed maintenance checklist: • Included date. • Documented whether maintenance or repairs were needed. • Signed the form.				
Student's Total Points					
Points Possible					
Final Score (Student's Total Points/ Possible Points)					

Name _____ **Date** _____ **Score** _____

WORK DOCUMENTATION

*Attach maintenance record form.

Instructor's/Evaluator's Comments and Suggestions:

_____

_____

_____

_____

_____

CHECK #1

Evaluator's Signature: Date:

CHECK #2

Evaluator's Signature: Date:

CHECK #3

Evaluator's Signature: Date:

ABHES Competency: VI.A.1.a.6.b Operate and maintain facilities and perform routine maintenance of administrative and clinical equipment safely

CAAHEP Curriculum: V.P.9 Perform routine maintenance of office equipment with documentation

Name _____ Date _____ Score _____

COMPETENCY ASSESSMENT

Procedure 46-1 Develop and Maintain a Policy Manual

Task: To develop and maintain a comprehensive, up-to-date policy manual of all office policies relating to employee practices, benefits, office conduct, and so forth.

Condition: Computer, three-ring binder, paper, standard policy format

Standards: Perform the Task within 20 minutes with a minimum score of _____ points.

Work Documentation: Printed policy manual entries

No.	Step	Points	Check #1	Check #2	Check #3
1	Following office format, developed precise, written office policies detailing all necessary information pertaining to the staff and their positions. Included benefits, vacation, sick leave, hours, dress codes, evaluations, rules of conduct, and grounds for dismissal.				
2	Identified procedures for reimbursing overtime, preventing discrimination and harassment, creating a safe workplace, and allowing for jury duty.				
3	Included a policy statement related to smoking and other substances.				
4	Identified steps to follow should an employee become disabled during employment.				
5	Determined what employee opportunities for continuing education would be reimbursed and included requirements for certification and licensures.				
6	Provided a copy of the policy manual for each employee.				
7	Reviewed and updated the policy manual regularly. Added or deleted items as necessary, dating each revision.				
Student's Total Points					
Points Possible					
Final Score (Student's Total Points/ Possible Points)					

Name _____ **Date** _____ **Score** _____

WORK DOCUMENTATION
*Attach printed policy manual entries.

_____

Instructor's/Evaluator's Comments and Suggestions:

_____

_____

_____

_____

_____

CHECK #1

Evaluator's Signature: Date:

CHECK #2

Evaluator's Signature: Date:

CHECK #3

Evaluator's Signature: Date:

ABHES Competency: VI.A.1.a.7.d Orient and train personnel

CAAHEP Curriculum: IV.P.4 Explain general office policies

Name _____ **Date** _____ **Score** _____

COMPETENCY ASSESSMENT

Procedure 46-2   Prepare a Job Description

Task: To develop a precise definition of the tasks assigned to a job, to determine the expectations and level of competency required, and to specify the experience, training, and education needed to perform the job for purposes of recruiting and performance evaluation.

Condition: Computer, three-ring binder, paper, standard job description format

Standards: Perform the Task within 20 minutes with a minimum score of _____ points.

Work Documentation: Printout of job description, or job description written in documentation area

No.	Step	Points	Check #1	Check #2	Check #3
1	Detailed each task that creates the job.				
2	Listed special medical, technical, or clerical skills needed.				
3	Determined the level of education, training, and experience required for the position.				
4	Determined where the job fits into the overall structure of the office.				
5	Specified any unusual working conditions (hours, locations, etc.) that may apply.				
6	Described career path opportunities.				
7	Reviewed and updated the policy manual regularly. Added or deleted items as necessary, dating each revision.				
Student's Total Points					
Points Possible					
Final Score (Student's Total Points/ Possible Points)					

Name _____   **Date** _____   **Score** _____

WORK DOCUMENTATION

Instructor's/Evaluator's Comments and Suggestions:

_____

_____

_____

_____

_____

CHECK #1

Evaluator's Signature: _____   Date:

CHECK #2

Evaluator's Signature: _____   Date:

CHECK #3

Evaluator's Signature: _____   Date:

ABHES Competency: VI.A.1.a.6.a Maintain physical plant

CAAHEP Curriculum: IV.P.4 Explain general office policies

Name _____ Date _____ Score _____

COMPETENCY ASSESSMENT

Procedure 46-3 Conduct Interviews

Task: To screen applicants for training, experience, and characteristics to select the best candidate to fill the position vacancy.

Condition: Interview questions; policy manual (for referencing); applicant's résumé, application, and cover letter

Standards: Perform the Task within 40 minutes with a minimum score of _____ points.

No.	Step	Points	Check #1	Check #2	Check #3
1	Reviewed résumés and applications received and selected candidates who had the skills being sought. Created an interview worksheet for each candidate, listing the points to cover, and identified who on staff would be part of the interview team.				
2	Screened the applicant over the phone.				
3	Conducted the in-office interview of the applicant: • Provided an overview about the practice and staff, describing the job and answering preliminary questions. • Asked questions about the applicant's work experience and educational background. • Informed the applicants when a decision would be made, and thanked each applicant for participating in the interview.				
4	Checked references of all prospective employees.				
5	Established a second interview for the qualified candidate if necessary.				
6	Confirmed accepted job offers in writing, specifying the details of the offer and acceptance, and notified all unsuccessful applicants by letter when the position was filled.				
	Student's Total Points				
	Points Possible				
	Final Score (Student's Total Points/ Possible Points)				

Name _____ **Date** _____ **Score** _____

Instructor's/Evaluator's Comments and Suggestions:

_____

_____

_____

_____

_____

CHECK #1

Evaluator's Signature: _____

Date: _____

CHECK #2

Evaluator's Signature: _____

Date: _____

CHECK #3

Evaluator's Signature: _____

Date: _____

ABHES Competency: VI.A.1.a.2.f Interview effectively; VI.A.1.a.2.i Recognize and respond to verbal and non-verbal communication; VI.A.1.a.2.k Principles of verbal and nonverbal communication; VI.A.1.a.2.l Recognition and response to verbal and non-verbal communication

CAAHEP Curriculum: IV.P.2 Report relevant information to others succinctly and accurately; IV.P.4 Explain general office policies

Name _____ Date _____ Score _____

COMPETENCY ASSESSMENT

Procedure 46-4   Orient Personnel

Task: To acquaint new employees with office policies, staff, what the job encompasses, procedures to be performed, and job performance expectations.

Condition: Policy manual

Standards: Perform the Task within 30 minutes with a minimum score of _____ points.

No.	Step	Points	Check #1	Check #2	Check #3
1	Toured the facilities and introduced the office staff. Assigned a mentor from the staff to help with the orientation.				
2	Completed employee-related documents and explained their purpose. Explained the benefits program.				
3	Presented the office policy manual and discussed the key elements. Reviewed federal and state regulatory precautions for medical facilities. Reviewed the job description.				
4	Explained and demonstrated procedures to be performed and the use of procedures manuals supporting these procedures.				
5	Demonstrated the use of any specialized equipment (such as time clocks, key entries, etc.). Medical equipment would be demonstrated by clinical staff.				
Student's Total Points					
Points Possible					
Final Score (Student's Total Points/ Possible Points)					

Name _____ **Date** _____ **Score** _____

Instructor's/Evaluator's Comments and Suggestions:

_____

_____

_____

_____

_____

CHECK #1

Evaluator's Signature: _____   Date: _____

CHECK #2

Evaluator's Signature: _____   Date: _____

CHECK #3

Evaluator's Signature: _____   Date: _____

ABHES Competency: VI.A.1.a.7.d Orient and train personnel

CAAHEP Curriculum: IV.P.4 Explain general office policies

Comprehensive Examination

1. Which term describes false and malicious writing about another that constitutes defamation of character?

    a. Slander

    b. Assault

    c. Libel

    d. Invasion of privacy

    e. Battery

2. When reviewing a résumé, the human resources manager docs NOT consider the applicant's:

    a. supplemental education

    b. unexplained gaps in employment

    c. training related to the position

    d. age, sex, and race

    e. previous experience

3. The standard of professional conduct for a certified medical assistant should be:

    a. in keeping with the AAMA Code of Ethics

    b. outlined by the provider or employer

    c. based on the Hippocratic oath

    d. in keeping with the AMA Principles of Medical Ethics

    e. determined by the state's medical practice act

4. After an interview, the applicant should:

    a. telephone to say thank you

    b. have his or her references call the interviewer

    c. telephone after three days to check the status of his or her application

    d. promptly send a follow-up letter

    e. send a lavish thank-you gift

5. A medical assistant must NEVER:

    a. perform a venipuncture

    b. perform a laboratory test

    c. imply that he or she is a nurse

    d. dispense a medication after a direct order from the provider

    e. give a medication after a direct order from the provider

6. Which legal principle is violated when a medical assistant practices outside of his or her training?

    a. Public d'uty

    b. Consent

    c. Privacy rights

    d. Confidentiality

    e. Standard of care

7. Which manner of dress is appropriate for an interview?

   a. A medical assistant's uniform

   b. Evening makeup

   c. Spectacular nail polish

   d. Casual clothing

   e. Neat business attire

8. Which statement accurately describes ethics?

   a. Ethics are a personal moral philosophy of right and wrong.

   b. Ethics are a code of minimal acceptable behavior.

   c. Ethics are the state's legal standards established for a profession.

   d. Ethics are the federal legal standards established for a profession.

   e. Ethics are standards for personal behavior as established by organized religions.

9. When stressed, we may exhibit all of the following EXCEPT:

   a. anxiety

   b. objective thinking

   c. depression

   d. anger

   e. irrational behavior

10. All of the following statements about Good Samaritan laws are true EXCEPT:

    a. These laws do not provide legal protection to on-duty emergency care providers.

    b. Providers must act in a reasonable and prudent manner.

    c. The conditions of these laws vary in each state.

    d. No matter what their level of training, providers must do everything for the patient.

    e. Health care providers are ethically, not legally, obligated to assist in emergency situations.

11. What is the purpose of the certification credential for medical assistants?

    a. The certification credential is required for graduation.

    b. The certification credential guarantees a job.

    c. The certification credential meets state registration requirements.

    d. The certification credential indicates a medical assistant's professional and technical competence.

    e. The certification credential meets state licensure requirements.

12. Consent for treatment may usually be given by:

    a. the patient's closest relative

    b. a patient in a mental institution

    c. any minor over 16

    d. the person accompanying the patient

    e. a legally competent patient

13. Who is the most important member of the health care team?

    a. The patient

    b. The provider

    c. The medical assistant

    d. The nurse

    e. The receptionist

14. All of the following cultural influences may affect communication EXCEPT:

    a. education

    b. sexual orientation

    c. ethnic heritage

    d. geographic location

    e. age

15. When the medical office wins in small claims court, the money is collected from the patient by:

    a. the bailiff

    b. the patient's insurance company

    c. the probate court

    d. the medical office

    e. the court-appointed collection agency

16. Which statement is accurate regarding the Americans with Disabilities Act (ADA)?

    a. The ADA applies only to medical practices and health care facilities.

    b. The ADA applies to all businesses.

    c. The ADA applies only to businesses with 15 or more employees.

    d. The ADA applies only to businesses with 50 or more employees.

    e. The ADA applies only to state and federal government agencies.

17. Which governmental agency requires employers to ensure employee safety concerning occupational exposure to potentially harmful substances?

    a. CDC

    b. HCFA

    c. OSHA

    d. USPS

    e. Department of Health and Human Services

18. The certifying board of which organization awards the CMA credential?

    a. AAMA

    b. AMT

    c. ABHES

    d. CAAHEP

    e. RMA

19. The certifying board of which organization awards the RMA credential?

   a. AAMA

   b. ABHES

   c. CAAHEP

   d. CMA

   e. AMT

20. Which of the following might be expected as an Asian expression of pain?

   a. Descriptive words such as "piercing" or "throbbing"

   b. A description of disturbances of the mind

   c. Ranking pain on a scale of 1 to 10

   d. Moaning and crying out

   e. Descriptive terms of body imbalance

21. How often must the CMA (AAMA) credential be renewed?

   a. Annually

   b. Every five years

   c. Biannually

   d. Every three years

   e. With every job change

22. What is the highest level in Maslow's hierarchy of needs?

   a. Safety needs

   b. Love needs

   c. Self-actualization

   d. Belongingness needs

   e. Esteem needs

23. Which of the following information is considered to be public domain?

   a. A person's sexual preference

   b. A person's police record

   c. A person's past drug addiction

   d. A person's HIV-positive status

   e. A person's alcoholism

24. The goal of the National Health Information Network is to create a:

   a. unified EMR for all health care facilities

   b. standard for computer hardware in health care facilities

   c. support network for health care facilities transitioning to EMR

   d. method of communicating EMR software program options

   e. system for exchange of health care information

25. Dr. Bennett's office will be switching to an EMR system. The office manager communicates to staff that they will be using a "remote hosted" system. This means that:

    a. the software will be run from a server in the office, which requires the purchase of only one software license

    b. the software will be installed on each individual computer, and each individual computer will require its own license

    c. the software is owned and maintained by another company, but the office will pay for the right to log in and use the system

    d. a software company will log in to the office computers in order to install and maintain the software

    e. the system will require the use of very complex hardware and additional training for staff

26. An individual who has done something that results in damage to another person or his or her property would be prosecuted under what type of law?

    a. Statute

    b. Case

    c. Breach of contract

    d. Tort

    e. Regulatory

27. Which of the following would NOT be considered an intentional tort?

    a. Defamation of character

    b. Invasion of privacy

    c. Assault

    d. Negligence

    e. Fraud

28. A patient who is undergoing a surgical procedure signs a consent for treatment. The consent would be referred to as a(n):

    a. expressed contract

    b. implied contract

    c. breach of contract

    d. tort contract

    e. consideration contract

29. Licensing for health care professionals, health department regulations, and regulations for mandatory reporting are all examples of:

    a. civil law

    b. administrative law

    c. criminal law

    d. negligent law

    e. contract law

30. A durable power of attorney document indicates:

    a. what type of medical treatment a patient wishes to have during end-of-life care

    b. who the patient would like to make decisions for him if he cannot make decisions himself

    c. what (if any) organs a patient would like to donate

    d. Do Not Resuscitate orders

    e. consent for surgical treatment

31. A medical professional who is convicted of nonfeasance would have:

    a. performed a treatment improperly

    b. performed an illegal act

    c. failed to perform necessary treatment

    d. violated confidentiality

    e. performed a duty outside of her scope of practice

32. Statutes of limitation apply to everything but:

    a. negligence

    b. fraud

    c. malfeasance

    d. dereliction of duty

    e. murder

33. Health care workers are mandatory reporters in all BUT which of the following situations?

    a. Child abuse

    b. Elder abuse

    c. Alcoholism

    d. Communicable diseases

    e. Death

34. Which of the following is true of HIPAA?

    a. Hospitals are prevented from releasing homicide or other crime-related information to law enforcement agencies.

    b. Students performing internships may not have access to computer systems in health care facilities.

    c. The HIPAA prevents health care facilities from sharing information with health care providers who are not their employees even when the information is essential for patient treatment.

    d. Health care facilities should appoint a privacy officer and adopt procedures for handling requests.

    e. HIPAA regulations do not apply to patients seeking care under government assistance programs.

35. The stage of grief in which patients attempt to make promises in order to change their situation would be considered:

    a. denial

    b. bargaining

    c. anger

    d. depression

    e. acceptance

36. End-of-life palliative care is most often provided by:

    a. hospice

    b. acute care hospitals

    c. rehabilitation hospitals

    d. skilled nursing facilities

    e. assisted living facilities

37. The AAMA code of ethics for medical assistants includes statements about each of the following EXCEPT:

    a. honor

    b. confidentiality

    c. continuing education

    d. improving community

    e. supervising provider

38. A medical office that transmits information over a wireless network must ensure that:

    a. the network allows staff to transmit information from home

    b. the network allows the provider to transmit information while doing patient visits at the hospital

    c. each staff member understands the encryption of the network

    d. the network meets HIPAA guidelines

    e. the network can be accessed by the appropriate insurance companies

39. Advanced Beneficiary Notices must be used for patients with what type of insurance?

    a. Medicaid

    b. Workers Compensation

    c. Medicare

    d. Blue Cross/Blue Shield

    e. TRICARE

40. Which of the following helps a medical assistant to manage time well?

    a. Reading email while answering patient calls

    b. Asking patients to jot down their complaints in their charts

    c. Asking patients to email rather than call with questions

    d. Asking front office staff to obtain patients' complaint

    e. Identifying priorities

41. Which of the following is NOT an important quality for a medical assistant?

    a. Ability to manage time efficiently

    b. Ability to delegate

    c. Initiative

    d. Flexibility

    e. Ability to work as a team member

42. Which of the following is an important aspect of verbal communication?

    a. Facial expressions

    b. Appearance

    c. Tone of voice

    d. Body language

    e. Gestures

43. The most important component of the message you communicate is:

    a. Perception of the person receiving the message

    b. Tone of voice

    c. The vocabulary used

    d. Facial expression

    e. Body language

44. Nancy, the medical assistant you work with, always changes the subject when you bring up topics that she does not want to discuss. This behavior would be considered:

    a. assertive

    b. passive

    c. aggressive

    d. professional

    e. passive-aggressive

45. Which of the following is NOT considered a part of negligence?

    a. Duty

    b. Dereliction

    c. Denial

    d. Direct cause

    e. Damages

46. The "base" of a medical word is called the:

    a. prefix

    b. suffix

    c. combining form

    d. root

    e. anatomical

47. The provider you are working with asks you to place a bandage just proximal to the knee. You would place the bandage:

    a. just below the knee

    b. on the front of the knee

    c. on the back of the knee

    d. just above the knee

    e. covering the entire knee area from top to bottom

48. You read a medical report that indicates that a provider made an incision from the superior to the inferior portion of the heart during a surgery. This means that the incision was made in the:

    a. frontal plane

    b. coronal plane

    c. transverse plane

    d. superior plane

    e. horizontal plane

49. The sac that covers the heart is referred to as the:

    a. pericardium

    b. epicardium

    c. endocardium

    d. myocardium

    e. mediastinum

50. The structure that is responsible for the formation of urine is the:

    a. medulla

    b. cortex

    c. nephron

    d. major calyx

    e. minor calyx

51. The congenital disorder that involves one or more vertebrae that do not close is called:

    a. cerebral palsy

    b. muscular dystrophy

    c. Tay-Sachs disease

    d. spina bifida

    e. hydrocele

52. Which of the following is a characteristic of a malignant tumor?

    a. Smooth borders

    b. Irregular shape

    c. Slow growth

    d. Well-differentiated cells

    e. Encapsulation

53. Muscular movements that are out of conscious control (e.g., the heart beating) are called:

    a. voluntary

    b. involuntary

    c. agonist

    d. antagonist

    e. synergistic

54. The type of joint that allows for the greatest range of motion is the:

   a. hinge

   b. suture

   c. pivot

   d. cartilaginous

   e. ball and socket

55. The portion of the brain that is responsible for higher thought processes such as logical thinking is the:

   a. parietal lobe

   b. frontal lobe

   c. occipital lobe

   d. temporal lobe

   e. cerebellum

56. An individual with a blood type of O positive is considered:

   a. a universal recipient

   b. ineligible to donate

   c. able to donate only to people with O positive blood

   d. able to donate only to people with only O negative blood

   e. a universal donor

57. The type of immunity that is developed from being vaccinated is:

   a. naturally acquired active immunity

   b. artificially acquired passive immunity

   c. artificially acquired active immunity

   d. naturally acquired passive immunity

   e. naturally acquired active passive immunity

58. An X-ray that is shot from the back of the person toward the front would be considered:

   a. AP

   b. lateral

   c. oblique

   d. PA

   e. transverse

59. Which of the following is NOT a portion of the large intestine?

   a. Duodenum

   b. Cecum

   c. Transverse colon

   d. Rectum

   e. Ascending colon

60. When performing screening, the medical assistant must:

    a. diagnose patients' symptoms

    b. prioritize patients' needs

    c. allow patients to determine their own needs

    d. schedule patients in the order in which they arrive

    e. evaluate patients' ability to pay

61. A person with a hypersensitivity to a bee sting may go into:

    a. cardiac arrest

    b. neurogenic shock

    c. anaphylactic shock

    d. seizures

    e. respiratory shock

62. All of the following statements about shock are accurate EXCEPT:

    a. There is inadequate circulation to body parts.

    b. The patient's body is kept warm to prevent chilling.

    c. The patient's pulse becomes rapid and weak.

    d. The medical assistant can administer medication as ordered by the provider.

    e. The patient's blood pressure increases.

63. Which of the following is a major disadvantage of NOT seeking care for an illness until it becomes very advanced?

    a. The patient does not have time to deal with death.

    b. Pain management and treatment may not work as well as they could have.

    c. The family can prepare without frightening the patient.

    d. Denial postpones the inevitable.

    e. The patient does not have time to create advance directives.

64. Redirecting a socially unacceptable impulse into one that is socially acceptable is called:

    a. regression

    b. repression

    c. projection

    d. sublimation

    e. denial

65. You are a medical assistant in an ambulatory care facility, and an emergency situation arises. What should you do first?

    a. Notify the provider.

    b. Give first aid.

    c. Assess the patient.

    d. Call 911.

    e. Evaluate the causes.

66. The act of evaluating the urgency of a medical situation and prioritizing treatment is known as:

    a. screening

    b. empathy

    c. trauma

    d. diagnosing

    e. sorting

67. Which condition is detected with the Mantoux test?

    a. HIV

    b. Syphilis

    c. PKU

    d. TB

    e. Infectious mononucleosis

68. Which of the following is used as a contrast medium for a radiographic lower GI examination?

    a. Air

    b. Iodine salts

    c. Water

    d. A barium swallow

    e. A barium enema

69. Which type of pathogen causes mumps, measles, and chicken pox?

    a. Bacteria

    b. Viruses

    c. Spirochetes

    d. Parasites

    e. Rickettsiae

70. Which body system does the acronym PERRLA refer to?

    a. Cardiovascular system

    b. Gastrointestinal system

    c. Nervous system

    d. Respiratory system

    e. Urogenital system

71. Which term means difficulty breathing?

    a. Apnea

    b. Bradypnea

    c. Tachypnea

    d. Eupnea

    e. Dyspnea

72. Which of the following statements is accurate regarding vitamins?

    a. Vitamins A, B, D, and E are fat soluble.

    b. Vitamins are needed in large quantities.

    c. Water-soluble vitamins are stored in fatty tissues.

    d. Vitamins are simple molecules.

    e. Vitamins B and C are water soluble.

73. Which statement is accurate regarding ventricular tachycardia?

    a. Ventricular tachycardia causes severe chest pain.

    b. Ventricular tachycardia is life threatening.

    c. Ventricular tachycardia is often seen in patients using depressants.

    d. Ventricular tachycardia has a cardiac cycle that occurs early.

    e. Ventricular tachycardia occurs in healthy people.

74. Which genetic disorder is characterized by mental retardation?

    a. Sickle cell anemia

    b. Huntington's disease

    c. Down's syndrome

    d. Cystic fibrosis

    e. Pernicious anemia

75. Which type of nutrient contains the most calories per gram?

    a. Carbohydrate

    b. Protein

    c. Mineral

    d. Fat

    e. Vitamin

76. Which term describes a reason why a medication should NOT be administered?

    a. Side effect

    b. Contraindication

    c. Potentiation

    d. Idiosyncratic

    e. Cross-tolerance

77. Robby is coming down with chicken pox but does not have any symptoms yet. He is now at the:

    a. acute stage

    b. convalescent stage

    c. declining stage

    d. incubation stage

    e. prodromal stage

78. Which of the following statements about medical asepsis hand washing is accurate?

    a. Medical assistants should turn the faucet on with a clean, dry paper towel.

    b. Medical assistants should hold their hands upward.

    c. Medical assistants should scrub up to their elbows.

    d. Medical assistants should touch only the inside of the sink with their hands.

    e. Medical assistants should turn off the faucet with a used paper towel.

79. Which of these positions is used for the treatment and examination of the back and buttocks?

    a. Trendelenburg

    b. Dorsal recumbent

    c. Lithotomy

    d. Supine

    e. Prone

80. Which term describes a woman who has never been pregnant?

    a. Multigravida

    b. Nullipara

    c. Nulligravida

    d. Multipara

    e. Primipara

81. Which infection control guidelines are used by all health care professionals for all patients?

    a. Body Substance Isolation guidelines

    b. Standard Precautions

    c. OSHA guidelines

    d. Transmission-Based Precautions

    e. Universal Precautions

82. All of the following are acceptable wrappings for autoclaving EXCEPT:

    a. plastic pouches

    b. muslin

    c. paper bags

    d. aluminum foil

    e. paper wrapping

83. The most common disorder of the urinary system is:

    a. renal calculi

    b. urinary tract infection

    c. glomerulonephritis

    d. cystitis

    e. pyelonephritis

84. Which of the following diseases is sexually transmitted?

    a. Pelvic inflammatory disease

    b. Cervical cancer

    c. Endometriosis

    d. Prostatitis

    e. Ovarian cancer

85. Which term describes an infection of the middle ear?

    a. Otitis externa

    b. Otalgia

    c. Otitis media

    d. Otorrhagia

    e. Otosclerosis

86. Which condition is commonly known as fainting?

    a. Tinnitus

    b. Singultus

    c. Bruit

    d. Syncope

    e. Vertigo

87. Which of the following is a progressive degenerative disease of the liver?

    a. Hepatitis A

    b. Cholecystitis

    c. Hepatomegaly

    d. Hepatitis B

    e. Cirrhosis

88. Which type of injection is made into the fatty layer just below the skin?

    a. Intramuscular

    b. Subcutaneous

    c. Intradermal

    d. Intravenous

    e. Intermuscular

89. An elevation of which blood cell count indicates the presence of inflammation in the body?

    a. Platelet count

    b. Erythrocyte sedimentation rate

    c. Hematocrit

    d. Total hemoglobin

    e. White blood cell differentiation

90. What condition is characterized by an abnormal thickening and hardening of the skin?

    a. Acne

    b. Melanoma

    c. Dermatophytosis

    d. Scleroderma

    e. Psoriasis

91. Who discovered penicillin?

    a. Sir Alexander Fleming

    b. Robert Koch

    c. Louis Pasteur

    d. Joseph Lister

    e. Edward Jenner

92. Homeostasis refers to what?

    a. A sterile environment

    b. A complete procedure

    c. Everyone getting along

    d. Internal equilibrium

    e. Rapid heart rate

93. The classification of drugs with the lowest potential of abuse is:

    a. Schedule IV

    b. Schedule I

    c. Schedule V

    d. Schedule II

    e. Schedule III

94. The provider you are working with asks you to provide a patient with samples of a new medication. By doing so, you are:

    a. prescribing medication

    b. administering medication

    c. compounding medication

    d. mixing medication

    e. dispensing medication

95. Which of the following is information about a medication that is NOT found in the PDR?

    a. Indications for use

    b. The shape of each pill

    c. Dosage and administration route

    d. Precautions

    e. Generic name

96. A drug that increases the effect of another has which type of effect?

    a. Local

    b. Remote

    c. Synergistic

    d. Systemic

    e. Topical

97. A medication that is ordered to be delivered in a sublingual route would be:

    a. placed in the cheek

    b. swallowed

    c. inserted into the rectum

    d. placed under the tongue

    e. placed on top of the tongue

98. A medication that is classified as an expectorant would have what effect?

    a. Dilate bronchi

    b. Prevent coughing

    c. Relax blood vessels

    d. Decrease nausea

    e. Increase the amount of mucus being expelled

99. A medication that increases the amount of urine excreted by the body would be classified as a(n):

    a. diuretic

    b. antiarrhythmic

    c. antiemetic

    d. vasopressor

    e. muscle relaxant

100. All of the following are part of a medication order EXCEPT:

    a. name of drug

    b. who dispenses the medication

    c. form of drug

    d. route of administration

    e. prescribing provider's signature

101. A prescription that indicates a medication should be administered "OD" would go where?

    a. Left eye

    b. Right ear

    c. Left ear

    d. Right eye

    e. In the nose

102. The metric prefix which refers to one-millionth of a unit is:

    a. milli

    b. kilo

    c. meter

    d. gram

    e. micro

103. Pediatric medication dosages are figured based on the child's:

    a. height

    b. age

    c. weight

    d. gender

    e. chest circumference

104. A patient weighs 130 pounds. The provider asked you to convert that weight into kilograms. You know that there are 2.2 pounds in 1 kilogram. How many kilograms does this patient weigh?

    a. 4.55 kg

    b. 59.09 kg

    c. 286 kg

    d. .07 kg

    e. 260 kg

105. Which of the following is NOT 1 of the 6 rights?

    a. Dose

    b. Provider

    c. Route

    d. Patient

    e. Drug

106. Parenteral medication is administered via:

    a. the mouth

    b. the rectum

    c. the skin

    d. inhalation

    e. an injection

107. The type of injection that is administered at a 90-degree angle is:

    a. subcutaneous

    b. intradermal

    c. intravenous

    d. inhaled

    e. intramuscular

108. Hypodermic needles are most appropriate for what?

    a. Venipuncture

    b. Aspirations

    c. Allergy injections

    d. Intramuscular and subcutaneous injections

    e. Insulin administration

109. Which of the following is NOT an appropriate injection site for an intramuscular injection?

    a. Dorsogluteal

    b. Biceps

    c. Ventrogluteal

    d. Deltoid

    e. Vastus lateralis

110. Which of the following points is the highest point in a normal ECG graph?

    a. P

    b. Q

    c. R

    d. S

    e. T

111. The yellow portion of the safety warning label indicates which of the following?

    a. Chemical instability

    b. Health hazard

    c. Fire hazard

    d. PPE requirements

    e. Biohazard level

112. A chemical that is extremely flammable would be given a safety rating of:

    a. 3

    b. 2

    c. 1

    d. 4

    e. 0

113. The component of blood that is responsible for clotting is:

    a. Erythrocyte

    b. Leukocyte

    c. Plasma

    d. Serum

    e. Thrombocyte

114. Which of the following substances is NOT a normal component of urine?

    a. Ammonia

    b. Blood

    c. Creatinine

    d. Urea

    e. Water

115. The type of urine sample that requires a patient to avoid eating and drinking prior to voiding is:

    a. 24-hour

    b. first-morning

    c. fasting

    d. random

    e. catheter collection

116. Which of the following is NOT a component of the physical examination of urine?

    a. Volume

    b. Color

    c. Unusual

    d. Specific gravity

    e. pH

117. Casts found in urine are formed from:

    a. carbohydrates

    b. lipids

    c. calcium

    d. proteins

    e. potassium

118. Exposing bacterial growth to an antibiotic in order to determine effective treatment of an infection is called:

    a. culturing

    b. taxonomy

    c. sensitivity testing

    d. inoculation

    e. Gram stain

119. The disease of the eye that is characterized by an elevated intraocular pressure is:

    a. cataract

    b. glaucoma

    c. macular degeneration

    d. amblyopia

    e. strabismus

120. The mineral that is important for the formation of bone tissue is:

    a. calcium

    b. potassium

    c. zinc

    d. iron

    e. magnesium

121. Which of the following is a type of bacteria?

    a. Streptococci

    b. Helminth

    c. Protozoa

    d. Tinea

    e. Scabies

122. Diseases caused by which type of pathogen are treated by antibiotics?

    a. Protozoa

    b. Fungi

    c. Bacteria

    d. Virus

    e. Parasite

123. Personal protective equipment should always be used in each of the follow situations EXCEPT:

    a. handling processing a urine specimen

    b. taking vital signs

    c. performing venipuncture

    d. assisting with surgical procedures

    e. disinfecting instruments

124. A worker who is exposed to bodily fluids through an accidental needlestick from a contaminated needle should immediately flush the area with:

    a. alcohol

    b. hydrogen peroxide

    c. betadine

    d. bleach

    e. water

125. Which immunization must be available free to all health care employees?

    a. Hepatitis A

    b. Hepatitis C

    c. Hepatitis B

    d. HIV

    e. TB

126. Use of alcohol-based hand rub is acceptable in which of the following situations?

    a. Before and after eating

    b. Before and after using the restroom

    c. After contact with body excretions

    d. After decontamination of a work area

    e. Following processing of microbiological specimens

127. Which of the following is NOT an OSHA requirement for housekeeping in a medical setting?

    a. Routine decontamination of reusable containers

    b. Double-bagged soiled linens

    c. Biohazard waste collected in impermeable red containers

    d. Sharps containers stored in an upright condition

    e. Alcohol-based hand rub available at all times

128. When performing CPR on an infant or child, circulation is checked by assessing pulse at which pulse point?

    a. Carotid

    b. Axial

    c. Femoral

    d. Brachial

    e. Dorsal pedis

129. The method used to clear an airway obstruction in an unconscious adult is:

    a. finger sweep

    b. back blows

    c. chest thrust

    d. 2 rescue breaths

    e. CPR

130. A burn that has penetrated to the bone would be considered:

    a. superficial

    b. partial thickness

    c. 100%

    d. full thickness

    e. 75%

131. Which of the following is NOT a step in controlling bleeding from an open wound on the arm?

    a. Applying direct pressure

    b. Elevating the arm

    c. Wrapping the wound tightly

    d. Applying pressure to the appropriate artery

    e. Disinfecting the area

132. Appropriate first aid for a patient with a case of acute frostbite would include:

    a. immersing the area in warm water

    b. warming the area by creating friction

    c. immediately raising the patient's core body temperature

    d. applying heavy moisturizing cream to the area

    e. immediately debriding necrotic tissues

133. Appropriate treatment for an acute sprain or strain would include all BUT which of the following?

    a. Ice

    b. Rest

    c. Compression

    d. Range of motion

    e. Elevation

134. A medication that is to be taken twice a day would be indicated as:

    a. qd

    b. tid

    c. qid

    d. bid

    e. od

135. Which type of manual identifies the specific methods for performing tasks?

    a. Policy

    b. Training

    c. Procedures

    d. Personnel

    e. Benefits

136. What is the primary purpose of managed care plans?

    a. To allow patients to manage their own care

    b. To control patients' access to providers

    c. To encourage patients to explore alternative medicine treatments

    d. To provide acute care only

    e. To provide comprehensive health care at a reasonable cost

137. How are claims managed when both parents are covered by health insurance?

    a. The father's plan is always primary.

    b. Claims for the family are paid according to the birthday rule.

    c. The mother's plan is always primary.

    d. Double benefits are paid for the children.

    e. The duplication of benefits rule is put into effect.

138. Why are accurate medical records legally important?

    a. Because they are needed to provide referrals

    b. Because they assist in controlling health care costs

    c. Because they aid in billing

    d. Because they are written documentation used to prove patient care

    e. Because they are essential to quality patient care

139. Which type of check is used most often for writing payroll checks?

    a. Voucher check

    b. Traveler's check

    c. Certified check

    d. Cashier's check

    e. Money order

140. What is the role of a computer firewall?

    a. A computer firewall limits potential damage from viruses.

    b. A computer firewall protects the computer in the event of a fire.

    c. A computer firewall does not allow outside computers access to your computer.

    d. A computer firewall allows outside access to an office computer but not to databases.

    e. A computer firewall prevents employees from surfing the Internet for personal reasons.

141. How should a letter that requires a written receipt be mailed?

    a. Registered mail

    b. Priority mail

    c. Third-class mail

    d. Certified mail

    e. First-class mail

142. Which of the following are used in conjunction with CPT codes?

    a. V Codes

    b. Preventive care codes

    c. Injury codes

    d. Modifiers

    e. E Codes

143. What must happen when more than one policy pays on a claim?

    a. Coinsurance

    b. Coordination of benefits

    c. Co-pay

    d. Deductible

    e. Exclusions

144. When alphabetizing and assigning units for filing order, titles are considered:

    a. as part of the last name

    b. as the first indexing unit

    c. as the third indexing unit

    d. as part of the patient's surname

    e. as a separate unit at the end

145. A person who is injured on the job may be covered by:

    a. workers' compensation

    b. CHAMPUS

    c. Medicaid

    d. disability insurance

    e. HCFA

146. Which of the following is an advantage of accepting credit cards in an ambulatory care setting?

    a. Maintaining patient confidentiality is not a problem.

    b. There are no fees to be paid by the practice.

    c. The money is available to the practice within one day.

    d. The money is usually available to the practice within 10 days.

    e. Accepting credit cards eliminates having to file insurance claims.

147. What is the key to having an effective scheduling system?

    a. Accommodating patient preferences

    b. Customizing the system to the type of practice

    c. Tailoring the system to provider preferences

    d. Accommodating the requirements of the insurance carriers

    e. Effectively monitoring the use of time versus the dollars produced

148. Which scheduling system assigns two patients to the same time?

    a. Clustering

    b. Stream

    c. Modified wave

    d. Double booking

    e. Open-hours

149. Which program provides health care coverage for low-income individuals?

    a. CHAMPUS

    b. Workers' compensation

    c. Medicare

    d. CHAMPVA

    e. Medicaid

150. Which of the following is a critical issue regarding the use of a fax machine in a medical office?

    a. The speed at which the machine works

    b. The time required to train personnel

    c. Compromised confidentiality due to access by unauthorized personnel

    d. The clarity of the documents received

    e. The volume of documents the machine can handle

151. Which of the following is used when there is not enough information to find a more specific code?

    a. NEC

    b. NOS

    c. CC

    d. V Codes

    e. E Codes

152. Which of the following tells the computer hardware what to do?

    a. Application software

    b. The motherboard

    c. The modem

    d. System software

    e. Servers

153. Which of the following conditions is most frequently related to the repetitive use of a computer?

    a. Eyestrain

    b. Fatigue

    c. Carpal tunnel syndrome

    d. Lower back pain

    e. Tension headaches

154. When seeking employment, a person who has job experience should use:

    a. a targeted résumé

    b. a functional résumé

    c. a complete résumé

    d. an Information Mapping résumé

    e. a chronological résumé

155. Which type of résumé highlights one's special qualities?

    a. Targeted

    b. Functional

    c. Chronological

    d. Concise

    e. Career oriented

156. Which statement is accurate regarding a cover letter?

    a. The cover letter may be addressed "To whom it may concern."

    b. The purpose of the cover letter is to ask for an interview.

    c. The cover letter includes résumé information.

    d. The cover letter should be bulleted.

    e. The cover letter should include a list of references.

157. Which of the following tasks is NOT assigned to the human resources manager?

    a. Creating office manuals

    b. Hiring and firing personnel

    c. Interpreting legal regulations

    d. Providing employee training

    e. Performing employee evaluations

158. Tiffany wants a well-paying position as a medical assistant. Which statement is accurate regarding her search?

    a. Every CMA (AAMA) is guaranteed a well-paying position.

    b. Using an employment agency is her most effective tool in finding a well-paying position.

    c. Networking is her most effective tool in finding a well-paying position.

    d. Running down all leads is her most effective tool in finding a well-paying position.

    e. Cold calling to offices that are not advertising will produce excellent leads.

159. Which federal law requires employers to verify the right of employees to work in the United States?

    a. Immigration Reform Act

    b. Equal Pay Act

    c. Civil Rights Act

    d. Fair Labor Standards Act

    e. Americans with Disabilities Act

160. Which of these interviewing tips is accurate?

    a. Think carefully before answering questions.

    b. Do not ask questions, as you may appear confused.

    c. Answer questions "off the cuff" so your responses do not seem rehearsed.

    d. Place your personal belongings—coat, purse, and so on—on the interviewer's desk.

    e. Give lengthy answers to all questions, even when you are not sure of the answer.

161. Which of the following statements about completing an employment application form is accurate?

    a. Write "See résumé" rather than repeating information.

    b. Using either a pen or pencil is acceptable.

    c. Try to complete the application without referring to your résumé.

    d. Complete the application quickly to demonstrate how well you work.

    e. Following instructions is very important.

162. Which of the following is the best networking resource for recruiting new personnel?

    a. Newspapers

    b. Family and friends

    c. Current employees

    d. Patients

    e. AAMA's national office

163. All of these interview questions are appropriate EXCEPT:

    a. "What is most important to you about this job?"

    b. "What is your clinical experience?"

    c. "Have you ever been bonded before?"

    d. "Do you have any health-related problems that might affect your job performance?"

    e. "Where did you go to school?"

164. Which of the following is NOT vital résumé information?

    a. Home address

    b. Current telephone number

    c. Education

    d. Date of birth

    e. Work experience

165. Which payroll forms must be submitted to the Social Security Administration each year?

    a. W-4

    b. W-2

    c. W-6

    d. 1099

    e. 941

166. A policy manual should include all of the following EXCEPT:

    a. employment practices

    b. insurance billing techniques

    c. wage and salary scales

    d. evaluation schedules

    e. continuing education policies

167. In order to track inventory in an office, the most appropriate type of software to use would be:

    a. word processing

    b. billing

    c. contact management

    d. spreadsheet

    e. EMR

168. When taking a telephone message, everything BUT the following should be included:

    a. full name of person leaving message

    b. reason for the call

    c. time and date of call

    d. expected action

    e. diagnosis of the patient the message is about

169. An office operating on a wave schedule will:

    a. have groups of patients arriving at relatively the same time throughout the day

    b. schedule two patients for the same appointment time

    c. schedule patients in specific time increments (e.g., every 15 minutes)

    d. allow for walk-in patients at any time

    e. provide "catch up" time for the provider

170. When scheduling an outpatient procedure, each of the following should be completed EXCEPT:

    a. obtaining necessary preauthorizations

    b. making arrangements with the facility

    c. notifying the patient of the arrangements

    d. determining and scheduling preprocedure testing

    e. precertifying the admission

171. A block letter style includes:

    a. centered paragraphs with all other components at the left margin

    b. all components starting at the left margin

    c. centered address and signature lines with paragraphs starting at the left margin

    d. centered address, signature line, and first paragraph

    e. all components centered

172. Source-oriented medical records are organized by the:

    a. cause of a patient's medical diagnosis

    b. location of a patient's medical record

    c. nature of a patient's complaint

    d. treatment methods being used

    e. professionals who have documented in the record

173. Each of the following is objective information EXCEPT:

    a. laboratory data

    b. diagnosis

    c. prescribed treatment

    d. patient's complaint

    e. exam findings

174. Color coding medical records assists with each of the following EXCEPT:

    a. increasing efficiency with filing

    b. increasing the ability to identify filing errors

    c. identifying a patient's diagnosis

    d. identifying patients who are due for a physical during a specific month

    e. removing inactive files

175. Tickler files are helpful in:

    a. sending billing notices

    b. scheduling the provider's time

    c. providing reminders for routine medical appointments

    d. submitting insurance claims

    e. processing payroll

176. Providers' fees are generally set by each of the following EXCEPT:

    a. reasonable

    b. insurance

    c. customary

    d. usual

    e. geographic region

177. Accounts receivable refers to:

    a. money collected by a practice during a day

    b. accounts turned over to a debt collection agency

    c. money owed by the practice

    d. money owed to a practice

    e. petty cash expenditures

178. Manually posting charges usually involves each of the following EXCEPT:

    a. day sheet

    b. ledger card

    c. account summary

    d. encounter form

    e. HCFA 1500

179. The Truth in Lending Act requires:

    a. lower interest rates for medical services

    b. an increased amount of time for repayment of medical loans

    c. use of an independent billing service

    d. accurate information regarding finance charges

    e. routine billing statements

180. Calls made to a patient's home in order to collect money owed to a practice are regulated by:

    a. the Truth in Lending Act

    b. CLIA

    c. the Fair Debt Collection Act

    d. OSHA

    e. AMA

181. Once an account has been submitted to a collection agency, the medical assistant should:

    a. discontinue sending statements to the patient

    b. continue to send routine billing statements to the patient

    c. send copies of billing statements to emergency contacts listed in the patient's chart

    d. file for legal action in small claims court

    e. telephone the patient in order to attempt to collect the debt

182. Best practices with manual bookkeeping involve all of the following EXCEPT:

    a. proficiency with 10-key typing

    b. using consistent methods

    c. writing with red ink

    d. writing numbers clearly

    e. double checking all math

183. In managing practice finances, an adjustment would be used for:

    a. recording payment

    b. recording charges

    c. indicating past due accounts

    d. indicating discounts or write-offs

    e. indicating accounts turned over to collections

184. When preparing a check to a supplier, the medical assistant should:

    a. verify the expense has been approved

    b. endorse with "for deposit only"

    c. reconcile the bank statement

    d. record the payment on the correct ledger card

    e. file a I-9 tax form

185. If an office determines it will accept personal checks as payment, it is important to:

    a. clearly post the policy

    b. implement use of a restrictive endorsement

    c. follow Truth in Lending guidelines

    d. verify policies with the practice's bank

    e. follow Fair Debt collection guidelines

186. Mrs. Jones's insurance requires that she pay for $400 of medical expenses before she is eligible for insurance payment for medical services. The $400 would be referred to as:

    a. a co-payment

    b. coinsurance

    c. a deductible

    d. a premium

    e. an exclusion

187. Mr. Johnson's insurance company has stated that it will not pay for treatment of his asthma because he was known to have the disease prior to the time when his policy was purchased. His asthma would be considered a(n):

    a. exclusion

    b. preexisting condition

    c. concurrent condition

    d. secondary diagnosis

    e. subjective condition

188. The type of Medicare coverage that provides benefits for inpatient medical care is:

    a. Medicare B

    b. Medicare D

    c. Medicare E

    d. Medicare A

    e. Medicare F

189. Most managed care organizations provide a capitated payment for services. This means that:

    a. a maximum payment for services is set

    b. patients must pay excess charges out of their own pocket

    c. they will not pay for services covered by another company

    d. the government sets the maximum allowed charge for a service

    e. patients' premiums will never change

190. RBRVS payment structures are based on all EXCEPT which of the following?

    a. Level of work

    b. Malpractice expenses

    c. Regional charges

    d. Diagnosis of patient

    e. Experience of the provider

191. E Codes in the ICD book are used to identify:

    a. wellness-related procedures

    b. cardiovascular diseases

    c. morphology

    d. neurological diseases

    e. accidents

192. V Codes in the ICD book are used to identify:

    a. accidents

    b. cardiovascular disease

    c. wellness-related procedures

    d. morphology

    e. neurological diseases

193. Which of the following would be considered a commercial form of health insurance?

    a. Medicare

    b. Medicaid

    c. CHAMPUS

    d. Blue Cross/Blue Shield

    e. Workers compensation

194. Patient Sally Kane arrives at your office as a new patient. While copying her insurance card you notice that she will need to pay 20 percent of the cost of the visit. That percentage is referred to as:

    a. co-payment

    b. coinsurance

    c. deductible

    d. premium

    e. exclusion

195. In order to accurately locate an ICD code, which section of the book would you use first?

    a. Volume II

    b. Volume I

    c. Volume III

    d. Volume IV

    e. Appendix

196. Which of the following is NOT a section in the CPT book?

    a. Anesthesia

    b. Surgery

    c. Pathology and Laboratory

    d. Rehabilitation

    e. Medicine

197. Deliberately billing a service at a higher level than what was completed would be considered:

    a. downcoding

    b. bundling

    c. unbundling

    d. upcoding

    e. proper procedure

198. A business letter sent from an office would be processed through which class of mail?

    a. Second class

    b. Third class

    c. First class

    d. Fourth class

    e. Priority mail

199. Hospital inpatient payments are based on:

    a. APG

    b. DRG

    c. Usual fees

    d. Reasonable fees

    e. Customary fees

200. Dr. Abernathy provides you with the growth chart appearing on the following page and asks you to explain it to the child's mother, who is concerned that the child is not as tall as other children his age. You would explain to the mother that:

    a. the child is actually slightly above average on the growth chart

    b. the child is actually slightly below average on the growth chart

    c. the child is actually well above average on the growth chart

    d. the child is actually well below average on the growth chart

    e. the child is of average height on the growth chart

CDC Growth Charts: United States

**Length-for-age percentiles:
Boys, birth to 36 months**

97th
95th
90th
75th
50th
25th
10th
5th
3rd

Age (months)

Birth 3 6 9 12 15 18 21 24 27 30 33 36

Published May 30, 2000.
SOURCE: Developed by the National Center for Health Statistics in collaboration with
the National Center for Chronic Disease Prevention and Health Promotion (2000).

SAFER · HEALTHIER · PEOPLE™